Neuroblastoma: Clinical and Biological Characteristics

Neuroblastoma: Clinical and Biological Characteristics

Edited by **Michael Jones**

hayle
medical

New York

Published by Hayle Medical,
30 West, 37th Street, Suite 612,
New York, NY 10018, USA
www.haylemedical.com

Neuroblastoma: Clinical and Biological Characteristics
Edited by Michael Jones

International Standard Book Number: 978-1-63241-287-4 (Hardback)

Printed in the United States of America.

Contents

Preface

Over the recent decade, advancements and applications have progressed exponentially. This has led to the increased interest in this field and projects are being conducted to enhance knowledge. The main objective of this book is to present some of the critical challenges and provide insights into possible solutions. This book will answer the varied questions that arise in the field and also provide an increased scope for furthering studies.

The book sets out to present the facts and contradictions of neuroblastoma. Tumors of neuroblastoma group are heterogeneous and their genomic/molecular properties are intimately associated with the prognosis of patients; certain children enjoy a distinguished clinical course post the surgery/biopsy alone, and others face a catastrophic result even after a thorough treatment. Latest advancement has also began unveiling crucial importance of cross-talking between neuroblastoma cells and their microenvironment in predicting clinical behaviors of individual cases. The biological and clinical characteristics of this disease are presented in this book by renowned investigators.

I hope that this book, with its visionary approach, will be a valuable addition and will promote interest among readers. Each of the authors has provided their extraordinary competence in their specific fields by providing different perspectives as they come from diverse nations and regions. I thank them for their contributions.

Editor

Neuroblastoma, Clinical

Clinical Presentation of Neuroblastoma

Josef Malis

Additional information is available at the end of the chapter

1. Introduction

Neuroblastoma is a cancer of the peripheral sympathetic nervous system, derived from embryonic neural crest cells (a neuroendocrine tumor) and is one of the few cancers known to undergo spontaneous regression from an undifferentiated state to a benign tumor.

Neuroblastoma is the most common extracranial solid tumor in children, accounting for 7% to 8% of all childhood cancers. The prevalence is about 1 case per 7,000 live births. This incidence is fairly uniform throughout the world, at least for industrialized nations. Neuroblastoma is slightly more common in boys than in girls, with a male-to-female sex ratio of 1.1 to 1 in most large studies [1]. While it accounts for 7% of all childhood malignancies, neuroblastoma accounts for 10% of childhood cancer mortality. Neuroblastoma is a pediatric neoplasm that is the most common cancer diagnosed during infancy. POG and CCG institutions from 1986 to 2001 showed a median age at diagnosis of about 19 months. In this cohort, 36% were infants, 89% were younger than 5 years, and 98% were diagnosed by 10 years of age. The distribution of cases by age shows that this is a disease of infancy and early childhood, with the highest number of cases diagnosed in the first month of life [2].

2. Current outcome

Patients with low- and intermediate-risk NBL have an overall survival rate exceeding 90% with a trend toward minimization of therapy [3,4,5]. Standard therapy for patients with high-risk NBL involves multi-agent chemotherapy induction, surgery and external beam radiotherapy, myeloablative consolidation with autologous hematopoietic stem cell recue and biologic agents, including the recent demonstration that GD2- directed immunotherapy combined with cytokines significantly improves survival. Despite these achievements, 50% of patients with newly diagnosed high-risk disease, and less than 10% of patients whose disease recurs, will survive [6].

3. General remarks

Neuroblastoma is very often called "enigmatic tumor" for its broad spectrum of clinical presentation, biological features and prognosis varying from clinically incidence benign to unresectable or metastic disease with very poor outcomes. Neuroblastomas can arise anywhere throughout the sympathetic nervous system, most common primary site is adrenal gland, followed by abdominal (extraadrenal), thoracic, cervical, and pelvic sympathetic ganglia. Neuroblastoma metastasizes to lymph nodes, bone marrow, bones (long bones, flat bone soft the scull, orbits), liver, and skin, rarely to lungs or brain. Widespread bone and bone marrow disease causes bone pain, which can lead to limping, or irritability in a younger child. There may be bone marrow replacement and symptoms such as anemia, bleeding, or infection. Skin involvement is seen almost exclusively in infants with INSS stage Ms (4S) tumors and is characterized by a variable number of nontender, bluish subcutaneous nodules.

Constitutional symptoms associated with disseminated disease may include failure to thrive and fever, the latter observed most often in the presence of extensive bone metastases [7]

Regional lymph node metastases are noted in up to 35% of patients with apparently localized tumors and 30% of patients with stage M (4) and Ms (4S) disease also have regional lymph node involvement. Spread of tumor to lymph nodes outside the cavity of origin is considered to be INSS stage 4 disease, but these patients may have a better outlook if there is no bone marrow, cortical bone, or other parenchymal organ involvement. [8,9]

Most primary tumors occur within the abdomen (65%), although the frequency of adrenal tumors is slightly higher in children (40%) compared with infants (25%). Infants also have more thoracic and cervical primary tumors. A primary tumor cannot be found in about 1% of patients.

4. Staging and stratification

The for decades used surgical-pathologic International Neuroblastoma Staging System (INSS) – Table 1 [10] has been recently replaced by the International Neuroblastoma Risk Group Staging System (INRGSS) [11]. The INRGSS uses radiologic features to distinguish locoregional tumors (Table 2) that do not involve local structures (INRGS L1) from locally invasive tumors (INRGS L2), exhibiting image defined risk factors (Table 3) [12]. Stages M and MS refer to tumors that are widely metastatic or have an INSS 4 and 4s pattern of disease, respectively. Neuroblastoma is classified into low-, intermediate-, or high-risk categories based upon clinical and biological features, with risk category correlating with outcome. The recently proposed INRG classification defines similar cohorts that will be used to assess clinical trial outcome. The International Neuroblastoma Response Criteria (INRC) provide a common basis for disease response comparisons across clinical trials [13]. Importantly, the INRC has limitations with respect to definitions of metastatic site response not measurable using anatomical imaging (bone and bone marrow). A National Cancer Institute-sponsored international meeting was held in 2012 to develop updated consensus response guidelines. Response components of a revised INRC will includeprimary tumor dimensions using anatomic imaging, and metastatic disease assessment using 123I-MIBG imaging and quantification of bone marrow disease.

Stage 1:	Localized tumor with complete gross excis ion, with or without microscopic residual disease; representative ipsilateral lymph nodes negati ve for tumor microscopically (nodes attached and removed with the primary tumor may be positive)
Stage 2A:	Localized tumor with incomplete gross excision; representative ipsilateral nonadherent lymph nodes negative for tumor microscopically
Stage 2B:	Localized tumor withor without komplete gross excision, with ipsilateral nonadherentlymph nodes positive for tumor. Enlarged contralateral lymph nodes must benegative microscopically
Stage 3:	Unresectable unilateral tumor infiltrating across the midline, with or without regional lymph node involvement; or localized unilateral tumorwith contralateral regional lymphnode involvement; or midline tumor with bilateral extensit by infiltration (unresectable) or by lymph node involvement
Stage 4:	Any primary tumor with dissemination to distant lymph nodes, bone, bone marrow, liver, skin, and/or other organs (except as defined for stage 4S)
Stage 4S:	Localized primary tumor (as defined for stage 1, 2A, or2B), with dissemin ation limited to skin, liver and/or bone marrow (limited to infants <1 year of age)

Table 1. International Neuroblastoma Staging System

Ipsilateral tumor extension within two body compartments

Neck-chest, chest-abdomen, abdomen-pelvis

Neck

    Tumor encasing carotid and/or vertebral artery and/or internal jugular vein

    Tumor extending to base of skull

    Tumor compressing the trachea

Cervico-thoracic junction

    Tumor encasing brachial plexus roots

    Tumor encasing subclavian vessels and/or vertebral and/or carotid artery

    Tumor compressing the trachea

Thorax

    Tumor encasing the aorta and/or major branches

    Tumor compressing the trachea and/or principal bronchi

    Lower mediastinal tumor, infiltrating the costo-vertebral junction between T9 and T12

Thoraco-abdominal

    Tumor encasing the aorta and/or vena cava

Abdomen/pelvis

    Tumor infiltrating the porta hepatis and/or the hepatoduodenal ligament

    Tumor encasing branches of the superior mesenteric artery at the mesenteric root

    Tumor encasing the origin of the coeliac axis, and/or of the superior

mesenteric artery

    Tumor invading one or both renal pedicles

    Tumor encasing the aorta and/or vena cava

    Tumor encasing the iliac vessels

    Pelvic tumor crossing the sciatic notch

Intraspinal tumor extension whatever the location provided that:

    More than one third of the spinal canal in the axial plane is invaded and/or the perimedullary leptomeningeal spaces are not visible and/or the spinal cord signal is abnormal

Infiltration of adjacent organs/structures

    Pericardium, diaphragm, kidney, liver, duodeno-pancreatic block, and mesentery

Conditions to be recorded, but not considered IDRFs

    Multifocal primary tumors

    Pleural effusion, with or without malignant cells

    Ascites, with or without malignant cells

Table 2. Image-defined risk factors (IDRFs)

L1:	Localized tumor not involving vital structures as defined by the list of image-defined risk factors and confined to one body compartment
L2:	Locoregional tumor with presence of one or more image-defined risk factors
M:	Distant metastatic disease (expect stage MS)
MS:	Metastatic disease in children younger than 18 months with metastases confined to skin, liver, and/or bone marrow

Table 3. International Neuroblastoma Risk Group Staging System

5. Sporadic and familiar neuroblastoma

Most neuroblastomas occur sporadically; around 1-2% are familial and associated with multiple primary tumours, usually occurring at <18 months of age. Familial disease has the same diverse clinical behaviour as somatic neuroblastoma, ranging from aggressive progression to spontaneous regression.11 Within the last 10 years significant advances have been in the understanding of hereditary neuroblastoma, with germline mutations in two genes ALK and paired homeobox 2b gene PHOX2B accounting for the majority of cases, which may present in the neonatal period. ALK mutations are now known to be the most now known common cause of hereditary neuroblastoma, and in familial neuroblastoma [14,15,16]

6. Associated conditions

Neuroblastoma can be associated with several inborn conditions, like Hirschsprung disease, congenital central hypoventilation syndrome (CCHS or Ondine's curse), neurofibromatosis type I, or Beckwith-Wiedemann syndrome

7. Clinical presentation

The presenting signs and symptoms of neuroblastoma are highly variable with a broad spectrum. Presenting symptoms of neuroblastoma depend on the location of the primary tumor, presence of metastatic lesions, systemic symptoms from catecholamine secretion. Weight loss and fever are present at advanced stages neuroblastoma.

8. Anatomical site of the primary tumour

8.1. Head and neck

Unilateral palpable mass developing in infants or in preschool age children, rarely are diagnosed in newborn mimicking cervical teratoma. [17]

Horners syndrome (ptosis, miosis, anophthalmos, anhydrosis). This syndrome is unilateral, Tatli reported a 28 old child with bilateral prosis [18]. Primary cervical neuroblastoma are ussually non agressive and thein prognosis is very good. But some are fatal - extremely rare case described Güzelmansur et al. – diagnosed prenatally with progression to brain. [19]

Orbit and eye exophthalmoses, periorbital ecchymoses (raccoon eyes), palpable masses, edema of conjunctiva, papilledema, strabismus, anisocoria. The periorbital ecchymoses can be present in about 20% of disseminated neuroblastoma. This clinical findings is related to obstruction of the palpebral ond orbita vessels by metastatic lesions within orbital bones. Frequently these children are investigated for an abuse or a trauma (basal skull fractures) [20,21]. Usually further systemic symptoms are present – weight loss, fever.

Opsoclonus also known as dancing-eye syndrome, presents in early childhood with opsoclonus (rapid, multidirectional, conjugate eye movements) usually associated with myoclonus, ataxia, and behavioral changes such as irritability and sleep problems.– opsoclonus-myoclonus syndrome (OMS) [22]

Chest Upper thoracic tumours: Primary thoracic tumors present as symptomatic masses or can be discovered incidentally when chest radiographs are obtained to evaluate patients for other reasons. High thoracic and cervical masses can be associated with Horner syndrome, which consists of unilateral ptosis, myosis, and anhydrosis. Occasionally, large thoracic tumors are associated with mechanical obstruction and resultant superior vena cava syndrome.

Lower thoracic tumours: usually no symptoms, usually accidental discovery on chest X-ray or thoracic CT performed for other reasons.

8.2. Abdominal neuroblastoma

About 60% of primary neuroblastomas arise in the abdomen, two thirds of them are from the adrenal glands (adrenal neuroblastoma), one third are from paravertebral ganglion (extraadrenal neuroblastoma). Only about one tenth of neuroblastoma are detected as an abdominal mass during a routine examination. The mass is ussually fixed,and firm.

Symptoms: abdominal pain or fullness, abdominal mass, or rarely intestinal obstruction, enlarged and/or displaced liver and spleen. Massive involvement of the liver with metastatic disease is particularly frequent in infants with stage Ms (4S) and may result in respiratory compromise (Pepper Syndrome). Occasionally, the size of primary or metastatic abdominal tumors can result in compression of venous and lymphatic drainage from the lower extremities, leading to scrotal and lower extremity edema. Rarely, patients will experience renin-mediated hypertension because of compromise of renal vasculature.

Hypertension, tachycardia, flushing, and sweating are uncommon symptoms because epinephrine is rarely released from most neuroblastomas, since they lack the enzyme necessary for synthesis.

Only about one tenth of neuroblastoma are detected as an abdominal mass during a routine examination. The mass is ussually fixed,and firm.

Spontaneous rupture from hemorrhage into the tumor occurs very rarely and only in rapidly growing tumors.

There is a small subgroup of abdominal neuroblastomas arising near to the aortic bifurcation (commonly called organ of Zuckerkandl, O. Z.) to assess their biologic outcome and problems in diagnosis and therapy. The organ of Zuckerkandl comprises of a small mass of chromaffin cells derived from neural crest located along the aorta, beginning cranial to the superior mesenteric artery or renal arteries and extending to the level of the aortic bifurcation or just beyond. When neuroblastoma arises these small organs, normally not visible on radiographs, then it could cause compression of bowel or urine bladder (constipation, enuresis) [23].

Paraspinal tumors in the thoracic, abdominal, and pelvic regions are able to invade the spinal canal through the neural foramina (dumbbell tumor) causing spinal cord compression and cause symptoms related to compression of nerve roots and spinal cord. The range of symptomatology includes subacute or acute paraplegia, bladder or bowel dysfunction, or less commonly radicular pain.

9. Paraneoplastic syndrome

Up to 2% of patients present with opsoclonus and myoclonus (OMS) (myoclonic jerking and random eye movements). Often have localized disease and a good long-term prognosis. Opsoclonus and myoclonus syndrome is manifested by rapid and chaotic eye movements, ataxia, and myoclonia. Most children with this syndrome have a favorable outcome with respect to their tumor, as this syndrome is correlated with an immune-mediated antitumor host response [24].

Autonomous tumor secretion of vasoactive intestinal peptide (VIP) is another paraneoplastic syndrome (Kerner-Morrison Syndrome) that is rarely associated with neuroblastoma. VIP secretion can cause abdominal distension and intractable secretory diarrhea with associated hypokalemia ; these symptoms usually resolve after removal of the tumor. chronic watery diarrhea preceded the diagnosis of the tumor; these patients were considered to have "Primary VIP secreting NTs."

10. Metastatic disease

NBL is associated with lymphatic and hematogenous metastatic disease.

Regional lymph node metastases are noted in 35% of patients with apparently localized tumors.

The most common sites for hematogenous spread are: bones (skull, long bones, ribs, vertebras),bone marrow, liver, skin and rarely brain or lungs.

Signs and symptoms of metastatic neuroblastoma include:

Pain and limping, sphenoid bone and retrobulbar tissue involvement causes orbital ecchymoses swelling and proptosis (raccoon face), infants present as irritable and fussy. Bone marrow involvement may result in pancytopenia. Respiratory distress may occur in young babies with Stage IVS (Ms) disease - due to enlarged liver. Skin or subcutaneous nodules are seen almost only in infants. These nodules are non-tender, bluish and mobile - called the "blueberry muffin sign".

Acknowledgements

This work was supported by the project for the conceptual development of research organization 00064203.

Author details

Josef Malis*

Dept. of Pediatric Oncology, University Hospital Motol and Charles University, Prague, Czech Republic

References

[1] Spix C, Pastore G, Sankila R, Stiller CA, Steliarova-Foucher E. Neuroblastoma incidence and survival in European children (1978–1997): report from the Automated Childhood Cancer Information System project. Eur J Cancer 2006;42:2081–91.

[2] Brodeur GM, Maris JM. Neuroblastoma. In: Pizzo PA, Poplack DG, eds. Principles and practice of pediatric oncology. 5th ed. Philadelphia PA: Lippincott Williams & Wilkins, 2006:933–970)

[3] Strother DR, London WB, Schmidt ML, et al. Outcome after surgery alone or with restricted use of chemotherapy for patients with low-risk neuroblastoma: Results of Children's Oncology Group study P964. J Clin Oncol 2012;30:1842–1848.;

[4] Baker DL, Schmidt ML, Cohn SL, et al. Outcome after reduced chemotherapy for intermediate-risk neuroblastoma. N Engl J Med 2010;363:1313–1323.;

[5] De Bernardi B, Mosseri V, Rubie H, et al. Treatment of localised resectable neuroblastoma. Results of the LNESG1 study by the SIOP Europe Neuroblastoma Group. Br J Cancer 2008;99:1027–1033).

[6] Matthay KK, Reynolds CP, Seeger RC, et al. Long-term results for children with high-risk neuroblastoma treated on a randomized trial of myeloablative therapy followed by 13-cis-retinoic acid: A children's oncology group study. J Clin Oncol 2009;27:1007–1013.)

[7] Garrett MB, Hogarty MD: Neuroblastoma In: Pizzo PA, Poplack D: Principles and Practice of Pediatric Oncology, pp. 884-886

[8] DuBois SG, Kalika Y, Lukens JN, et al. Metastatic sites in stage IV and IVS neuroblastoma correlate with age, tumor biology, and survival. J Pediatr Hematol Oncol 1999;21:181–189.

[9] Brodeur GM, Pritchard J, Berthold F, et al. Revisions of the international criteria for neuroblastoma diagnosis, staging, and response to treatment. J Clin Oncol 1993;11:1466–1477.

[10] Monclair T, Brodeur GM, Ambros PF, et al. The International Neuroblastoma Risk Group (INRG) staging system: An INRG Task Force report. J Clin Oncol 2009;27:298–303].

[11] Cecchetto G, Mosseri V, De Bernardi B, et al. Surgical risk factors in primary surgery for localized neuroblastoma: The LNESG1 study of the European International Society of Pediatric Oncology Neuroblastoma Group. J Clin Oncol 2005;23:8483–8489.

[12] Dubois SG, London WB, Zhang Y, et al. Lung metastases in neuroblastoma at initial diagnosis: a report from the International Neuroblastoma Risk Group (INRG) project. Pediatr Blood Cancer 2008;51:589–592

[13] Mosse YP, Laudenslager M, Longo L, et al. Identification of ALK as a major familial neuroblastoma predisposition gene. Nature 2008;455(7215):930e5.

[14] Chiarle R, Voena C, Ambrogio C, Piva R, Inghirami G. The anaplastic lymphoma kinase in the pathogenesis of cancer. Nat Rev Cancer 2008;8:11e23.

[15] Trochet D, Bourdeaut F, Janoueix-Lerosey I, et al. Germline mutations of the paired-like homeobox 2B (PHOX2B) gene in neuroblastoma. Am J Hum Genet 2004;74:761e4

[16] Gorincour G, Dugougeat-Pilleul F, Bouvier R, Lorthois-Ninou S, Devonec S, Gaucherand P, Pracros JP, Guibaud L. Prenatal presentation of cervical congenital neuroblastoma Prenat Diagn. 2003 Aug;23(8):690-3

[17] Tatli B, Saribeyoğlu ET, Aydinli N, Calişkan M, Anak S. Neuroblastoma: an unusual presentation with bilateral ptosis. Pediatr Neurol. 2004 Apr;30(4):284-6.)

[18] Güzelmansur I, Aksoy HT, Hakverdi S, Seven M, Dilmen U, Dilmen GFetal cervical neuroblastoma: prenatal diagnosis. Case Report Med. 2011;2011:529749. Epub 2011 Aug 4

[19] Gumus K: A child with raccoon eyes masquerading as trauma.. Int Ophthalmol. 2007 Dec;27(6):379-81. Epub 2007 May 30

[20] Ahmed S, Goel S, Khandwala M, Agrawal A, Chang B, Simmons IG: Neuroblastoma with orbital metastasis: ophthalmic presentation and role of ophthalmologists Eye (Lond). 2006 Apr;20(4):466-70

[21] Brunklaus A, Pohl K: Outcome and Prognostic Features in Opsoclonus-Myoclonus Syndrome From Infancy to Adult LifePediatrics Vol. 128 No. 2 August 1, 2011 pp. e388 -e394

[22] Berdon WE, Stylianos S, Ruzal-Shapiro C, Hoffer F, Cohen M.: Neuroblastoma arising from the organ of Zuckerkandl: an unusual site with a favorable biologic outcome. Pediatr Radiol. 1999 Jul;29(7):497-502

[23] Mitchell WG, Davalos-Gonzalez Y, Brumm VL, et al. Opsoclonus-ataxia caused by childhood neuroblastoma: developmental and neurologic sequelae. Pediatrics 2002; 109:86–98

[24] Bourdeaut F, de Carli E, Michon J: VIP Hypersecretion as Primary or Secondary Syndrome in Neuroblastoma:Retrospective Study by the Socie'te' Franc,aise des Cancers de l'Enfant (SFCE)Pediatr Blood Cancer 2009;52:585–590

A Novel Diagnostic Tool for Therapy Stratification of Neuroblastoma: Preoperative Analysis of Tumor Biology Using Circulating Tumor-Released DNA in Serum

Shigeki Yagyu, Tomoko Iehara and Hajime Hosoi

Additional information is available at the end of the chapter

1. Introduction

Neuroblastoma (NB) patients fall into two clinically distinct subgroups; a low-risk subgroup and a high-risk subgroup. These subgroups are correlated with the age of onset [1], the extent of the disease (International Neuroblastoma Staging System) [2], pathological findings (International Neuroblastoma Pathological Criteria) [3], and genomic changes in NB tumors as represented by *MYCN* gene amplification (MNA) [4, 5]. Above all, the patterns of genetic changes can predict the subgroups of NB [6]. The low-risk, favorable NBs have mitotic disorders, and are characterized by near triploid karyotypes with whole chromosomal gains. On the other hand, the high-risk, unfavorable NBs exhibit genetic instability, and are characterized by chromosomal structural changes, including deletion of 1p or 11q, unbalanced gain of 17q, and/or MNA. MNA is the most powerful prognostic factor identified so far, and is useful regardless of the tumor stage. In the recent studies, the 5-year event free survival of patients who had NB tumors with MNA was 53% for localized NB [7] and 29% for all NBs [8], even with intensive, multimodal treatment. On the other hand, NB without *MYCN* amplification (non-MNA) falls into another two clinically distinct subgroups: a low-risk subgroup with overall survival rates of more than 95% without any intensive therapy, and a high-risk subgroup with overall survival rates of less than 40% despite the use of dose-intensive, multimodal therapy. In the high-risk non-MNA group, the development of NB depends on factors other than MNA, such as the expression profiles of other genes [9], aberrant hypermethylation of tumor suppressor genes [10], and chromosomal loss of heterozygosity (LOH) [11]. To determine the stratification of NB patients more precisely with regard to the treatment approach, a screen for these genetic aberrations should be performed before the initial treatment. Indeed, in the INRG staging system, routine assessments of MNA and 11q loss were required for the therapeutic stratification of NB [8]. Currently, genetic alterations in NB tumors are clinically evaluated by interphase dual-color fluorescence in situ hybridization (I-FISH), array comprehensive genomic hybridization (aCGH), PCR and multiple ligation probe amplification (MLPA) [12]. However, the evaluation of tumor-related genetic aberrations requires a fresh tumor sample, which is often difficult to obtain due to the frequent occurrence of life-threatening conditions in NB patients.

Recent improvements in molecular techniques such as PCR have made it possible to detect small amounts of cell-free DNA in the serum and plasma of patients with various diseases, including cancers. In particular, tumor-derived cell-free DNA has attracted attention as a novel genetic marker for cancer. Other improvements in molecular techniques have enabled the evaluation of tumor-related genetic aberrations using small amounts of cell-free DNA in the serum. NB has been detected with several tumor-related genetic alterations, such as RAS mutations [13], or TP53 mutations [14], microsatellite instability [15], gene amplification [16, 17], aberrant promoter hypermethylation [18, 19], and allelic gain and loss of oncogenes [15, 20, 21].

We have been attempting to establish a preoperative risk stratification system for NB based on a serum-based assay system for *MYCN* gene amplification, aberrant promoter hyperme-thylation, and chromosomal loss of 11q. These less invasive techniques are clinically useful for the preoperative risk stratification of NB patients, because genomic changes in the tumor correlate with the tumor behavior, survival outcome, and response to therapy of NB patients. In this paper, we provide an update on the novel serum-based system for evaluating genetic aberrations for the risk stratification of patients with NB, including our recent studies.

2. Methods and results

Serum samples were collected from the patients with NB before initial treatment. Cellular components were immediately removed from the collected sera immediately by centrifugation or filtration. DNA fragments were purified from 200µl of serum according to manufacturer's protocol and were used for further genetic analysis as mentioned below.

2.1. Detection of amplified *MYCN* gene in the sera of NB patients

The *MYCN* oncogene can be detected in the serum of patients with MNA-NB. We previously established a system for quantitatively evaluating system of *MYCN* gene copy number using serum DNA of NB patients [17]. We simultaneously quantified the dosages of the *MYCN* gene located on 2p24 as a target, and the *NAGK* gene located on 2p12 as a reference by real-time PCR using DNA samples obtained from paired serum and tumor samples before the initial treatment. Also, we evaluated the *MYCN* gene copy number to obtain the *MYCN/NAGK* ratio. The *MYCK/NAGK* ratios of serum DNA and tumor DNA were strongly correlated, and the serum *MYCN/NAGK* ratio in the MNA group was significantly higher than the ratio in the non-MNA group. Notably, the sensitivity and specificity of the serum *MYCN/NAGK* ratio as a diagnostic test were both 100% when the serum *MYCN/NAGK* ratio cutoff was set at 10.0

(Figure 1). We also reported that the serum-based *MYCN* status was an indicator of therapeutic efficacy. Among six MNA patients whose clinical courses were followed, the serum ratios decreased to within the normal range in the patients in remission (n=3), whereas the ratios increased to high levels in the patients who relapsed (n=2) or failed to achieve remission (n=1). These data strongly suggested that the serum-based quantitative *MYCN* status was a useful tool for preoperatively determining the stratification for therapy and for the evaluation of therapeutic efficacy during the course of treatment, when tumor cells were not available for a molecular analysis. Considering that it is often impossible to obtain tumor samples from patients with advanced NB for biological studies due to their life-threatening conditions, these data may have important clinical implications.

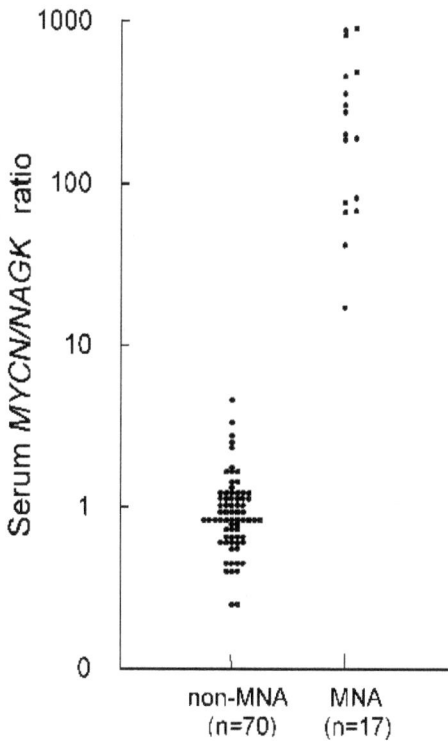

Figure 1. A scatter plot of serum *MYCN/NAGK* ratio according to tumor *MYCN* status. The serum *MYCN/NAGK* ratio was significantly (p<0.001) higher in the MNA group (median, 199.32; range, 17.1 to 901.6; 99% CI, 107.0 to 528.7) than in the non-MNA group (median, 0.87; range, 0.25 to 4.6; 99% CI, 0.82 to 1.26; Mann-Whitney *U* test). Adopted from Ref. [17]

Combaret et al., who first reported the existence of the *MYCN* gene in the sera of NB patients confirmed our data using a European cohort and the same method that we used. Also, they indicated that the sensitivity of serum-based *MYCN* status depends on the stage of NB and is lower for patients with locoregional NB [22]. Indeed, they analyzed 10 serum samples obtained at diagnosis from MNA-NB patients with INSS stages 1 and 2, and 16 serum samples from MNA-NB patients with INSS stage 3 disease, and revealed that only one of 10 patients with stage 1 and 2 disease, and 12 of the 16 INSS patients with stage 3 disease showed high levels of circulating *MYCN* DNA sequences (10% and 75% sensitivity, respectively). In contrast, significant levels of circulating *MYCN* DNA sequences were detected in the patients with stage 4 disease and MNA (85% sensitivity).

We also confirmed the sensitivity and specificity of serum MNA analysis using 148 samples obtained from NB patients with various INSS stages in two Japanese cohorts other than ours and a cohort from the Children Oncology Group. A sub-group analysis according to INSS stages revealed that the sensitivities and specificities were not statistically different (67% and 95%, respectively, in stages 1 and 2, 92% and 86% in stage 3, and 87% and 97% in stage 4), although the number of each group was not statistically sufficient (p=0.48 for sensitivity, p=0.68 for specificity, chi-squared test) (our unpublished data). Accordingly, the serum *MYCN/NAGK* ratio would be a specific tool for the prediction of tumor *MYCN* amplification in patients with NB regardless of tumor stage, even though the sensitivity of serum MNA analysis showed a tendency to be low among the patients with INSS stages 1 and 2. Indeed, for most therapeutic regimens, primary radical resection is recommended for localized non-MNA NB. Moreover, up-front surgical resection is not indicated for advanced localized NB, including tumors with MNA. Therefore, knowing the preoperative serum-based *MYCN* status should result in better decision-making, especially for localized NB. As mentioned above, circulating tumor-derived cell-free DNA could be detected in the serum of cancer patients regardless of the tumor stage. Therefore, it was of interest to determine whether the serum-based *MYCN* status was also useful to determine the risk classification for localized NB. Being able to determine the *MYCN* status of NB patients from a blood sample would be very useful for cases who cannot provide tumor samples for a molecular analysis.

2.2. Detection of methylated DNA fragments in the sera of NB patients

It is important to have additional biomarkers with prognostic value for the management of non-MNA cases of NB because some cases without MNA also have a poor prognosis. Recent studies have revealed that epigenetic alterations, such as silencing of tumor suppressor genes by aberrant hypermethylation of the promoter, often play important roles in the pathogenesis and progression of NB. A positive correlation has been found between the hypermethylation of the promoters of these genes and a poor prognosis, thus suggesting that hypermethylation influences the phenotype of neuroblastoma.

We previously revealed that the aberrant hypermethylation in the promoter region of the *DCR2* gene in serum is a potent prognostic factor especially in non-MNA NB [18]. *DCR2* (decoy receptor 2) is a tumor necrosis factor alpha receptor superfamily gene, and is negatively associated with tumor necrosis factor-related apoptosis-inducing ligand (TRAIL)-induced apoptosis, because it lacks an intracellular death domain [23]. In NB tumors, the methylation profile of *DCR2* has been found to be drastically different and independent of the *MYCN* status

[10, 24, 25]. Moreover, *DCR2* methylation was found to be associated with rapidly progressing tumors and a reduced overall survival [10]. Using the methylation-specific real-time PCR analysis we established [18], the aberrant hypermethylation in the promoter region of *DCR2* gene could also be detected in the serum DNA, and strongly correlated with the expression in the tumor. The 5-year event-free survival and overall survival of NB patients with methylated *DCR2*, as detected by a serum-based assay, were significantly poorer than those of NB patients with unmethylated *DCR2* [18] (Figure 2). These observations indicated that the serum-based *DCR2* methylation status could help predict the prognosis of NB patients, especially those without MNA. Additionally, the serum-based *DCR2* methylation status can distinguish patients with a poor outcome within the non-MNA group, and may allow for a new type of risk stratification for patients with non-MNA NB in future trials.

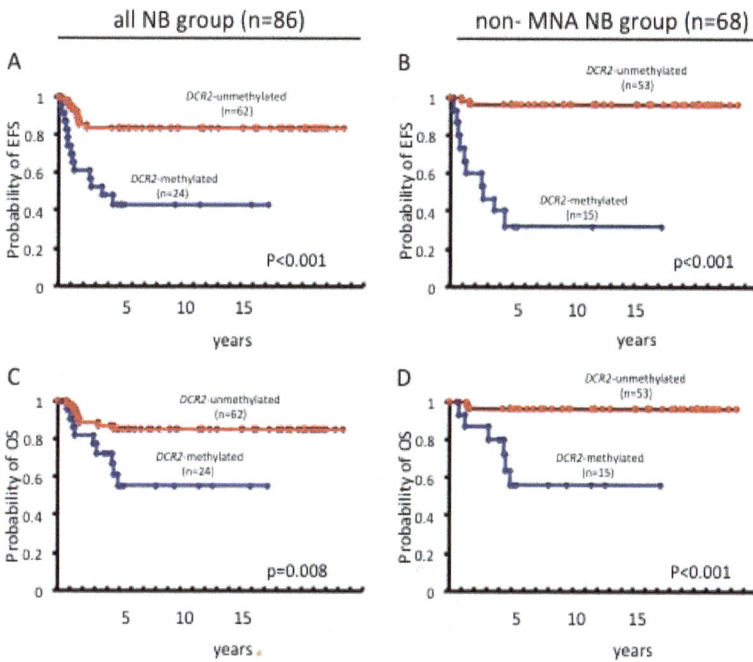

Figure 2. Event-free and overall survival for patients with neuroblastoma according to the serum-based *DCR2* methyl-ation status. A: Event-free survival in all patients with neuroblastoma: methylated (n = 24) and unmethylated (n = 62); P < 0.001. B: Event-free survival in patients with non-MNA neuroblastoma: methylated (n = 15) and unmethylated (n = 53); P < 0.001. C: Overall survival in all patients with neuroblastoma: methylated (n = 24) and unmethylated (n = 62); P = 0.008. D: Overall survival in patients with non-MNA neuroblastoma: methylated (n = 15) and unmethylated (n = 53); P < 0.001. Adopted from Ref. [18]

RASSF1A is hypermethylated in 93-94% of NB primary tumors and in 100% of relapsed tumors [19, 26]. *RASSF1A* hypermethylation in tumors appears to be a relatively early event in NB tumorigenesis, as it is usually detectable in early stage tumors. On the other hand, *RASSF1A* methylation was detected in the serum from only 25% of NB patients, and methylated *RASSF1A* was more frequently detectable in the serum of advanced NB patients than in those with early stage NB, although the *RASSF1A* methylation status in NB tumors was not significantly different between patients with advanced and early stage NB. These discrepancies in the sensitivities between serum-based and tumor-based methylation assays could be explained by the smaller quantity of DNA released from a small tumor burden. Nevertheless, this serum-based *RASSF1A* methylation assay should help to determine the appropriate risk classification.

2.3. Detection of chromosomal loss and gain in the serum DNA of NB patients

Chromosomal gain and/or loss are frequently observed in NB as mentioned above. Among the various unbalanced chromosomal aberrations, 17q gain is the most frequent chromosomal aberration, and correlates with a poor outcome [27]. The loss of 11q is also a strong prognostic factor that can be used in addition to MNA [11], and routine assessment of the 11q status, as well as MNA, is required for therapeutic stratification of NB in the INRG staging system [8].

Some groups, including ours, have developed serum-based assays to detect chromosomal gain and/or loss in NB using various techniques. Combaret et al. reported a serum-based detection system for 17q gain [20]. They simultaneously quantified the gene dose of MPO (17q.23.1) and survivin (17q25) as targets, and p53 as a reference, by quantitative real-time PCR using 142 serum samples. They revealed that the serum-based determination of 17q gain had good specificity (94.4%) and sensitivity (58.8%) in patients who were less than 18 months old ($p<0.001$), while this approach showed moderate specificity (71.4%) and sensitivity (51.2%) in patients over 18 months of age. In a subset analysis according to the stage of NB, the sensitivity of serum-based 17q gain determination tended to increase with the stage of the disease. On the other hand, for metastatic NB, the sensitivity of the test never exceeded 60%, which is lower than the results achieved by the analysis of the serum-based *MYCN* status.

We developed an assay for detecting chromosomal aberration of 11q, using a different method that doesn't use quantitative real-time PCR. Previous studies have revealed the presence of a smallest region of overlap (SRO), which is a common region of deletion in all NB cases with 11q loss. By targeting some polymorphic markers in the SRO of 11q (most of which are located in 11q23), allelic loss could be detected using serum DNA as well as tumor DNA of NB patients [21] (Figure 3). Using this technique, the sensitivity and specificity of the results between the serum- and tumor-based 11q loss analyses were both 100%, although a further study is needed to confirm of these findings because of the limited number of cases that were analyzed.

3. Discussion

In a large-scale randomized trial of children with high-risk NBs [28], the *MYCN* status was unknown in 27% of the children. In a clinical setting, some life-threatening cases with a huge mass or hepatomegaly (hepatic metastasis in stage 4s) received chemotherapy and/or radio-

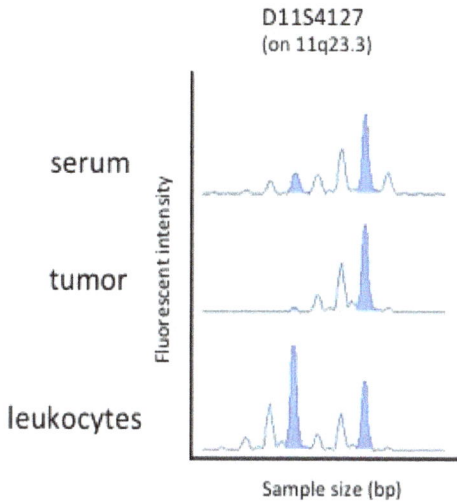

Figure 3. Representative case of 11q loss. The results of 11q microsatellite analysis were shown. This case was a neuroblastoma categorized into low-risk subgroup (INSS stage2, *MYCN* non-amplified NB, Shimada: Favorable Histology). Complete resection after initial diagnosis was performed without any additional chemotherapy. Relapse at bone and bone marrow 1 year after resection was observed, and he died of disease 3year after relapse. Microsatellite analysis were performed using his serum, tumor and leucocyte DNA, and STS marker D11S4127 located on 11q 23.3. Non-tumor DNA purified from leukocytes has two fluorescent peaks (shown in blue), whereas in tumor and serum DNA, one of the peaks is reduced, suggesting the existence of 11q loss. Adopted from Ref. [21].

therapy based on elevated tumor markers and positive MIBG scintigraphy, prior to tumor biopsy without evaluation of the *MYCN* status. The serum-based assays described above will be most useful when a primary tumor biopsy is not possible and when genetic information will influence the risk grouping and treatment allocation of the NB patients.

In Japan, infantile NB cases were formerly subclinically detected by mass-screening. Most of these cases showed a good prognosis and were recommended to undergo a reduced regimen, including the "wait-and-see" approach. However, we and others demonstrated that MNA was strongly correlated with a poor prognosis even in infantile, localized NB [7, 29]. The serum-based MNA status has considerable prognostic value for infantile NB cases. Indeed, the serum-based MNA status of NB patients has considerable prognostic value, especially in cases less than 18 months of age (our unpublished data).

On the other hand, most of the infantile, localized NB patients did not have MNA. In the Cooperative German Neuroblastoma NB95 and NB97 trials, some localized patients without MNA did not receive chemotherapy after biopsy and showed spontaneous regression [30]. Considering the clinical behavior of non-MNA NB, an early and non-invasive system for detecting genetic alterations besides MNA is needed to help select the appropriate therapy. In other words, combined preoperative assessments of MNA and 11q loss using serum DNA will make it possible to safely perform risk-adapted therapy according to the INRG staging system

[8]. Particularly, preoperative serum-based MNA and 11q loss detection can be useful for cases that are in INRG stages L2 and MS, which have a wide range of clinical outcomes and potential therapeutic strategies depending on the existence of MNA and 11q loss. Further, we may be able to select infants with NB who truly need to receive treatment including surgical treatment, intensive chemotherapy, and even radiotherapy from infants with NB who do not need to require any treatment by using our technique.

In conclusion, serum-based, less invasive molecular analysis can provide much better clinical information to determine the optimal therapeutic strategy for NB patients. Prospective validation in a large cohort will be needed to confirm the utility of these tools for assessing biological risk. Serum-based, surgery-free, rapid, sensitive, and specific genetic assessments have great potential to provide a personalized, risk-adapted therapy for patients with NB.

Author details

Shigeki Yagyu, Tomoko Iehara and Hajime Hosoi*

Department of Pediatrics, Graduate School of Medical Science, Kyoto Prefectural University of Medicine, Kyoto, Japan

References

[1] London, W. B, Castleberry, R. P, Matthay, K. K, et al. Evidence for an age cutoff greater than 365 days for neuroblastoma risk group stratification in the Children's Oncology Group. (2005). , 2005, 23-6459.

[2] Brodeur, G. M, Pritchard, J, Berthold, F, et al. Revisions of the international criteria for neuroblastoma diagnosis, staging, and response to treatment. (1993). , 1993, 11-1466.

[3] Peuchmaur, M, Amore, d, & Joshi, E. S. VV et al. Revision of the International Neuroblastoma Pathology Classification: confirmation of favorable and unfavorable prognostic subsets in ganglioneuroblastoma, nodular. (2003). , 2003, 98-2274.

[4] Brodeur, G. M, Seeger, R. C, Schwab, M, et al. Amplification of N-myc in untreated human neuroblastomas correlates with advanced disease stage. (1984). , 1984, 224-1121.

[5] Seeger, R. C, Brodeur, G. M, Sather, H, et al. Association of multiple copies of the N-myc oncogene with rapid progression of neuroblastomas. (1985). , 1985, 313-1111.

[6] Brodeur, G. M. Neuroblastoma: biological insights into a clinical enigma. (2003). , 2003, 3-203.

[7] Bagatell, R, Beck-popovic, M, London, W. B, et al. Significance of MYCN amplifica-
     tion in international neuroblastoma staging system stage 1 and 2 neuroblastoma: a
     report from the International Neuroblastoma Risk Group database. (2009). , 2009,
     27-365.

[8] Cohn, S. L, Pearson, A. D, London, W. B, et al. The International Neuroblastoma Risk
     Group (INRG) classification system: an INRG Task Force report. (2009). , 2009,
     27-289.

[9] Ohira, M, Oba, S, Nakamura, Y, et al. Expression profiling using a tumor-specific
     cDNA microarray predicts the prognosis of intermediate risk neuroblastomas.
     (2005). , 2005, 7-337.

[10] Banelli, B, & Gelvi, I. Di Vinci A et al. Distinct CpG methylation profiles characterize
     different clinical groups of neuroblastic tumors. (2005). , 2005, 24-5619.

[11] Attiyeh, E. F, London, W. B, Mosse, Y. P, et al. Chromosome 1p and 11q deletions
     and outcome in neuroblastoma. (2005). , 2005, 353-2243.

[12] Ambros, P. F, Ambros, I. M, Brodeur, G. M, et al. International consensus for neuro-
     blastoma molecular diagnostics: report from the International Neuroblastoma Risk
     Group (INRG) Biology Committee. (2009). , 2009, 100-1471.

[13] Anker, P, Lefort, F, Vasioukhin, V, et al. K-ras mutations are found in DNA extracted
     from the plasma of patients with colorectal cancer. (1997). , 1997, 112-1114.

[14] Kirk, G. D, Lesi, O. A, Mendy, M, et al. ser) TP53 mutation in plasma DNA, hepatitis
     B viral infection, and risk of hepatocellular carcinoma. (2005). , 2005, 24-5858.

[15] Nawroz, H, Koch, W, Anker, P, et al. Microsatellite alterations in serum DNA of
     head and neck cancer patients. (1996). , 1996, 2-1035.

[16] Combaret, V, Audoynaud, C, Iacono, I, et al. Circulating MYCN DNA as a tumor-
     specific marker in neuroblastoma patients. (2002). , 2002, 62-3646.

[17] Gotoh, T, Hosoi, H, Iehara, T, et al. Prediction of MYCN amplification in neuroblas-
     toma using serum DNA and real-time quantitative polymerase chain reaction.
     (2005). , 2005, 23-5205.

[18] Yagyu, S, Gotoh, T, Iehara, T, et al. Circulating methylated-DCR2 gene in serum as
     an indicator of prognosis and therapeutic efficacy in patients with MYCN nonampli-
     fied neuroblastoma. (2008). , 2008, 14-7011.

[19] Misawa, A, Tanaka, S, Yagyu, S, et al. RASSF1A hypermethylation in pretreatment
     serum DNA of neuroblastoma patients: a prognostic marker. (2009). , 2009, 100-399.

[20] Combaret, V, Brejon, S, Iacono, I, et al. Determination of 17q gain in patients with
     neuroblastoma by analysis of circulating DNA. (2011).

[21] Yagyu, S, Iehara, T, Gotoh, T, et al. Preoperative analysis of 11q loss using circulating tumor-released DNA in serum: a novel diagnostic tool for therapy stratification of neuroblastoma. (2011). , 2011, 309-185.

[22] Combaret, V, Hogarty, M. D, London, W. B, et al. Influence of neuroblastoma stage on serum-based detection of MYCN amplification. (2009).

[23] Srivastava, R. K. TRAIL/Apo-2L: mechanisms and clinical applications in cancer. (2001). , 2001, 3-535.

[24] Yang, Q, Kiernan, C. M, Tian, Y, et al. Methylation of CASP8, DCR2, and HIN-1 in neuroblastoma is associated with poor outcome. (2007). , 2007, 13-3191.

[25] Van Noesel, M. M, Van Bezouw, S, Salomons, G. S, et al. Tumor-specific down-regulation of the tumor necrosis factor-related apoptosis-inducing ligand decoy receptors DcR1 and DcR2 is associated with dense promoter hypermethylation. (2002). , 2002, 62-2157.

[26] Michalowski, M. B, De Fraipont, F, Plantaz, D, et al. Methylation of tumor-suppressor genes in neuroblastoma: The RASSF1A gene is almost always methylated in primary tumors. (2008). , 2008, 50-29.

[27] Lastowska, M, Cotterill, S, Pearson, A. D, et al. Gain of chromosome arm 17q predicts unfavourable outcome in neuroblastoma patients. U.K. Children's Cancer Study Group and the U.K. Cancer Cytogenetics Group. (1997). , 1997, 33-1627.

[28] Matthay, K. K, Villablanca, J. G, Seeger, R. C, et al. Treatment of high-risk neuroblastoma with intensive chemotherapy, radiotherapy, autologous bone marrow transplantation, and 13-cis-retinoic acid. Children's Cancer Group. (1999). , 1999, 341-1165.

[29] Iehara, T, Hosoi, H, Akazawa, K, et al. MYCN gene amplification is a powerful prognostic factor even in infantile neuroblastoma detected by mass screening. (2006). , 2006, 94-1510.

[30] Hero, B, Simon, T, Spitz, R, et al. Localized infant neuroblastomas often show spontaneous regression: results of the prospective trials NB95-S and NB97. (2008). , 2008, 26-1504.

Neuroblastoma, Biology - 1

Chapter 3

Neurotrophin and Neurotrophin Receptor Involvement in Human Neuroblastoma

Pierdomenico Ruggeri, Antonietta R. Farina,
Lucia Cappabianca, Natalia Di Ianni, Marzia Ragone,
Stefania Merolle, Alberto Gulino and
Andrew R. Mackay

Additional information is available at the end of the chapter

1. Introduction

Neuroblastoma (NB) is an embryonic tumour that originates from cells of the neural crest (NC) arrested in their differentiation at different stages along the sympatho-adrenal lineage and, less frequently, from precursors of sensory neurons [1, 2]. As a consequence, NB can occur throughout the sympathetic chain from thoracic, abdominal and pelvic sites to the adrenal medulla, which accounts for the majority of NBs. Consistent with this, NBs exhibit a high degree of genetic heterogeneity and biological variability, including differences in catechola-mine expression, according to their differentiation state along the sympathoadrenal lineage, with a small number of primitive midline and spinal NBs that do not secrete catecholamines considered to be of dorsal root sensory origin [1, 2].

Sympathetic nervous system development is orchestrated by neurotrophins (NT) and their respective neurotrophin receptors (NTR), which exhibit subtle temporal and spatial changes in expression that are critical for the delamination, migration, proliferation, survival, differ-entiation and apoptotic programs of NC lineages that form the fully differentiated and functional sympathetic nervous system. Not surprisingly NBs, consistent with their origin and particular differentiation state at the time of transformation, exhibit a variety of different patterns of NT and NTR expression. A great deal of research has focussed on characterising and exploiting these different patterns of expression for potential prognostic and therapeutic benefit. Recent studies have led to exciting new developments in understanding how block-ages in sympathetic differentiation promote NB and how NBs utilise different patterns of NT and NTR expression to select a more malignant, stress-resistant, invasive, genetically unstable, stem cell-like phenotype. Furthermore, they have also identified novel potential therapeutic targets and characterised patterns of NT/NTR expression of value in prognosis and therapeutic choice. In this chapter therefore, we will review the origins of NB during neural crest migation and sympathetic nervous system development, introduce NTs and NTRs and describe their roles NC and sympathetic nervous system development, examine patterns of NT/NTR expression in NB, review their potential roles in regulating spontaneous NB regression and metastatic NB progression, and discuss potential therapeutic ways to target the NT/NTR system in NB.

2. Formation of the neural crest, neural crest cell delamination and migration

NBs originate from NC cells (NCC) during sympathetic nervous system development. In this section therefore, we will briefly describe the natural history of neural crest, sensory dorsal root and sympathetic nervous system development, focussing attention on the sympatho-adrenal neuroblast lineage, which is responsible for generating neuroendocrine chromaffin tissues, SIF and ganglion cells, and in particular the adrenal medulla within which the majority (40-50%) of NBs develop [2, 3].

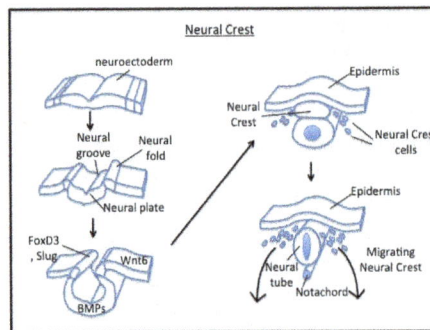

Figure 1. Formation of the Neural Crest and Neural Crest cell migration

During the 3rd week of human embryonic development the intra-embryonic mesoderm differentiates into paraxial, intermediate and lateral plate portions. The paraxial mesoderm organises into primitive segmented somites and the lateral plate mesoderm splits into somatic (parietal) and splanchnic (visceral) layers. This event occurs in a BMP-induced Notch-dependent "clock" and Wnt-dependent "wave" manner in a rostral to caudal gradient of FGF [2, 4-6] and results in the simultaneous formation of Somite pairs either side of the forming neural tube, in a head to tail direction along the entire length of the embryo, with each new somite forming on the caudal side of an existing somite. Somites further differentiate into dermomyotome and sclerotome structures that will eventually provide the cells for skin, muscle and skeletal formation. Contemporarily, the embryonic neuroectoderm undergoes progressive indentation to form the neural groove, neural folds and neural plate. This neurulation process causes the fusion of opposing neural folds at the future upper cervical level, which progresses in both rostral and caudal directions, eventually resulting in continuity between neural and squamous surface ectoderm. This event separates the presumptive epidermis from the neural plate, which in turn forms the distinct and separate columnar cellular structure of the Neural Tube. Interaction between the neural plate and presumptive epidermis is regulated by Wnts, BMPs and FGFs and results in mesenchymal transformation of the epithelial cells that line the margins of the neural fold. These cells organise between the epidermis and neural tube to form the transient Neural Crest (NC) embryonic structure [2, 6] (Fig. 1).

NC cells (NCC) delaminate from the NC and migrate initially in a ventrolateral manner and later in a dorsolateral direction, relative to the somites. Ventrolateral NCC migration occurs in chain-like manner [7] between the somites and neural tube and the rostral half of each somite [8]. NCC initially migrate through the inter-somitic boundary before switching to a sclerotome pathway controlled by semaphorin and its receptor neuropilin, with the entire dermomyotome repulsing neuropilin positive trunk NCC [9] (Fig. 2).

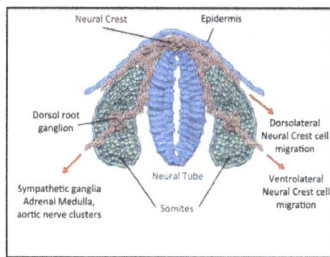

Figure 2. Neural Crest cell ventrolateral and dorsolateral migration

Dorsolateral NCC migration occurs between the developing dermis and the dorsal dermomyotome boundary [8, 10]. During NCC migration cells receive signals from adjacent structures that initiate a series of differentiation processes that will eventually lead to differentiation-commitment and specific cell fates at different locations. This process provides a wide variety of differentiated tissues, including: epidermal pigment cells (melanocytes); dorsal root, sympathetic and parasympathetic ganglia, neurons and plexuses; neuroglial and Schwann cells; endocrine/paracrine cells of the adrenal medulla, carotid body and organ of Zuckerland; cartilage and bones of the facial and ventral skull; corneal endothelium and stroma; tooth papillae; dermis, smooth muscle and adipose tissue of the head and neck;

connective tissue of the salivary, lachrymal, thymus, thyroid and pituitary glands and connective tissue and smooth muscle in arteries of aortic origin (Fig. 3).

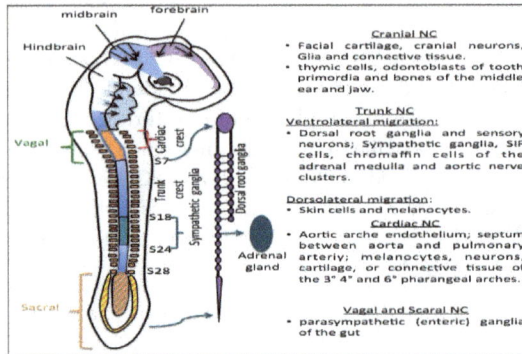

Figure 3. Neural crest cell destinations during embryonic development

3. The sympathetic nervous system

The vertebrate nervous system is composed of the central (CNS) and peripheral (PNS) nervous systems, the former comprised of the brain and spinal cord and the latter comprised of ganglia and associated plexuses that innervate and connect visceral organs and other tissues to the CNS.

The PNS is divided into the somatic and autonomic nervous systems, the former responsible for skeletal muscle function and the latter for innervation of visceral organs [11, 12]. The autonomic nervous system is further subdivided into sympathetic (SNS) and parasympathetic (PSNS) nervous systems, which are often antagonistic. Motor outflow from both systems is formed by serially connected neurons that initiate with pre-ganglionic neurons of the brain stem or spinal chord, which synapse with ganglia and post ganglion neurones outside the CNS. Parasympathetic ganglia lie close to or within the organs they innervate, whereas sympathetic ganglia lie at some distance from their target organ. Both have sensory fibres that feedback information concerning organ function to the central nervous system [11, 13].

The NC is fundamental for SNS formation. Pluripotent migratory NCC progenitors delaminate from the NC and migrate in a vetrolateral direction through the rostral half of each somite. NCC remaining within somites coalesce to form paraspinal dorsal root ganglia, which contain the nerve bodies of afferent spinal nerves responsible for relaying sensory information into the CNS. NCC that exit somites ventrolaterally initially lose segmental organisation, mix adjacent to the dorsal aorta then re-segregate to form sympathetic ganglia, helping to explain sympathetic ganglia heterogeneity [7]. At this point cells initiate differentiation that is responsible for the eventual formation of sympathetic ganglia, associated sympathetic neurones and

Schwann cells, small intensely fluorescent (SIF) cells and chromaffin cells of the adrenal medulla and extra adrenal paraganglia (Fig. 4). Together, these components form the neuro-endocrine SNS, which consists of preganglionic neurones that exit from spinal chord ventral routes of the 12 thoracic and 3 lumbar spinal segments that synapse with neurons of the sympathetic ganglia or specialised chromaffin cells of adrenal medulla and paraganglia. Sympathetic ganglia include paravertebral and prevertebral ganglia, with pairs of paraverte-bral ganglia each side of the vertebra interconnected to form the sympathetic chain. Normally, there are 21 to 22 pairs of paravertebral sympathetic ganglia, 3 cervical, 10-11 thoracic, 4 lumbar, 4 sacral and a single ganglion impar in front of the coccyx. Cervical superior, middle and stellar ganglia innervate viscera of the head and neck, thoracic ganglia innervate viscera of the trunk, and lumbar/sacral ganglia innervate the pelvic floor and lower limbs. Sympathetic ganglia also innervate blood vessels, muscle, skin, erector pilli and sweat glands [11, 13].

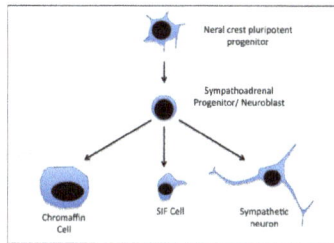

Figure 4. Cell types generated from differentiated sympathoadrenal neuroblast progentitors

In general, preganglionic neurons utilise acetylcholine as the major neurotransmitter, whereas post-ganglionic neurons are noradrenergic and utilise noradrenalin as the major neurotrans-mitter, combined with specific neuropeptide transmitters (e.g. neuropeptide Y, somatostatin, vasointestinal peptide and calcitonin related peptide), utilised in an organ-specific manner. Under normal conditions the sympathetic nervous system provides local adjustments (e.g. sweating) and relax adjustment to the cardiovascular system. Under conditions of stress, the entire SNS can activate to induce the "fight or flight" response, during which adrenalin released from the adrenal gland leads to rapid increases in heart rate, cardiac output, skeletal muscle vasodilation, cutaneous and gastrointestinal vasoconstriction, pupil dilation, bronchial dilation and pili-erection, in preparation for imminent danger [11, 13].

3.1. Sympatho-adrenal progenitors, SIF and Chromaffin cells of the neuroendocrine SNS

The vast majority (40-50%) of NBs arise from neuroblastic NCCs within the developing adrenal gland [2, 3]. Therefore, a description of normal adrenal gland development is also warranted at this point.

The fully developed functional adrenal gland is composed of cortex and medulla. The adrenal medulla is composed of neuroendocrine-differentiated chromaffin, SIF and ganglion cells, which are also present in extra-adrenal paraganglia of the carotid body and organ of Zuckerland [14]. Chromaffin and SIF cells, characterised by their affinity from chromium salts, are closely related to sympathetic neurons and, like sympathetic neurons, synthesise, store, uptake and release catecholamines and express enzymes for noradrenalin synthesis including tyrosine hydroxylase (TH) and dopamine-β-hydroxylase (DBH). Unlike sympathetic neurons, chromaffin cells also synthesise, store and release adrenalin and retain their capacity proliferate but do not produce axons or dendrites [15]. Adrenal and extra-adrenal chromaffin tissues, like sympathetic ganglia, are innervated by pre-ganglionic neurones originating from the spinal chord [16]. Chromaffin, SIF and sympathetic neurons exemplify the wide spectrum of sympathoadrenal cell types that originate from NCC [17].

Chromaffin and SIF cells differentiate from pluripotent NCC progenitors that delaminate from the NC at the "adreno-medullary" somite level (somites 18-24 in avian development) [18]. These cells migrate ventrolaterally initially between Somite dermomyotome and sclerotome then through the rostral sclerotome mesenchyme to arrive at para-aortic sites [18-20]. At these sites, NCC mix, re-segregate and coalesce to form sympathetic ganglia. At the same time, NCC derived from the "adreo-medullar" somite region coalesce adjacent to the adrenal cortex anlage then invade the anlage in considerable numbers, initially in a nerve fibre-independent then nerve fibre-dependent manner [21], in a Sox transcription factor-dependent manner [22]. Once within the adrenal primordium, NCCs form rosettes, nests and nodules along nerve fibres, proliferate and initiate pheo-chromoblast differentiation. This process continues throughout foetal development and into the neonatal period, providing differentiated Chromaffin and SIF adrenal medulla cell populations. In humans, the gestational period between 17 and 20 weeks is critical for adrenal sympathetic component development, with neuroblastic NCC proliferation peaking during this period in terms of maximal nodule size and number, waning thereafter. Neuroblastic nodules tend to disappear during the third trimester and are usually absent at birth. However, nodules that continue to grow and persist into neonatal life are not infrequent and have been classified as *in situ* NB. A sizeable number of these NBs spontaneously regress and are likely, therefore, to represent delayed differentiation in addition to neoplastic transformation [23].

Chromaffin cells, SIF cells and sympathetic neurons develop from catecholaminergic sympathoadrenal (SA) progenitors [18, 24, 25] and their formation involves BMP signalling [18, 26-28]. However, the classical concept that a common SA lineage acquires neuronal and catecholaminergic traits prior to migration to secondary sympathetic ganglia and adrenal sites [24, 25] has now been discounted, as chromaffin cells undergo catecholaminergic differentiation within the adrenal anlage and not within primary sympathetic ganglia, and do not express neuronal markers at the onset or even following induction of TH expression [29, 30]. Therefore, sympathetic neuronal and chromaffin lineages must separate upstream prior to catecholaminergic differentiation, despite evidence of sympathoadrenal marker expression in some migrating cells [22, 24, 30], and enter the adrenal primordium as undifferentiated Sox10 expressing NCC [22, 30]. Indeed, chromaffin and sympathetic neurones originate at the same axial level from common NC progenitors but differ in the time of catecholaminergic differentiation [18]. Furthermore, NCC populations migrating to the adrenal anlage and within the adrenal medulla exhibit heterogeneity, and consist of SOX10/Phox2B/p75NTR, SOX10/ p75NTR and PHox2B/p75^{NTR} sub-populations [22].

3.2. Transcriptional regulation of sympathoadrenal differentiation

Chromaffin and sympathetic neuron differentiation is regulated by BMP-induced transcription factors Phox2B, Mash-1, Insm1, Hand2 and Gata 2/3 [31]. Knockout technology has identified a fundamental role for Phox2B in chromaffin and sympathetic neuronal differentiation [18], with Phox2B knockout increasing neuron but not chromaffin precursor death. This not only relates to specific cell traits but also differences in environment and migration [32, 33], and confirms that adrenal anlage are colonised by undifferentiated NCC progenitors. Knockout technology has also characterised a role for Mash-1 as an accelerator of sympathetic neuronal and chromaffin differentiation [34, 35], a role for Insm-1 as a regulator of catecholamine synthesising enzyme expression and, therefore, endocrine differentiation [36, 37], a role for Hand2 in the induction and maintenance of noradrenergic differentiation [38, 39] and a role for Gata3 in the differentiation of both sympathetic ganglia and chromaffin cells [31, 40].

It has now been confirmed that adrenal cortex glucocorticoids are not responsible for chromaffin cell differentiation [41] but they do, however, regulate postnatal chromaffin cell survival and phenyl ethanolamine N-methyl transferase expression [30, 42]. The adrenal cortex is also dispensable for chromaffin differentiation, which is also found in extra-adrenal neuroendocrine tissue, but may regulate adrenal chromaffin cell numbers and associated vascularity [30, 43]. Within the adrenal gland, hypoxia has recently been shown to promote chromaffin/SIF cell differentiation from neuroblasts [44-46].

4. Neurotrophins and neurotrophin receptors in neural crest, sympathetic nervous system and adrenal development

Neurotrophins (NTs) and NT receptors (NTRs) are critical for the development and maintenance of the vertebral CNS and PNS [47-50], NTs and NTRs are also expressed by human NBs and have been implicated in both NB regression and malignant progression. In this section, therefore, we will introduce NTs and NTRs and describe their potential involvement in normal SNS and adrenal development.

4.1. Neurotrophins (NTs)

NTs are a family of growth, differentiation, survival and apoptosis-inducing factors that are involved in many aspects of nervous system development, maintenance and function. They comprise four structurally related basic 115-130 amino acid containing polypeptides, nerve growth factor (NGF), brain-derived growth factor (BDNF), and the neurotrophins 3 (NT-3) and 4/5. NGF was first NT to be described and purified from the mouse salivary gland [51]. This was followed by the discovery of BDNF, NT-3 and NT-4/5 some 30 years later [52-54].

NTs exhibit close structural homology, with the exception of NT4/5 that exhibits only 50% homology to the others NTs, and all contain six conserved cysteines that form structurally important disulphide bridges [55, 56]. NTs are expressed by both neuronal and non-neuronal cells as pre-NTs and are converted to pro-NTs upon signal peptide removal. This can occur within the endoplasmic reticulum (ER), in which NTs are converted to mature-NTs by furins. Alternatively, NTs are transported to the cell surface and released following signal peptide removal as pro-NTs. Secreted pro-NTs, which also exhibit biological activity, are converted to mature NTs by enzymes including plasmin and the matrix metalloproteinases MMP-7 and MMP-9 [56-58]. Within the extracellular environment, pro- and mature NTs form homo-dimers and bind specific receptors to induce an array of biological activities, including cell migration, proliferation, survival, differentiation, apoptosis and neuronal synapse/junction plasticity, depending upon the cell population, receptor expression and activation status [57, 60]. The human *NGF* gene localises to chromosome 1p13.1 [61], the human *BDNF* gene localises to chromosome 11p13 [62], the human *NT-3* gene localises to chromosome 12p13 [62] and the human *NT4/5* gene localises to chromosome 19q13.3 [63]. Since the discovery of NTs, their respective receptors have been identified and many of their roles in nervous system development and function have been elucidated.

4.2. NT receptors

4.2.1. Tropomyosin-related kinases TrkA, TrkB and TrkC

The family of NT receptors includes the tropomyosin-related tyrosine kinases TrkA, TrkB and TrkC [64]. TrkA is the preferred receptor of mature NGF but also binds the mature neurotrophin NT-3 [64, 65]. Identified following the discovery of the first tumour-associated TrkA oncogene [64, 66, 67], the 25kb human *TrkA* gene maps to chromosome 1q21-22 and is organised into 17 exons [68-70]. TrkA proteins are expressed either as the fully spliced gp140kDa TrkAII receptor, alternatively spliced TrkA L0 and L1 variants that exhibit differential exon 2-4 use [71], the TrkAI variant that exhibits exon 9 skipping [72] or the TrkAIII variant, which exhibits in-frame skipping of exons 6 and 7 combined with exon 9 omission [73]. TrkA L0 (exons 2, 3 and 4 alternatively spliced) and TrkA L1 (exons 2 and 3 alternatively spliced) are expressed during rat development [71] as truncated receptors with in-frame deletions of leucine-rich sequences encoded within exons 2-4 [68]. Since, TrkA leucine rich sequences may modulate ligand binding [74], these variants may exhibit altered ligand-binding activity similar to analogous alternative TrkB splice variants [75]. TrkAI (exon 9 exclusion) and TrkAII (exon 9 inclusion) splice variants [72] are expressed as cell surface transmembrane receptors and exon 9 omission does not result in ligand-independent receptor activation. TrkAI and TrkAII variants bind NGF and NT3 [72, 76] but TrkAII exhibits higher levels of NT-3-mediated activation when co-expressed with the low affinity neurotrophin receptor CD271/p75^{NTR} [76]. TrkAII is predominantly expressed within the nervous system, whereas TrkAI expression predominates in the thymus [72].

TrkAIII was identified as an unexpected RT-PCR product in primary human NBs [73]. This variant exhibits exon 6 and 7 skipping plus exon 9 omission, resulting in the in-frame deletion of amino acids 192-284 that encode the D4 extracellular immunoglobulin-like domain, several functional N-glycosylation sites and introduces a valine substitution at the novel exon 5/8 splice junction [73]. In addition to being expressed by primary human NBs, TrkAIII is also developmentally regulated and is detected from stages E13-E18 of mouse embryonic development and is also expressed by immature thymocytes within the developing thymus [73, 77]. Unlike fully spliced TrkA receptors, TrkAIII is not expressed at the cell surface but is retained within intracellular membranes of the endoplasmic reticulum (ER), GN and ER/GN intermediate compartment (ERGIC) [73, 78, 79], within which it exhibits interphase-restricted spontaneous ligand-independent activation [73, 78, 79].

TrkB is the preferred receptor of BDNF but also binds NT-4/5 [65, 80-82]. The 590kb human *TrkB* gene maps to chromosome 9q22 and contains 24 exons [70, 83]. In addition to fully spliced gp145kDa TrkB, eight TrkB variant isoforms have been described, including a gp95kDa C-terminal truncated receptor that lacks the tyrosine kinase and Shc binding domains; a C-terminal truncated receptor that lacks the tyrosine kinase domain but retains the Shc binding site; a C-terminal truncated receptor that lacks exons 23 and 24 but retains tyrosine kinase activity and four N-terminal truncated receptors that exclude combinations of exons 1-5 and upstream signal sequence [75, 83-85]. The *TrkB* gene has also been reported to encode up to 100 different transcripts ranging from 0.7-9kb, at least 36 of which can be translated into functional TrkB proteins [85-87]. Both full length and C-terminal truncated TrkB receptors are expressed in the brain and share 100% extracellular domain homology, consisting of 5 highly glycosylated extracellular binding domains (D1-5) [75, 85, 86].

TrkC binds NT-3 and no other NT [88]. The 387kb human *TrkC* gene maps to chromosome 15q25 and is organised into 18 exons [70] and six TrkC isoforms have been described. In addition to the fully spliced gp145kDa receptor, these isoforms include C14/K2, C25/K3 and C39 variants which contain 14, 25 and 39 additional amino acid insertions between kinase subdomains VII and VIII, downstream of the TDYYR motif of the putative Trk receptor family autophosphorylation site [89] and NC1/T1 and NC-2/T2 non-catalytic variants truncated in the tyrosine kinase domain by short C-terminal sequences [90-92]. Full-length TrkC receptors are expressed during development, whereas truncated receptors predominate in later life in post mitotic cerebellar granule neurons and young stem cell-derived differentiated neurons but not in proliferating neural stem cells. TrkC NC1/T1 and NC2/T2 variants do not support NT-induced neuritogenesis, suggesting that TrkC variants could exert different roles during nervous system development [90, 93].

4.2.2. CD271/p75 neurotrophin receptor

The p75 neurotrophin receptor (CD271/p75^{NTR}) is a member of the tumour necrosis factor (TNFR)/FAS receptor superfamily and binds all NTs in pro-form with high affinity and mature NGF with low affinity [94, 95]. The 3.4kb *CD271/p75^{NTR}* gene is organised into 5 exons and maps to chromosome 17q21-q22 [96]. In addition to the fully spliced 75kDa CD271/p75^{NTR} receptor, a truncated alternative s-p75^{NTR} splice variant has been described that is devoid of exon III. S-p75^{NTR} lacks the NT binding domain, does not bind NTs and is expressed by several neural tissues [97]. The fully spliced CD271/p75^{NTR} extracellular-domain contains four 40-

amino acid repeats with 6 cysteine residues at conserved positions that are required for NT binding, a serine/threonine-rich region, a single transmembrane domain and a 155-amino acid cytoplasmic domain, which does not exhibit catalytic activity. CD271/p75[NTR] acts either as an independent NT receptor, a NT receptor complex with Sortilin or a co-receptor for TrkA, and is involved in regulating death, differentiation or survival signals [94, 98]. The CD271/P75[NTR] receptor is devoid of intrinsic catalytic activity, indicating that signalling from this receptor must depend upon intracellular interactors [99, 100].

4.2.3. Sortilin

Sortilin is a member of the Vps10p domain-containing transmembrane proteins that binds both mature NGF and the neurotrophins NGF, BDNF and NT-3 in pro-form [98, 101, 102]. The 7kb human *Sortilin* gene localises to chromosome 1p13.3 and is expressed as a gp95-100kda glycoprotein [103, 104]. Sortilin co-expression with CD271/p75[NTR] results in the formation of a co-receptor complex that augments affinity for proNGF and acts principally as an inducer of apoptosis [105].

4.3. NT receptor structure and ligand binding

All three Trk receptors share significant sequence homology and a conserved domain organization. This organization comprises from N-terminus to C-terminus of five extracellular domains, a transmembrane region and the intracellular kinase domain.

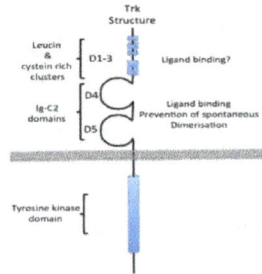

Figure 5. NT receptor structure and ligand binding domains

The first three extracellular domains consist of a leucine-rich region (D-2) flanked by two cysteine-rich regions (D-1 and D-3), and domains 4 and 5 are immunoglobulin-like domains. Studies on TrkB and TrkC have shown that D-5 is sufficient for the binding of ligands and is responsible for binding specificity [106-109], although the D-4 domain, leucines and cysteine clusters may regulate ligand binding [55, 73]. Receptor transmembrane and juxta-membrane regions are critical for signal internalisation and transduction. The intracellular tyrosine-rich carboxyl terminal cytoplasmic domain exhibits tyrosine kinase activity upon ligand-mediated activation and is responsible for propagating post-receptor signal transduction [74, 107, 110-114]. The immunoglobulin-like D4 and D5 domains stabilise receptors in monomeric form and prevent spontaneous receptor oligomerisation and activation. Deletions, chimeric receptors and point mutations that disrupt the structure of the first (D4) and second (D5) immunoglobulin-like domains result in ligand-independent spontaneous receptor activation and the acquisition of oncogenic activity [73, 110, 115] (Fig. 5).

CD271/p75^{NTR} receptors modulate the affinity and enhance the specificity of TrkA for NGF, and TrkB for BDNF, with optimal affinity reflecting the ratio of Trk to CD271/p75^{NTR} receptors [116-118]. In contrast, CD271/p75^{NTR} reduces TrkAI activity in response to NT-3 and TrkB activity in response to NT-3 and NT-4/5 [76, 119, 120]. The CD271/p75^{NTR} receptor analogue neurotrophin-related homolog-2 (NRH2) that is expressed by neural cells, also interacts with TrkA to promote high affinity NGF binding [121].

4.4. NT receptor signalling

In the absence of ligand, Trk receptors are maintained as inactive oligomers [120], concentrated within caveolin and cholesterol-containing cell membrane caveolae invaginations, which also contain components of the Ras signalling pathway [122]. Receptor oligomers are maintained in an inactive state by mature extracellular domain N-glycosylation, intact D4 and D5 domains and by receptor-associated protein tyrosine phosphatases (PTPases) [110, 123-126]. Upon ligand binding, oligomeric Trk receptors dimerize, alter their conformation and acquire tyrosine kinase activity, facilitated by temporary inactivation of receptor-associated PTPases, which results in auto- and trans-phosphorylation of receptor tyrosine residues Y490, Y670, Y674/675, Y751 and Y785, in TrkA and their equivalents in TrkB and TrkC. These tyrosines act as phosphorylation-dependent binding sites for a variety of signalling proteins, including the adapters Shc and FRS-2; Grb-2 and SOS; the IP3K subunit p85α and PLCγ. These interactions, which are modulated by CD271/p75^{NTR}, provide avenues for signal transduction through RAS/MAPK, IP3K/Akt/NF-κB and PKC pathways that mediate NT effects upon migration, proliferation, survival, differentiation and apoptosis [73, 111, 127-141]. Cell surface Trk localisation and NT-mediated Trk activation also involves interaction with the heat shock protein chaperone Hsp90 [78].

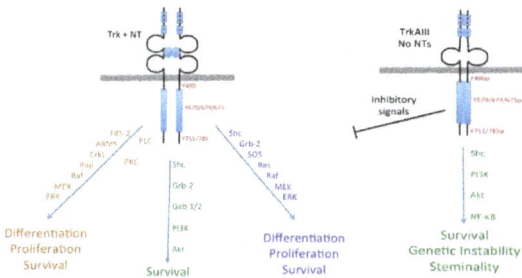

Figure 6. Trk receptor signalling and outcome

Trk receptors activated by NTs use two main pathways to activate MAPKs. The first pathway involves Shc, Grb-2, SOS, Ras and Raf, and the second pathway involves CrkL, Rap and Raf [142, 143]. Trk activation of MAPK is now considered to depend not only upon the phosphorylated Trk Y490 tyrosine residue [144, 145] but also the ankyrin repeat-rich membrane spanning protein ARMS, acting through CrkL [146, 147]. MAPKs activate CREB transcription factors to promote differentiation and survival [148-150]. Trk activation of PI3K/Akt signalling occurs through Shc/Grb-2 and Gab-1 and induces pro-survival signals [73, 151, 152], resulting from the phosphorylation of Bad and activates the pro-survival transcription factor NF-κB [73, 153, 154]. PLCγ is activated as a consequence of being recruited to the phosphorylated Trk tyrosine Y785 [73, 132] and provides additional differentiation and survival signals that involve MAPK [155] (Fig. 6).

The alterative TrkAIII splice variant, in contrast to other Trk receptors (see above), is not expressed at the cell surface but accumulates within intracellular membranes. Intracellular TrkAIII does not bind extracellular NTs and is prone to spontaneous ligand-independent intracellular activation [73, 78, 79]. In contrast to ligand activated cell surface TrkA signalling, spontaneously active TrkAIII signals through PI3K/Akt/NF-κB but not Ras/MAPK, resulting in increased survival and the induction/maintenance of a stem cell-like undifferentiated phenotype [73, 78, 79, 156] (Fig. 6).

An additional feature of TrkA receptors is retrograde transport signalling within the cell. This depends upon receptor/ligand interaction, internalisation and retrograde transport of activated receptors, resulting in signal transduction within the cell body. Sympathetic neurons most dramatically illustrate this activity, with retrograde transport of NGF-activated TrkA occurring along the axonal length to the neuronal cell body. This phenomenon involves ubiquitin mediated receptor internalisation through interaction with CD271/p75[NTR] and TRAF6, receptor endocytosis within clatherin-coated vesicles and receptor endocytosis facilitated by the endocytosis inducing protein EHD4/Pincher [157-159]. In addition, immature Trk receptors also localise to intracellular membranes of the Golgi Network (GN) and can be trans-activated by agonists of the G-protein linked A_{2A} adenosine receptors, potentially through the non-receptor tyrosine kinase Src [160, 161], providing evidence for intracellular neurotrophin-independent Trk activation. Post receptor signal transduction from GN-associated TrkA differs from cell surface-activated TrkA, by signalling through IP3K/Akt but not RAS/MAPK, which results in NF-κB transcription factor activation, inducing a more stress-resistant phenotype, not dissimilar to that induced by the intracellular alternative TrkAIII splice variant [73, 124, 160]. TrkA localisation to the GN may not only reflect transient passage of de-novo synthesised receptors but also alterations in receptor extracellular domain N-glycosylation and folding.

CD271/p75[NTR] receptors regulate cell survival, apoptosis, differentiation and proliferation. CD271/p75[NTR] is a positive modulator of Trk-mediated survival, and within this context, it is likely that CD271/p75[NTR] does not directly bind NTs in competition with Trks [162] but acts as a co-receptor, interacting with Trk dimers ligated to active NTs, refining receptor specificity (e.g. increasing specificity for NGF, while restricting NT-3 binding) [163]. This may be responsible for shifting NT dependence during development coincident with CD271/p75[NTR]

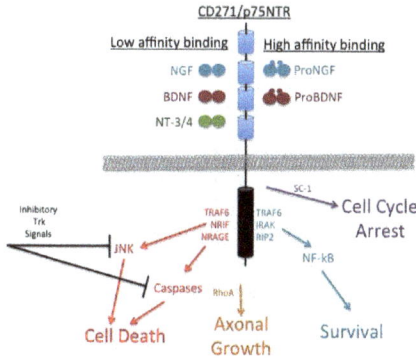

Figure 7. CD271/p75^{NTR} receptor signalling and outcome

expression, which is exemplified by the shift from NT-3/TrkC to NGF/TrkA dependence observed during SNS development [164]. CD271/p75^{NTR} may also influence Trk signalling by binding of the Shc adapter, which also binds to activated Trk, to augment or inhibit Trk signalling [165, 166], and in Trk-complexed form may result in different signalling to that from Trk dimers alone [147], resulting in differences in capacity to complete differentiation programs [167] (Fig. 7).

As a pro-apoptotic receptor CD271/p75^{NTR} also exhibits Trk-independent activity. The cytoplasmic tail of CD271/p75^{NTR} contains death domains and its role in apoptosis has been clearly demonstrated in CD271/p75^{NTR} exon 3 knockout mice [168]. CD271/p75^{NTR} exon 3 knockout mice combined with TrkA knockout mice have highlighted the dual function for CD271/p75^{NTR} in refining innervation and eliminating neuronal excess during early development and later in neuronal survival [169, 170]. Apoptosis induced by CD271/p75^{NTR} involves JNK, phosphorylated c-jun, p53, Bad, Bim and activated caspases [168, 169, 171-174]. Apoptosis induced by CD271/p75^{NTR} may also involve β-secretase-mediated release of the intra-cytoplasmic domain, its subsequent nuclear transport and potential involvement in transcriptional regulation, together with TRAF6, NRAGE, NADE, NRIF and SC-1. TRAF6 interaction with NRIF has been implicated in the generation of death signals through the activation of JNK [169, 175]. NRAGE interaction with CD271/p75^{NTR} is involved in inducing cell death through JNK and caspase activation, and is blocked by TrkA [176]. A role for NADE in CD271/p75^{NTR}-mediated apoptosis, involving NGF but not BDNF or NT-3, has been reported [177], whereas CD271/p75^{NTR} interaction with SC-1 has been implicated in cell cycle arrest via transcriptional repression of cyclins [178] (Fig. 7). Further advances in the understanding of this effect have come with the observation that inactive pro-form NT precursors bind CD271/p75^{NTR} receptors with high affinity and trigger apoptosis at far lower concentrations than active counterparts, which bind with low affinity (Lee et al., 2001). Up to 60% of NTs released by cells are proform [56]. Indeed proNGF induces death in CD271/p75^{NTR} expressing cells, highlighting an opposite effect to activated NGF in cells, including sympathetic neurones [56]. The capacity of proNGF to activate CD271/p75^{NTR} but not TrkA is now known to depend upon Sortilin, a 95kDa member of the Vps10p-domain receptor family [98, 101]. In this interaction, complexes between CD271/ p75^{NTR} and Sortilin are augmented by proNGF, which simultaneously binds both receptors to induce apoptosis. Thus Sortilin acts as an essential co-receptor capable of switching cells that co-express TrkA and CD271/p75^{NTR} from survival to apoptosis.

CD271/p75^{NTR} receptors, therefore, promote either survival or death in response to NTs, depending upon NT status and the cellular context. Survival through CD271/p75^{NTR} receptors involves NF-κB activated through TRFA6, p62, Interleukin-1 receptor-associated kinase IRAK and receptor interacting protein RIP2 [179]. CD271/p75^{NTR} promotion of axon growth involves neurotrophin-mediated dissociation of axonal growth inhibitory complexes between CD271/p75^{NTR} and the G-protein Rho [180]. Furthermore, the proteolytic shedding of cell surface CD271/p75^{NTR} releases an intracellular domain that moves to the nucleus and may act as a transcription factor [181].

4.5. Trks A and C are dependence receptors

A classical concept is that NT activation of Trk receptors inhibits default apoptotic programs to promote NT-dependent survival [134]. This concept is considered to involve PI3K/Akt/NF-κB signalling and induction of Bcl-2 inhibitor of mitochondrial apoptosis. In this mechanism, NT depletion results in the turning-off of PI3K/Akt signalling, which reduces Bad phosphorylation and releases it from the chaperone 14-3-3. This results in Bcl-2 and Bcl-XL sequestration [182, 183], reduces FOX03A phosphorylation resulting in nuclear translocation, induces pro-apoptotic FAS, Trail, Puma and BIM transcription [184-188], abrogates CREB and NF-κB survival signals [189, 190] and activates pro-apoptotic JNK, inducing BIM expression [188], which together trigger apoptosis (Fig. 8).

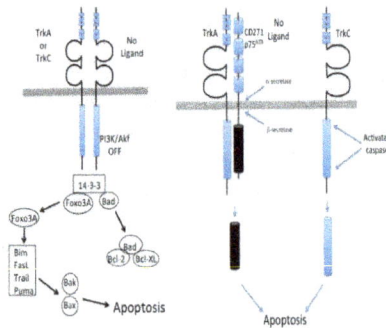

Figure 8. TrkA and TrkC receptors and Apoptosis

Recently, however, both TrkA and TrkC have also been characterised as true dependence receptors. In one study, TrkC but not TrkA or TrkB triggered apoptosis in the absence of NT-3 in a variety of cell lines by an activated caspase-dependent cleavage mechanism, releasing a pro-apoptotic intracellular TrkC domain capable of inducing caspase-9 dependent death [191].

In a separate study, TrkA and TrkC but not TrkB induced apoptosis in neurons differentiated from stable transfected embryonic stem cells and promoted loss of all TrkA and TrkC but not TrkB transfected cells with associated loss of nervous system at E13.5 during mouse embryonic development, through a CD271/p75^{NTR} -mediated mechanism, in which CD271/p75^{NTR} is recruited as a "hired killer" [192]. Therefore in the absence of ligand, TrkC acts directly as a death receptor and TrkA death receptor activity appears to depend upon CD271/p75^{NTR}, whereas TrkB does not exhibit death receptor activity (Fig. 8)

5. NTs and NTRs in sympathetic nervous system development

5.1. TrkC and NT–3

TrkC is the only NT receptor expressed during early embryogenesis. During avian development TrkC expression coincides with neurulation and is detected in both neural tube and neural plate anlage [193, 194]. TrkC is also expressed in hindbrain rhombomeres 3 and 5. This, however, does not associate with lateral NCC migration, suggesting that either TrkC positive NCC cells die prior to NCC migration or that they migrate away from these regions. NT-3 expression is low at this time and the recent characterisation of TrkC as pro-apoptotic dependency receptor, supports the former hypothesis [191, 192]. Neither TrkC nor NT-3 knockout prevent neurulation but do result in neuronal loss from sympathetic ganglia [195-197], indicating that TrkC/NT-3 interactions are not required for neurulation but are required for later stages of SNS development. Consistent with this, the NT-3 protein is detected at later developmental stages. There have been no reports concerning the expression of alternative TrkC isoforms during early development.

During PNS formation, TrkC is expressed by neurogenic pre-migratory and migrating NCC subsets [194, 198, 199] and TrkC/NT-3 interactions are required prior to NCC arrival at destination [200]. Indeed, NT-3 acts as a NCC survival factor and promotes NCC proliferation in the presence of somites [201]. Furthermore, somites express NT-3 during this period [198, 202], sympathetic neuroblasts and neurons also express TrkC and NT-3, NT-3 is expressed by non-neuronal sympathetic cells [194, 199, 203], and NT-3 and TrkC expression during this time is stimulated by neuroregulin, PDGF and CNTF [204]. NT-3 in sympathetic tissues increases mature neuron numbers by promoting the survival of proliferating neuroblast and their subsequent differentiation, without directly effecting proliferation [205]. This temporary effect subsequently declines with a switch to NGF-dependence [206], associated with reduced TrkC expression and the induction of TrkA and later CD271/p75^{NTR} expression [204, 207]. NT-3 continues to be expressed by both sympathetic neural and non-neural cells [198, 199, 204], by adult non-neural cells [208] and TrkA expression is regulated in part by NT-3 [207]. Therefore, NT-3 acts as both a survival and differentiating factor through TrkA, eventually rendering differentiating post-mitotic neurons dependent upon NGF produced by effector tissues. NT-3, at this stage, acts as an autocrine interim and not peripherally derived paracrine factor, corroborated by the lack of target innervation at this time [207]. In support of this, NT-3 knockout mice exhibit sympathectomy [106, 197, 209-212] caused principally by neuroblast apoptosis, which is partially rescued by exogenous NGF [212]. In the adult, NT-3 continues to be expressed by a wide range of tissues [202, 203, 213, 214] and, together with NGF, continues to be important for post-natal sympathetic neuron survival [214, 215]. Consistent with this, exogenous NT-3 promotes target organ sympathetic innervation in NT-3 knockout animals [211, 212], suggesting that the switch from NT-3 to NGF dependence observed in sympathetic neurons *in vitro* [216] does not actually occur *in vivo*. This may relate to environmental differences, corroborated by the mitogenic effect of NT-3 on neuroblasts *in vitro* [201] but not *in vivo* [217], the susceptibility of TrkC transcription to environmental factors and also by the capacity of NT-3 to bind and activate TrkA receptors, and in particular TrkAII [76]. This helps to explain how NT-3 rescues NGF-dependent neurons from NGF depletion and *vice versa* and is consistent with the characterisation of TrkA as a functional NT-3 receptor *in vivo*. However, one difference between these two NTs is that exogenous NGF but not NT-3 induces sympathetic ganglia hyperplasia [218].

NT-3 released from effector tissues and acting through TrkA also promotes sympathetic innervation of target organs [202, 213, 214, 219, 220]. In support of this, effector tissue elimination induces the death of innervating neurons, which cannot be completely reversed by exogenous NGF alone, and adult sympathetic neurons expressing TrkA are immunoreactive for both NGF and NT-3 [49, 221, 222]. Therefore, NT-3 plays an important role throughout sympathetic neuron life-cycle from neuroblast to neuron, acting initially through the TrkC receptor as an autocrine/paracrine factor stimulator of migration and survival in proliferating sympathetic neuroblasts and later as a paracrine promoter of sympathetic neuron differentiation, survival and target organ innervation acting through the TrkA receptor. CD271/p75^{NTR} is also required for optimal neurotrophin sensitivity since CD271/p75^{NTR} deficient dorsal root and sympathetic neurons exhibit reduced sensitivity to NGF [223].

During sympathoadrenal development, progenitors switch from being dependent upon NT3 and TrkC to dependence upon NGF and TrkA, through an intermediate stage of combined TrkA and TrkC expression. In murine thoracic sympathetic ganglia TrkC expression alone is detected at E14-15, whereas both TrkA and TrkC expression are detected at E16.5-17 and only TrkA at E19.5 [224]. Interestingly, sympathetic chromaffin tissues of the adrenal medulla and paraganglia, which form in parallel to sympathetic ganglia, exhibit differences in NT receptor expression consistent with upstream progenitor separation. This difference is characterised by the expression of TrkC but not TrkA by NCCs migrating into the adrenal anlage, at times when TrkC expression is lost in associated with the induction of TrkA expression by NCCs within sympathetic ganglia [225].

5.2. TrkA and NGF

Unlike TrkC, TrkA is not expressed during neurulation, NC development or NCC dorsolateral or vetrolateral migration. In rodent development, TrkA is detected at E12.5 within sensory cranial and spinal dorsal root ganglia and subsequently in the paravertebral sympathetic ganglia [226]. NGF is expressed during the mid-stage of development initiating within CNS structures then within PNS structures at later stages of development [227, 228]. Within the developing adrenal gland NGF exhibits a brief period of post-natal expression, whereas NT-3 is expressed by both the developing and adult adrenal gland [229]. This suggests that TrkA/ NGF interactions are of transient importance in adrenal gland development. Consistent with this, both TrkA and NGF knockout mice exhibit a relatively normal adrenal medulla chromaffin cell content, although cholinergic innervation of pre-ganglionic origin is lost in TrkA knockout animals [230], and both chromaffin and SIF cells express TrkA but do not depend upon NGF for survival. Normal NCC progenitors entering the developing adrenal glands express TrkC and begin to express TrkA upon seeding under the influence of the adrenal environment. This event may depend upon NT-3 and/or NT4/5 expressed by the adrenal cortex anlage, with subsequent chromaffin/SIF differentiation and survival regulated by these NTs. In contrast, sympathetic neurones in paravertebral sympathetic ganglia, despite their common origin, express TrkA and require NGF for their development, differentiation and survival [229-231]. In support of this, NGF neutralising antibodies do not delay adrenal development nor induce chromaffin cell degeneration [232]. Differences between human and rodent adrenal development include observations that the adult rat adrenal cortex but not medulla express TrkB or TrkC [229, 230], whereas TrkA immunoreactivity is restricted to the adrenal cortex and TrkC immunoreactivity to the adrenal medulla with no TrkB immunoreactivity detected in the human adult adrenal glands [233]. Interestingly, stress induces a massive release of NGF from salivary glands, which targets adrenal chromaffin cells inducing marked adrenal medullary hyperplasia and catecholamine synthesis through enhanced TH and BDH expression [234-236]. In chromaffin tissues, sympathoadrenal cells of the carotid body express NGF and TrkA, providing an autocrine/ paracrine mechanism [237]. Pre-natal and post-natal differentiating and differentiated chromaffin cells express TrkA mRNA within the adrenal medulla [238], which increases with development, at times when NGF expression is all but absent [229]. TrkA knockout eliminates the acetylcholine positive component but does not influence chromaffin content of the adrenal medulla [230], indicating that chromaffin cells, unlike their sympathetic neuronal cousins, do not depend upon NGF/TrkA interactions for survival [232, 239]. Chromaffin cells do, however, respond to NGF with acute hyperplasia [235] and eventual neuronal differentiation [240, 241]. In rodents, immature sympathoblasts within sympathetic ganglia cells express TrkA from E14 onwards and express CD271/p75^{NTR} from E16 to birth, in association with acquisition of NGF-responsiveness [242]. Differentiated neurons within sympathetic ganglia express TrkA but not NGF [208].

5.3. TrkB, BDNF and NT4/5

TrkB, like TrkA, is also not expressed during neurulation but is expressed by motor progenitors in hindbrain rhombomere 2 at later stages 9-10 and 12, during avian development, either side of the floor plate in the caudal midbrain, extending through the hindbrain and into the spinal chord [193]. Alternative TrkB splice variant expression has not been assessed during early development.

Following neurulation, TrkB expression is detected within motor neuron progenitors of the ventral neural tube and corresponds to BDNF expression by elements within dorsal neural tube, which coordinate motor neuron development [243]. Consistent with this, both TrkB and

BDNF knockout mice exhibit the loss of motor and sensory neurons from dorsal root, trige-minal, nodose/petrosal, vestibular, and geniculate ganglia [244].

During SNS development, TrkB exhibits expression restricted to sub-populations of pre-ganglionic cells [230, 245], and sympathoblasts within coalescing sympathetic ganglia, which exhibit transient TrkB expression prior to differentiating [225]. Sympathoblasts that express TrkB within coalescing sympathetic ganglia are non-proliferating but do proliferate in response to BDNF *in vitro*, suggesting that the concentration of BDNF within coalescing sympathetic ganglia is sub-threshold at this time [225]. Pre-ganglionic cells respond to BDNF expressed and release by effector tissues, resulting in pre-ganglionic innervation [230]. Within the adrenal gland, chromaffin cells express NT4/5 but not TrkB, which is weekly expressed by the adrenal cortex, providing a neurotrophic source for extra-adrenal TrkB expressing pre-ganglionic neurons located in spinal chord segments T7-T10. Thes cells use adrenal medullary NT-4/5 to project axons into the adrenal medulla in a TrkB-dependent manner [230]. BDNF, on the other hand, is expressed by sympathetic neurones and regulates sympathetic synaptic complexity [246].

The fact that NT4/5 but not TrkB is expressed within the developing adrenal medulla [230, 238, 247] has prompted hypotheses that medullary NT-4/5 may also ligate and activate TrkA receptors expressed by adrenal medullary neuroblasts and chromaffin cells [63, 80, 229, 230]. However, adrenal medullary chromaffin tissues do exhibit rapid stress-induced TrkB expres-sion, which facilitates the adrenal catecholamine response to stress-induced elevation of blood bourn BDNF [248].

5.4. CD271/P75^{NTR}

CD271/p75^{NTR} is a neural crest marker that is expressed by NC crest stem cells during early development, by NC stem cells in peripheral neural tissues during late development after NCC migration has ceased, and by nerve associated post natal and adult NC stem cells [249]. CD271/p75^{NTR} expressing adult NC stem cells have been identified as a potential origin for adult tumours of the PNS and NC, including adult NB [249, 250]. Within the human foetal adrenal medulla, CD271/p75^{NTR} immunoreactivity is detected in nerve fibres and primitive neuroblast clusters, and in the adult adrenal medulla is detected in nerve fibres, ganglion cells and connective tissue cells of septi but not chromaffin cells [251, 252]. CD271/p75^{NTR} is required for normal sympathetic neuronal death and the death of damaged neurons [253-255]. CD271/p75^{NTR} knockout alters synapses within sympathetic ganglia and reduces sympathetic target organ innervation, consistent with its function in enhancing NT-responsiveness [223, 256].

6. Neurotrophins and neurotrophin receptors in human neuroblastoma

6.1. TrkA and NGF expression in NB

The cloning of the TrkA receptor in 1991 [113] initiated the study of TrkA expression in human NBs [257]. This initial report detected an inverse relationship between TrkA mRNA levels and N-myc amplification and expression, with low to no TrkA mRNA expression associated with poor prognosis. This salient study not only implicated Nmyc in the repression of TrkA expression but also reported moderate to high TrkA expression in non-Nmyc amplified disease. The inverse relationship between Nmyc amplification and expression, low TrkA expression and advanced stage disease has now been confirmed by many studies, and it is generally accepted that low TrkA expression combined with Nmyc amplification and expression characterises unfavourable NB and carries poor prognosis [156, 257-270]. In support of this, NBs that form in the root ganglia of Nmyc transgenic mice also exhibit reduced TrkA expression [271]. Nmyc amplified NBs, however, also exhibit heterogeneity [272] and a small number of these tumours exhibit high TrkA expression and favourable histology [270], suggesting that the relationship between NMYC and TrkA in NB is not always straightforward.

Adding to the observation that moderate to high TrkA levels associate with non-Nmyc amplified NB [257, 258], Shimada and colleagues extended the clinical relationship between TrkA expression in NB to include outcome, prognostic significance, biological relevance and histopathological status. They reported that TrkA expression could not distinguish prognostic groups but could distinguish between Nmyc amplified (low TrkA) and non-Nmyc (high TrkA) amplified NB, between Nmyc amplified NB with favourable (high TrkA) and unfavourable (low TrkA) histology, but could not distinguish between non-Nmyc amplified NB with favourable histology (moderate to high TrkA) and unfavourable histology (moderate to high TrkA) [270]. This contrasts with some reports [257, 258, 264] but not others [263]. Adult NBs are aggressive non-Nmyc amplified tumours that express high TrkA levels and in such bear similarity to non-Nmyc amplified paediatric NBs [156, 268, 273].

Low TrkA expression by Nmyc amplified NBs may relate to an origin along the sympathoadrenal lineage within non-TrkA expressing NCC subpopulations that colonize coalescing sympathetic ganglia, paraganglia and adrenal medulla anlage during development [225]. Alternatively, reduced TrkA expression in Nmyc amplified NBs may occur post transformation, since Nmyc represses TrkA transcription by promoting TrkA promoter methylation and TrkA promoter methylation is detected in Nmyc amplified NBs [274, 275].

Moderate to high TrkA levels in non Nmyc-amplified NBs may also relate to cellular origin within undifferentiated TrkA expressing NCC subpopulations of the sympathetic chain and adrenal primordia [225, 276], or may also occur post-transformation, regulated by NTs, growth factors and/or cytokines [277-279].

Despite elevated TrkA expression in advanced stage non-Nmyc amplified and in a small subgroup of Nmyc amplified NBs with favourable histology [270], full length TrkA exhibits a tumour suppressor function in NB models, suggesting that defects in TrkA receptor signalling occur in NB [280]. Consistent with this, TrkA gene transfection in the absence of CD271/ p75^{NTR} restores NGF responsiveness to NB cells, inducing either neuronal differentiation, growth arrest and/or apoptosis in response to NGF [73, 281-284]. Differentiation induced by NGF in TrkA transfected NB cells involves insulin growth factor II [285], RET [286], c-Src [287], protein kinase C-ε [288] and Ras/MAPK/Erk signalling [289, 290], and associates with reduced angiogenic factor expression and angiogenesis resulting in reduced tumorigenic activity [291,

292]. Furthermore, full length TrkA does not promote genetic instability [73, 293] or invasive behaviour of NB cells [294]. Apoptosis induced by TrkA in NB cells is p53-dependent [295], involves the cerebral cavernous malformation 2 protein, CCM2 [296], ERK and caspase-7, and can also be augmented by NGF [297]. As stated above, TrkA may also acts as a true dependency receptor, recruiting CD271/p75[NTR] as a hired killer to promote apoptosis in the absence of NGF [192]. TrkA responsiveness and specificity for NTs is optimised by CD271/p75[NTR], which in its own right acts as a Fas-like apoptosis receptor in response to pro-NTs, supporting the hypothesis that NBs that coexpress TrkA and CD271/p75[NTR] are favourable tumours that carry good prognosis [298, 299]. It should be noted, however, that metastatic bone marrow NB infiltrates induced in SCID mice express TrkA [300] and human NB metastatic bone marrow infiltrates express CD271/p75[NTR] [301].

Although, TrkA gene rearrangements have not been described in NB, a c.1810 C>T TrkA polymorphism has been detected in approximately 9% of NB, with potential to predict disease relapse in non-Nmyc amplified NB [302].

6.2. The alternative TrkAIII splice variant in NB

Anomalies of TrkA expression that do not support an exclusively tumour suppressing role for TrkA in NB, include moderate to high TrkA expression reported in non-Nmyc amplified advanced stage, metastatic unfavourable NBs. These reports may be explained by TrkAIII expression [73], an increase in which was originally reported in advanced stage NB [73], and later confirmed [156, 303, 304]. Recently, TrkAIII expression in a cohort of 500 NBs was found to be significantly higher in high TrkA expressing unfavourable NBs compared to high TrkA expressing favourable NBs (p<0.0001) and to correlate with worse prognosis [156]. Furthermore in the latter study, TrkAIII promoted a cancer stem cell NB phenotype [156], helping to explain high TrkA levels in unfavourable non-Nmyc amplified NB, adult NB and a subset of relapsing NBs [73, 156, 270, 303, 304]. In support of this, gene-based outcome prediction studies focussed on exon-specific expression, have identified a TrkA splicing difference between stage I and stage IV non-Myc amplified NBs [305, 306], and an exon gene array analysis using TrkAI/II specific primers, excluding TrkAIII, reported to provide a significant prognostic and predictive statistical advantage, associating high TrkAI/II expression with better prognosis in NB [307].

TrkAIII represents a developmental and stress-regulated TrkA isoform [73, 77] that exhibits spontaneous ligand-independent activation and oncogenic activity in NB models [73, 78, 79] and promotes a nestin, CD117, CD133 and Sox2 positive NB stem cell phenotype [156]. In contrast to full length TrkA, TrkAIII does not restore NGF responsiveness to NB cells nor induce NB cell differentiation or apoptosis [73, 78, 79] but interfers with NGF/TrkA signalling through Ras/MAPK, augments genetic instability by promoting centrosome amplification [79] and promotes angiogenesis by altering the equilibrium between MMP-9, VEGF and thrombospondin, through IP3K/Atk. Together these phenomena promote NB cell xenograft primary [73] and metastatic tumorigenic activity [308]. Furthermore, TrkAIII increases NB cell resistance to stress, doxorubicin and geladanamycin-induced cytotoxicity [73, 78, 79].

TrkAIII expression in human NB cells is regulated by hypoxic stress [73] and by agents that promote stress within the endoplasmic reticulum (unpublished observations). TrkAIII signalling through IP3K/Akt but not Ras/MAPK, combined with interference in NGF/TrkA signalling, would permit tumours to override NT-dependence, whilst promoting survival and staminality to provide a selective advantage [73, 78, 79]. Therefore, TrkAIII expression in non-Nmyc amplified NBs may parallel the selective advantage provided by BDNF/TrkB in Nmyc amplified NBs [309-313], and NT-3/TrkC in a subgroup of advanced stage NBs [314].

It remains to be determined whether TrkAIII can counteract the pro-apoptotic effects of the Sortlin-CD271/p75^{NTR} complex in the presence of pro-NTs or prevent CD271/p75^{NTR}-mediated apoptosis in the absence of NTs.

6.3. CD271/ p75^{NTR} expression in NB

The CD271/p75^{NTR} low affinity nerve growth factor receptor is a neural crest stem cell marker [249, 250, 315] and is expressed by neural crest-derived melanoma and NB cancer stem cells [250, 316, 317]. In a model of non-Nmyc amplified NB cancer staminality, self replicating CD133, CD271/p75^{NTR} positive clonogenic stem cells produce both a non-malignant fibromuscular lineage and a malignant neuronal (N)-type cell lineage defective in terminal neuronal differentiation. Although Trk expression in this NB population remains to be determined, CD271/p75^{NTR} positive self-replicating neural stem cells have been shown to express TrkA, TrkAIII, TrkB and TrkC [73, 318].

Consistent with a restricted pattern of CD271/p75^{NTR} expression in NB, primary human NBs have been reported to not express CD271/p75^{NTR} [252, 259, 319] or to express variable levels of CD271/p75^{NTR} [251, 319], which either correlate [259] or don't correlate with TrkA expression [259, 264]. Indeed, differences in CD271/p75^{NTR} co-expression with TrkA have been associated with survival, with the co-expression of CD271/p75^{NTR} and TrkA in NB associated with a 100% survival probability, TrkA expression in the absence of CD271/p75^{NTR} with a 62.3% (intermediate) survival probability and no TrkA or p75^{NTR} expression with a 0% probability of survival [259]. Consistent with this, a lack of CD271/p75^{NTR} expression has been reported in Nmyc amplified and undifferentiated NB [252, 319, 321] and high CD271/p75^{NTR} expression reported in more favourable differentiating NBs, ganglioneuromas and ganglioneuroblastomas [251, 252, 299, 320]. However, despite the general concept that high level CD271/p75^{NTR} expression associates with favourable NB behaviour and outcome [259, 264, 322], CD271/ p75^{NTR} expression characterises GD2 positive stage IV metastatic bone marrow NB infiltrates [301] and aggressive adult NBs [268, 323].

Consistent with a general association with favourable NB, CD271/p75^{NTR} exhibits a tumour suppressor role in NB models, promoting differentiation, apoptosis and reducing tumorigenic activity [299, 324, 325]. Differentiation promoted by CD271/p75^{NTR} depends upon the molecular context and may involve an IP3K-Akt-mediated BcL-X-dependent survival pathway [326, 327] or a TrkA-dependent pathway, in which CD271/p75^{NTR} plays a subtle but critical role in optimising and prolonging NGF-mediated TrkA activation [328-331]. Indeed, mutation of CD271/p75^{NTR} within a TrkA context results in proliferation and not differentiation in response to NGF [332]. Coexpression studies in NB cells have also indicated that, in response to NTs,

CD271/p75[NTR] alone induces mild differentiation, TrkA alone causes a more marked differentiation and coexpression an even more marked and rapid differentiation [333].

CD271/p75[NTR] can acts as either an anti-apoptotic or pro-apoptotic factor, depending upon the molecular context. At low TrkA to CD271/p75[NTR] ratios the anti-apoptotic activity of NGF requires binding to CD271/p75[NTR], whilst at higher TrkA to CD271/p75[NTR] ratios involves a mechanism independent of CD271/p75[NTR] binding [334]. Conversely, NGF also induces apoptosis in NB cells with a high CD271/p75[NTR] to TrkA ratios [335]. In the absence of NTs and TrkA, CD271/p75[NTR] induces apoptosis and inhibits NB tumorigenic activity [299, 336-338]. It has been reported that apoptosis, induced by non-ligated CD271/p75[NTR] is inhibited by non-ligated TrkA but this may reflect spontaneous activation of overexpressed TrkA [337]. Furthermore, agents such as prion proteins activate CD271/p75[NTR] to promote apoptosis in NB cells via NF-κB [339]. In the absence of spontaneous TrkA activation and NT expression, however, the coexpression of CD271/p75[NTR] and TrkA promotes more marked apoptosis [333]. In the presence of BDNF CD271/p75[NTR] interaction with TrkB promotes NB cell proliferation and survival, through RAS/MAPK and PI3K/AKT/NF-κB [322]. These reports suggests that CD271/p75[NTR] is a pivotal regulator of the disparate behaviour of TrkA and TrkB expressing NBs, exhibiting capacity to enhance differentiation and apoptotic responses in TrkA expressing NBs and enhance proliferation and survival responses in TrkB expressing NBs, by increasing receptor sensitivity to low NT concentrations and blocking responses to promiscuous NTs.

CD271/p75[NTR] also interacts with Sortilin and other proteins, complicating potential responses to both pro- and active NTs. The CD271/p75[NTR]-Sortilin co-receptor complex augments affinity for proNGF and induces apoptosis [105, 340]. Furthermore, CD271/p75[NTR] also interacts with NRIF, TRAF, NRAGE and MAGE proteins to promote apoptosis [340-342].

With respect to the regulation of CD271/p75[NTR] expression in NB, Nmyc acts as a transcriptional repressor of CD271/p75[NTR] expression by promoting promoter methylation [274]. This effect can be reversed by HDAC inhibitors, resulting in the resoration of NGF-mediated apoptosis [274]. This novel pathway, detected in Nmyc amplified NB, may help to explain the inverse relationship between CD271/p75[NTR] and Nmyc expression detected in human Nmyc amplified NBs and in root ganglia NBs in Nmyc transgenic mice [271, 343]. The histone methyltransferase EZH2A has also been reported to repress CD271/p75[NTR] providing an additional Nmyc-independent CD271/p75[NTR] transcriptional repressing mechanism that may contribute to the genesis and maintenance of undifferentiated CD271/p75[NTR] negative NBs [344].

At the therapeutic level, CD271/p75[NTR] protects NCC and NB cells from apoptosis induced by antimitotic agents [345], and histone deacetylase inhibitors induce NB cell apoptosis and restore CD271/p75[NTR] and TrkA expression [274, 346].

6.4. TrkB and BDNF in NB

Fully spliced TrkB is expressed by a subpopulation of Nmyc amplified NBs [311, 347-349]. Despite observations that Nmyc alone is insufficient to induce TrkB expression [348], TrkB expression in NB exhibits a positive correlation with Nmyc amplification and expression [309, 311, 347, 348, 350]. TrkB expression is stimulated by activated c-erbA in NB cells, unveiling a potential oncogenic receptor tyrosine kinase-mediated mechanism for promoting TrkB expression [351]. Aggressive unfavourable Nmyc amplified NBs also express BDNF, which when coexpressed with TrkB provides an autocrine/paracrine survival mechanism in tissues that do not express NTs [309-313]. Recently, BDNF variants encoding exons 4, 6 and 9 have been associated with unfavourable NB outcome [312, 313].

TrkB expression by sympathoblasts subpopulations during SNS development provides a potential origin for TrkB expressing NBs. However, this population proliferates in response to BDNF *in vitro* but does express BDNF *in vivo* [225, 245], suggesting that BDNF expression may be acquired at a later stage. TrkB transcription in NB cells is also up regulated by hypoxia inducible factor-1, providing a potential epigenetic mechanism through which tumour-associated hypoxia could augment TrkB expression [352].

In contrast to signals from NGF-activated TrkA, which induces NB cell differentiation and growth arrest [73, 324, 353, 354], BDNF activation of TrkB induces partial differentiation in the absence of growth arrest, through Ret tyrosine kinase [354-357]. BDNF activation of TrkB increases NB cell survival [358], resistance to chemotherapeutic agents [358-363], augments invasive capacity [294] in cooperation with c-Met [364] and galectin-1 [365], promotes angiogenesis and angiogenic factor expression [292, 350, 366], augments genetic instability [293] (Schulte et al., 2008) and increases metastatic behaviour by inhibiting anoikis [367]. In contrast, NB cells expressing truncated TrkB lacking the tyrosine kinase domain, display a more differentiated phenotype [311] and this receptor is more frequently detected in ganglioneuroblastomas and ganglioneuromas. Consistent with this, truncated TrkB overexpression in NB cells promotes differentiation suggesting that this receptor variant promotes a more benign phenotype [368]. Oxidative stress up-regulates the expression of full length TrkB relative to the truncated isoform, providing an additional epigenetic mechanism for regulating TrkB involvement in NB [369].

6.5. TrkC and NT3 in NB

TrkC is expressed by migrating NCC progenitors, sympathoblasts and sympathetic neurons [194, 201, 203], providing many potential origins for TrkC expressing NBs. High level TrkC expression in low stage NBs is associated with favourable outcome (309, 310, 349, 353, 370-372], and is often accompanied by TrkA expression [257, 258, 309]. Recently, however, a subset of advanced stage IV NBs has been identified that exhibit high level NT-3 and TrkC co-expression, providing an autocrine/paracrine survival and proliferation mechanism for selecting these NBs in tissues that do not express NT-3 [314]. This expression pattern bears close similarity to migrating, proliferating NCC sympathoblasts prior to sympathetic neuronal differentiation, which also coexpress NT-3 and TrkC [194, 201, 203], identifying a potential origin for this NB subset. TrkC expression in NB, like that of TrkA, inversely correlates with Nmyc amplification and expression, and Nmyc amplified NBs either do not express TrkC at all, or express truncated TrkC [371, 372]. With the exception of NBs that coexpress NT3 and TrkC [314], the co-expression of TrkC, TrkA and CD271/p75^NTR in NB carries the best prognosis and associates more frequently with spontaneous regression, differentiation and chemo-responsiveness [100, 258, 259, 333, 370, 371]. The *TrkC* gene, however, encodes multiple NT-3 receptors with distinct biological properties and substrate specificities [89, 373] and, although *TrkC* gene rearrangements in NB have not been reported, the effect of differential TrkC isoform expression in NB remains to be elucidated.

Association between high TrkC expression and favourable NB outcome, in the absence of NT-3 [333, 371], is consistent with pro-apoptotic TrkC dependency receptor function, which promotes apoptosis in the absence of CD271/p75^{NTR} and NT expression [191, 192]. Furthermore, NT-3 activation of TrkC induces NB cell differentiation [374] and the co-expression of TrkC with CD271/p75^{NTR} lowers tumorigenic potential and tumour growth [375] but may protect NB cells from doxorubicin and cisplatin cytotoxicity [375].

With respect to the transcriptional regulation of TrkC, Nmyc silencing increases TrkC expression in human NB cells [376], corroborating the inverse relationship reported for TrkC expression and Nmyc amplification [371,372]. TrkC expression, furthermore, is abrogated by the activation of c-erbA, providing a potential oncogenic tyrosine kinase-mediated mechanism for repressing TrkC expression in NB [351]. Retinoic acid induces TrkC expression in human NB cells, restoring NT-3-dependent differentiation [152]. Retinoids also induce the expression of microRNAs-9, 125a and 125b that repress truncated kinase domain-deleted TrkC, resulting in altered growth and highlighting a role for the truncated TrkC receptor in the regulation of NB growth and differentiation [377]. MiR-151-3p represses full length TrkC expression, whereas miRs-128, 485-3p, 765 and 768-5p repress truncated TrkC expression in NB cells [378], indicating that full length and truncated TrkC receptors are regulated by different miRs, linking NT-mediated processes to miR expression in NB.

6.6. General considerations on NT and NTR expression patterns in NB

The concept that different NT and NTR receptor expression profiles characterise NB subsets and that these differences are involved in divergent NB behaviour and therapeutic susceptibility, continues to evolve with potential to improve prognosis and therapeutic choice, whilst identifying novel potential therapeutic targets.

The hypothesis that high TrkA, high TrkC and/or high CD271/p75^{NTR} expression always associate with low disease stage and better prognosis in NB is clearly not the case. Moderate to high levels of TrkA, TrkC and/or CD271/p75^{NTR} can also characterise advanced stage and relapsing non-Nmyc amplified NBs and a subset of Nmyc amplified NB with favourable histology (see section 6.1). However, high TrkB expression appears to distinguish advanced stage Nmyc amplified from non-Nmyc amplified NB and carries poor prognosis associated with potential therapeutic resistance (see section 6.4). It is also now apparent that NTRs can be expressed as different isoforms with altered biological activity and can interact with one other and with a variety of ancillary proteins to modulate function (see section 6.3), complicating prognosis and potential therapeutic outcome, as outlined below (Fig. 9).

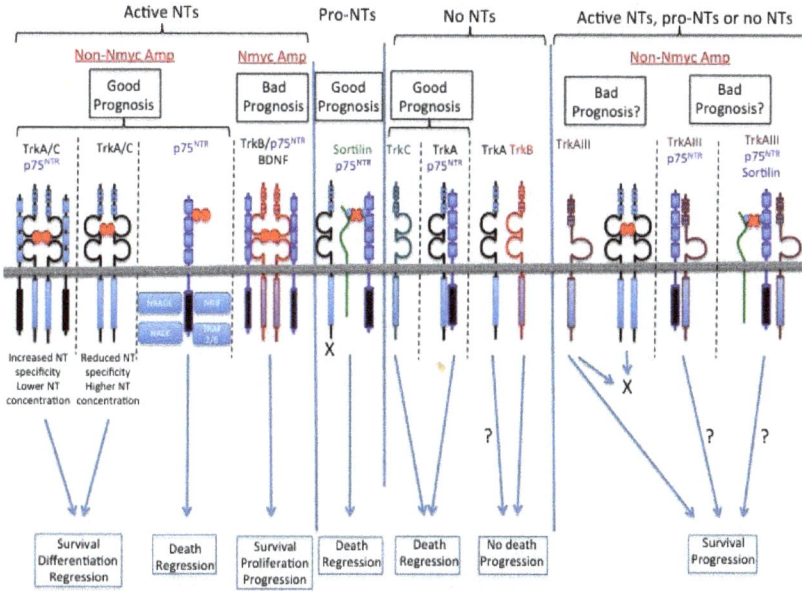

Figure 9. Different combinations, potential outcomes and prognosis of NTs and NTRs in NB

NTR expression in low stage non-Nmyc amplified NB characterised by the coexpression of TrkA and CD271/p75^{NTR} may carry the best prognosis. These tumours may terminally differentiate in response to NGF (TrkAI) or NT-3 (TrkAII), or undergo TrkA and/or CD271/ p75^{NTR}–mediated apoptosis in the absence of NTs, depending upon the CD271/p75^{NTR} to TrkA expression ratio. Furthermore, the coexpression of Sortilin in these tumours would extend apoptotic potential to include pro-NTs (see Sections 4.2.1-4.2.4). NBs that express TrkA but not CD271/p75^{NTR} may have a worse prognosis, as they require higher NT concentrations for TrkA activation and signalling and would also respond to promiscuous NTs potentially with a response of proliferation, survival and/or partial differentiation. In the absence of CD271/ p75^{NTR}, these NBs would neither exhibit TrkA dependency receptor-mediated apoptosis nor Sortilin-CD271/p75^{NTR} complex-mediated apoptosis in response to pro-NTs.

NBs that co-express TrkC and CD271/p75^{NTR} but not TrkA or TrkB, may have better prognosis with potential to differentiate in response to NT-3 but alternatively could proliferate and survive in response to NT-3, complicating prognosis. NT-3 is rarely expressed in NBs, increasing the potential for TrkC dependency receptor-mediated apoptosis, in the presence or absence of CD271/p75^{NTR} (see Sections 4.5 and 6.3). The coexpression of Sortilin with CD271/p75^{NTR} in these NBs would increase apoptotic potential to include a response to pro-NTs (see Sections 4.2.3 and 6.3). Advanced stage NBs coexpressing TrkC and NT-3 would be expected to carry worse prognosis as a result of this autocrine survival and proliferation mechanism that may also extend to NBs expressing TrkC but not NT-3 in tissues that express NT-3, and could be further optimised by co-expression of CD271/p75^{NTR} (see Section 6.3).

High levels of BDNF and TrkB expression in Nmyc-amplified NBs, in the absence of TrkA, TrkC and CD271/p75^{NTR}, carries the worse prognosis as a result of autocrine/paracrine BDNF-mediated TrkB activation, which would be expected to promote proliferation, survival and metastatic capacity. Furthermore in the absence of BDNF, TrkB would not be expected to promote apoptosis, as TrkB does not act as a dependence receptor (see Sections 6.4). As with other Trk receptors, TrkB co-expression with CD271/p75^{NTR} would be expected to optimise NT-specificity and responsiveness, which would be expected to further promote aggressive bahaviour in TrkB expressing NBs.

NBs that express CD271/p75^{NTR} but not Trks may carry better prognosis, as they would be expected to respond to active NTs with an apoptotic response and if co-expressed with Sortilin in the absence of Trks, would also be expected to exhibit an apoptotic response to pro-NTs, which comprises up to 50% of secreted NTs (see Sections 4.2.2 and 6.3).

Non-Nmyc amplified NBs that express TrkAIII may carry worse prognosis, as spontaneous TrkAIII activation would override NT-dependency, provide a selective growth advantage in tissues including those that do not express NTs, promote NB cell stamilality, survival, angiogenesis and genetic instability, resulting in a more tumorigenic, metastatic and stress-resistant phenotype (see Sections 4.2.1 and 6.2). Although it remains to be elucidated whether TrkAIII may interfere with CD271/p75^{NTR} –mediated apoptosis in the presence or absence of Sortilin, its expression in NB may represent the biological equivalent to BDNF/TrkB expression in Nmyc amplified NB and TrkC/NT3 expresssion in a subset of advanced stage NBs, as an indicator of poor prognosis.

7. Potential therapeutic approaches

7.1. Trk kinase inhibitors

Trk kinase inhibitors would be more suitable for use in advanced stage Nmyc amplified TrkB expressing NBs and advanced stage unfavourable non-Nmyc amplified NBs that express the TrkAIII oncogene but may also reduce survival in NBs expressing full length TrkA and TrkC and their corresponding NTs.

Therapeutic Trk kinase inhibitors include the selective Trk kinase inhibitors AZ-23 and AZ623, which inhibit Trk kinase activity at low nanomolar concentrations. AZ-23 has shown efficacy following oral administration in a TrkA-driven mouse allograft NB model [379], whereas AZ623 inhibits BDNF-mediated signalling and NB proliferation, and when combined with topotecan prolongs the inhibition of tumour regrowth and reduces chemo and radio thera-peutic resistance [380, 381]. Lestaurtinib (CEP-701) is a small-molecule receptor tyrosine kinase inhibitor that competitively inhibits ATP binding to the Trk kinase domain at nanomolar concentrations. This compound not only inhibits the tyrosine kinase activities of full-length Trk receptors but also inhibits the kinase activity of the alternative TrkAIII splice variant [73,

78,79]. Lestaurtinib inhibits NB growth *in vitro* and *in vivo*, and substantially enhances the efficacy of conventional chemotherapy, such as 13-cis-retinoic acid, ferenteride and bevacizumab, presumably by inhibiting autocrine TrkB/BDNF [382-384] and/or spontaneous TrkAIII activity [73]. Lestaurtinib is an active metabolite of the Trk kinase inhibitor CEP-751, and is more suitable for clinical trials, as it can be administered orally [384, 385]. These Trk tyrosine kinase inhibitors not only target tumour promoting effects of Trk receptor activation but also Trk-mediated chemotherapeutic resistance, which has been attributed not only to TrkB [348, 358-363] but also to TrkC [375], fully spliced TrkA [375] and TrkAIII [73, 78, 79]. CEP-701 synergises with retinoids in the treatment of NB by inhibiting TrkB activity [386].

Nifutimox, a drug used for years to treat Chagas disease, is also currently in clinical trials for refractory or relapsed NB, and has been shown to suppress TrkB-mediated Akt activation and induce caspase-dependent apoptosis of NB cells *in vitro* and *in vivo* [387].

7.2. TrkAIII inhibitors

Tyrosine kinase inhibitors K252a and CEP-701 inhibit TrkAIII tyrosine kinase activity. TrkAIII activity is also inhibited by the Hsp90 inhibitor geladanamycin and its clinically relevant analogues 17-AAG and 17-DMAG, and by the ARF inhibitor Brefeldin A (BFA) [78, 79]. CEP701 inhibits TrkAIII activity and TrkAIII-induced centrosome amplification at nanomolar concentrations, whereas BFA reversibly inhibits spontaneous TrkAIII activation in association with disruption of the Golgi Network and the endoplasmic reticulum/Golgi Network intermediate compartment [78, 78]. Geldanamycin and its analogues reversibly inhibit TrkAIII tyrosine kinase activity and reduce proliferation of TrkAIII expressing NB cells *in vitro* [78]. Inhibitors of TrkAIII activity, however, do not inhibit TrkAIII expression nor promote TrkAIII elimination but cause retention within the endoplasmic reticulum, with potential to induce an ER stress response. This may help to explain the high level of resistance to GA-mediated cytotoxicity exhibited by TrkAIII but not TrkAI transfected NB cells, despite inhibition of TrkAIII activity [78, 79]. This suggests that, in addition to other off target effects, reversible TrkAIII tyrosine kinase inhibitors may increase stress-resistance by promoting TrkAIII-ER retention and inducing an ER stress response. Consistent with this, geldanamycin selects slow growing TrkAIII expressing NB cells from mixed populations, with TrkAIII re-activation post drug-removal, suggesting a mechanism for potential post therapeutic relapse [78]. To counter this, we have also developed a specific peptide nucleic acid (PNA) inhibitor of TrkAIII expression based upon the novel exon 5/8 splice junction (TrkAIII PNA conjugate (KKAA)$_4$-GGCCGGGA-CAC) [78, 79] for use in combination with with TrkAIII tyrosine kinase inhibitors, to maximise therapeutic efficacy.

7.3. Agents that conserve Trk tyrosine phosphorylation and facilitate signal transduction

TrkA activation and signal transduction is fundamental for NB differentiation and the loss of TrkA expression or defective activation and/or signalling probably contributes to NB pathogenesis. Agents that optimise TrkA activation and facilitate subsequent signal transduction may, therefore, overcome defective TrkA signalling and restore differentiation and/or apoptotic responses to NTs. In this context, a novel cyclophane compound CPPy, with low toxicity, has been shown to facilitate NGF-induced TrkA signal transduction through RAS/ MAPK and to induce NB differentiation [388]. Since, $CD271/p75^{NTR}$ optimizes TrkA responses to NTs and augments NT specificity, agents such as CPPy may be particularly useful in NBs that express TrkA but not $CD271/p75^{NTR}$.

7.4. DNA methylation and HDACs inhibitors

Recent reports have identified promoter methylation as an important mechanism in the transcriptional repression of TrkA and $CD271/p75^{NTR}$ in NB [274, 389, 390]. Therapies that reverse or inhibit DNA methylation may, therefore, be useful in malignant NBs to restore the expression of favourable NB genes. In support of this, the DNA methylation inhibitor 5-aza-2'-deoxycytidine and histone deacetylase inhibitors 4-phenylbutyrate, trichostatin A and Romidepsin, have been shown to restore TrkA and $CD271/p75^{NTR}$ expression in NB cells, decrease proliferation, reduce tumorigenicity and promote caspase-dependent apoptosis [291, 346, 390]. Romidepsin is presently in clinical trials [346].

7.5. Liposome targeting of TrkB expressing cells

Considering the importance of TrkB in advanced stage Nmyc amplified NB, a recent report has characterised liposomes that target TrkB expressing cells, providing the opportunity to deliver nanotherapeutic cargos to TrkB expressing cells within NBs [392].

8. Concluding remarks

The complex nature of NT and NTR expression during normal development of the sympathetic nervous system is reflected in the different patterns of NT and NTR expression exhibited by human NB, which is consistent with their NCC origin at different stages along the differentiating sympathoadrenal lineage. The different biological potentials of TrkA, TrkB, TrkC, $CD271/p75^{NTR}$ and Sortilin receptors expressed alone or in different combinations, range from promotion of proliferation and/or differentiation to survival and/or apoptosis and to chemotherapeutic resistance. This complexity is increased by the potential of each receptor to be expressed as a functionally altered alternative splice variant, the recent characterisation of TrkA and TrkC as true dependency receptors, and the pro-apoptotic behaviour of the $CD271/p75^{NTR}$ -Sortilin complex, providing an exciting array of new potential ways to restore and/or modulate Trks, $CD271/p75^{NTR}$ and Sortilin behaviour for therapeutic purposes, based upon accurate characterisation of NT and NTR expression profiles in individual tumours.

Acknowledgements

This work was supported by grants form PRIN, AIRC and the Maugieri Foundation.

Author details

Pierdomenico Ruggeri[1], Antonietta R. Farina[1], Lucia Cappabianca[1], Natalia Di Ianni[1], Marzia Ragone[1], Stefania Merolle[1], Alberto Gulino[2,3] and Andrew R. Mackay[1]

1 Department of Applied Clinical and Biotechnological Science, University of L'Aquila, Coppito II, L'Aquila, Italy

2 Department of Molecular Medicine, University of Rome "La Sapienza", Rome, Italy

3 Neuromed Institute, Pozzilli, Italy

References

[1] Voorhess, M. L. & Gardner, L. S. (1961). Urinary excretion of neurepinephrine and 3-methoxy-4-hydroxy mandelic acid by children with neuroblastoma. *Journal of Clinical and Endocrinological Metabolism*, 21, 321-355.

[2] Jiang, M.; Stanke, J. & Lahti, J. M. (2011). The connections between neural crest development and neuroblastoma. *Current Topics in Developmental Biology*, 94, 77-127.

[3] Fisher, J. P. H. & Tweddle, D. A. (2012). Neonatal neuroblastoma. *Seminars in Fetal and Neonatal Medicine*,17,207-215.

[4] Endo, Y.; Osumi, N. & Wakamatsu, Y. (2002). Bimodal functions of Notch-mediated signalling are involved in neural crest formation during avian ectoderm development. *Development*, 129, 863-873.

[5] Cornell, R. A. & Eisen, J. S. (2002). Delta/Notch signaling promotes formation of zebrafish neural crest by repressing Neurogenin 1 function. *Development*, 129, 2639-2648.

[6] Kalcheim, C. & Burstyn-Cohen, T. (2000). Early stages of neural crest ontogeny: formation and regulation of cell delamination. *International Journal of Developmental Biology*, 49, 105-116.

[7] Kasemeier-Kulesa, J. C.; Kulesa, P. M. & Lefcort, F. (2005). Imaging neural crest cell dynamics during formation of dorsal root ganglia and sympathetic ganglia. *Development*, 132, 235-245.

[8] Gammill, L. S. & Roffers-Agarwal, J. (2010). Division of labour during trunk neural crest development. *Developmental Biology*, 344, 555-565.

[9] Schwarz, Q.; Maden, C. H.; Davidson, K. & Ruhrberg, C. (2009). Neuropilin-mediated neural crest cell guidance is essential to organise sensory neurons into segmented dorsal root ganglia. *Development*, 136, 1785-1789.

[10] Anderson, D. J. (2000). Genes, lineages and the neural crest a speculative view. *Philosophical Transactions of the Royal Society of Biological Sciences*, 355, 953-964.

[11] McCorry, L. K. (2007). Physiology of the autonomic nervous system. *American Journal of Pharmaceutical Education*, 71, 1-11.

[12] Young, H. M.; Cane, K. N. & Anderson, C. R. (2011). Development of the autonomic nervous system: a comparative view. *Autonomic Neuroscience: Basic and Clinical*, 165, 10-27.

[13] Janig, W. & Habler, H. J. (2000). Specificity in the organisation of the autonomic nervous system: a basis for precise neural regulation of homeostatic and protective body functions. *Progress in Brain Research*, 122, 351-367.

[14] Shepard, D. M. & West, G. B. (1952). Noradrenalin and accessory chromaffin tissue. *Nature*, 170, 42-43.

[15] Tischler, A. S.; Ruzicka, L. A. & Riseberg, J. C. (1992). Immunocytochemical analysis of chromaffin cell proliferation *in vitro*. *Journal of Histochemistry and Cytochemistry*, 40, 1043-1045.

[16] Schober, A. & Unsicker, K. (2001). Growth and neurotrophic properties regulating development and maintenance of sympathetic preganglionic neurons. *International Review of Cytology*, 205, 37-76.

[17] Unsicker, K. & Kriegelstein, K. (1996). Growth factors in chromaffin cells. *Progress in Neurobiology*, 48, 307-324.

[18] Huber, K.; Kalcheim, C. & Unsicker, K. (2009). The development of the chromaffin cell lineage from the neural crest. *Autonomic Neuroscience: Basic and Clinical*, 151, 10-16.

[19] Loring, J. F. & Erickson, C. A. (1987). Neural crest cell migratory pathways in the trunk of the chick embryo. *Developmental Biology*, 121, 220-236.

[20] Teillet, M. A.; Kalcheim, C, Le Dourain, N. M. (1987). Formation of the dorsal root ganglia in the avian embyo: segmental origin and migratory behaviour of neural crest progenitor cells. *Developmental Biology*, 120, 329-347.

[21] Waring, H (1935). The development of the adrenal gland of the mouse. *Quarterly Journal of Microscopic Science*. Vol. LXXVIII.

[22] Reiprich, S.; Stolt, C. C.; Schreiner, S.; Parlato, R. & Wegner, M. (2008). SoxE proteins are differentially required in mouse adrenal gland development. *Molecular and Cellular Biology*, 19, 1575-1586.

[23] Shimada, H. (2005). In situ neuroblastoma: An important concept related to the natural history of neural crest tumors. *Pediatric and Developmental Pathology*, 8, 305-306.

[24] Anderson, D. J. & Axel, R. (1986). A bipotential neuroendocrine precursor whose choice of cell fate is determined by NGF and glucocorticoids. *Cell*, 47, 1079-1090.

[25] Anderson, D. J.; Carnahan, J. F.; Michelsohn, A. & Patterson, P. H. (1991). Antibody markers identify a common progenitor to sympathetic neurons and chromaffin cells in vivo and reveal the timing of commitment to neuronal differentiation in the sympathoadrenal lineage. *Journal of Neuroscience*, 11, 3507-3519.

[26] Reissmann, E.; Ernsberger, U.; Francis-West, P. H.; Rueger, D.; Brickell, P. M. & Rohrer, H. (1996). Involvement of bone morphogenetic protein-4 and bone morphogenetic protein-7 in the differentiation of the adrenergic phenotype in developing sympathetic neurons. *Development*, 122, 2079-2088.

[27] Shah, N. M.; Groves, A. K. & Anderson, D. J. (1996). Alternative neural crest cell fates are instructively promoted by TGFbeta superfamily members. *Cell*, 85, 331-343.

[28] Bilodeau, M. L.; Boulineau, T.; Greulich, J. D.; Hullinger, R. L. & Andrisani, O. M. (2001). Differential expression of sympathoadrenal lineage determining genes and phenotypic markers in cultured primary neural crest cells. *In Vitro Cellular and Developmental Biology: Animal*, 37, 185-192.

[29] Ernsberger, U.; Esposito, L.; Partimo, S.; Huber, K.; Franke, A.; Bixby, J. L.; Kalcheim, C. & Unsicker, K. (2005). Expression of neuronal markers suggests heterogeneity of chick sympathoadrenal cells prior to invasion of the adrenal anlagen. *Cell and Tissue Research*, 319, 1-13.

[30] Gut, P.; Huber, K.; Lohr, J.; Bruhl, B.; Oberle, S.; Treier, M.; Ernsberger, U.; Kalcheim, C. & Unsicker, K. (2005). Lack of an adrenal cortex in Sf1 mutant mice is compatible with the generation of and differentiation of chromaffin cells. *Development*, 132, 4611-4619.

[31] Moriguchi, T.; Lim, K. C. & Engel, J. D. (2007). Transcription factor networks specify sympathetic and adrenal chromaffin cell differentiation. *Functional Developmental Embryology*, 1, 130-135.

[32] Pattyn, A.; Morin, X.; Cremer, H.; Goridis, C. & Brunet, J. F. (1999). The homeobox gene Phox2B is essential for the development of autonomic neural crest derivatives. *Nature*, 399, 366-370.

[33] Brunet, J. F. & Pattyn, A. (2002). Phox2 genes-from patterning to connectivity. *Current Opinions in Genetic & Development*, 12, 435-440.

[34] Guillemont, F.; Lo, L. C.; Johnson, J. E.; Auerbach, A.; Anderson, D. J. & Joyner, A. L. (1993). Mammalian achaete-scute homolog 1 is required for the early development of olfactory and autonomic neurons. *Cell*, 75, 463-476.

[35] Hirsch, M. R.; Tiveron, M. C.; Guillemont, E.; Brunet, J. F. & Goridis, C. (1998). Control of noradrenergic differentiation and Phox2a expression by MASH1 in the central and peripheral nervous system. *Development*, 125, 599-608.

[36] Mellitzer, G.; Bonne, S.; Luco, R. F.; Van de Casteele, M.; Lenne-Samuel, N.; Collombat, P.; Mansouri, A.; Lee, J.; Lan, M.; Pipeleers, D.; Nielsen, F. C.; Ferrer, J.; Gradwohl, G. & Heimberg, H. (2006). 1A1 in NGN-3-dependent and essential for differentiation of the endocrine pancreas. *EMBO Journal*, 25, 1344-1352.

[37] Gierl, M. S.; Karoulias, N.; Wende, H.; Strehle, M. & Birchmeier, C. (2006). The zinc finger factor Insm1 (IA-1) is essential for the development of pancreatic beta cells and intestinal endocrine cells. *Genes and Development*, 20, 2465-2478.

[38] Morikawa, Y.; D'Atreaux, F.; Gershon, M. D. & Cserjesi, P. (2007). Hand2 determines the noradrenergic phenotype in the mouse sympathetic nervous system. *Developmental Biology*, 307, 114-126.

[39] Schmidt, M.; Lin, S.; Pape, M.; Ernsberger, U.; Stanke, M.; Kobayashi, K.; Howard, M. J.; and Rohrer, H. (2009). The bHLH transcription factor Hand2 is essential for the maintenance of noradrenergic properties in differentiated sympathetic neurons. *Developmental Biology*, 15, 191-200.

[40] Tsarovina, K.; Pattyn, A.; Stubbusch, J.; Muller, F.; van der Wees, J.; Schneider, C.; Brunet, J-F. & Rohrer, H. (2004). Essential role of GATA transcription factors in sympathetic neuron development. *Development*, 131, 4775-4786.

[41] Finotto,S.; Kriegelstein, K.; Schober, A.; Diemling, F.; Lindner, K.; Bruhl, B.; Beier, K.; Metz, J.; Garcia-Arraras, J. E.; Roig-Lopez, J. L.; Monighan, P.; Schmid, W.; Cole, T. J.; Kellendonk, C.; Tronche, F.; Schutz, G. & Unsicker, K. (1999). Analysis of mice carrying targeted mutations of the glucocorticoid receptor gene argues against an essential role for glucocorticoid signalling for generating adrenal chromaffin cells. *Development*,126,2935- 2944.

[42] Parlato, R.; Otto, C.; Tuckermann, J.; Stotz, S.; Kaden, S.; Grone, H. J.; Unsicker, K. & Schutz, G. (2009). Conditional inactivation of glucocorticoid receptor gene in dopamine-beta-hydroxylase cells impairs chromaffin cell survival. *Endocrinology*, 150, 1775-1781.

[43] Lohr, J.; Gut, P.; Karch, N.; Unsicker, K. & Huber, K. (2006). Development of adrenal chromaffin cells in Sf1 heterozygous mice. *Cell and Tissue Research*, 325, 437-444.

[44] Wassberg, E.; Hedborg, F.; Skoldenberg, E.; Stridsberg, M. & Christofferson, R. (1999). Inhibition of apoptosis induces chromaffin differentiation and apoptosis in neuroblastoma. *American Journal of Pathology*, 154, 395-403.

[45] Hedborg, F.; Ulleras, E.; Grimelius, L.; Wassberg, E.; Maxwell, P. H.; Hero, B.; Berthold, F.; Schilling, F.; Harms, D.; Sabdstedt, B. & Franklin, G. (2003). Evidence for hypoxia-induced neuronal-chromaffin metaplasia in neuroblastoma. *FASEB Journal*, 17, 598-609.

[46] Hedborg, F.; Fischer Colbrie, R.; Ostlin, N.; Sandstedt, B.; Tran, M. G. B. & Maxwell, P. H. (2010). Differentiation in neuroblastoma: diffusion-limited hypoxia induces

neuro-endocrine secretory protein 55 and other markers of a chromaffin phenotype. *PloS ONE* 5, e12825.

[47] Bibel, M. & Barde, Y-A. (2000). Neurotrophins: key regulators of cell fate and cell shape in the vertebrate nervous system. *Genes and Development*, 14, 2919-2937.

[48] Kaplan, D. R. & Miller, F. D. (2000). Neurotrophin signal transduction in the nervous system. *Current Opinions in Neurobiology*, 10, 381-391.

[49] Oppenheim, R. W. (1991). Cell death during development of the nervous system. *Annual Reviews in Neuroscience*, 14, 453-501.

[50] Ernsberger, U. (2009). Role of neurotrophin signalling in the differentiation of neurons from dorsal root ganglia and sympathetic ganglia. *Cell and Tissue Research*, 336, 349-384.

[51] Levi-Montalcini, R. & Brooker, B. (1960). Excessive growth of the sympathetic ganglia evoked by a protein isolated from mouse salivary glands. *Proceeding of the National Acadamy of Science. USA*, 46, 373-384.

[52] Leibrock, J.; Lottspeich, F.; Hohn, A.; Hofer, M.; Hengerer, B.; Masiakowski, P.; Thoenen, H. & Barde, Y-A. (1989). Molecular cloning and expression of brain-derived neurotrophic factor. *Nature*, 341, 149-152.

[53] Ernfors, P. C.; Ibanez, F.; Ebendal, T.; Olson, L. & Persson, H. (1990). Molecular cloning and neurotrophic activities of a protein with similarities to nerve growth factor: developmental and topographical expression in the brain. *Proceeding of the National Acadamy of Sciences, USA*, 87, 5454-5458.

[54] Hallbook, F.; Ibanez, C. F. & Persson, H. (1991). Evolutionary studies of the nerve growth factor family reveal a novel member abundantly expressed in Xenopus ovary. *Neuron*, 6, 845-858.

[55] McDonald, N. Q.; Lapatto, R.; Murray-Rust, J.; Gunning, J.; Wlodawaer, A. & Blundell, T. L. (1991). New protein fold revealed by a 2.3-A resolution crystal structure of nerve growth factor. *Nature*, 354, 411-414.

[56] Lee, R.; Kermain, P.; Teng, K. K. & Hempstead, B. L. (2001) Regulation of cell survival by secreted neurotrophins. *Science*, 294, 1945-1948.

[57] Thoenan, H. (1999). Neurotrophins and neuronal plasticity. *Science*, 270, 593-598.

[58] Le, A. P. & Friedman, W. J. (2012). Matrix metalloproteinase-7 regulates cleavage of pro- nerve growth factor and is neuroprotective following Kainic acid-induced seizures. *Journal of Neuroscience*, 32, 703-712.

[59] Lu, B. & Figurov, A. (1997). Role of neurotrophins in synapse development and plasticity. *Reviews in Neuroscience*,8, 1-12

[60] Lu, B.; Pang, P. T. & Woo, N. H. (2005). The yin and yang of neurotrophin action. *Nature Reviews in Neuroscience*, 6, 603-614.

[61] Dracopoli, N. C. & Meisler, M. H. (1990). Mapping the human amylase gene cluster on the proximal short arm of chromosome 1 using a highly informative (CA)n repeat. *Genomics*, 7, 97-102.

[62] Maisonpierre, P. C.; Le Beau, M. M.; Espinosa, R 3rd.; Ip, N. Y.; Belluscio, L.; de la Monte, S. M.; Squinto, S.; Furth, M. E. & Yancopoulos, G. D. (1991). Human and rat brain-derived neurotrophic factor and neurotrophin-3 gene structures, distributions, and chromosomal localizations. *Genomics*, 10, 558-568.

[63] Ip, N. Y.; Ibanez, C. F.; Nye, S. H.; McClain, J.; Jones, P. F.; Gles, R.; Belluscio, L.; Le Beau, M. M.; Espinosa, R 3rd. & Squinto, S. P. (1992). Mammalian neurotrophin-4: structure, chromosomal localization, tissue distribution, and receptor specificity. *Proceeding of the National Academy of Sciences, USA*, 89, 3060-3064.

[64] Patapoutian, A. & Reichardt, L. F. (2001). Trk receptors: mediators of neurotrophin action. *Current Opinions in Neurobiology*, 11, 272-280.

[65] Klein, R.; Jing, S.; Nanduri, V.; O'Rourke, E. & Barnacid, M. (1991). The trk proto-on-cogene encodes a receptor for nerve growth factor. *Cell*, 65, 198-197.

[66] Martin-Zanca, D.; Hughes, S. H. & Barbacid, M. (1986). A human oncogene formed by the fusion of truncated tropomyosin and protein tyrosine kinase sequence. *Nature*, 319, 743-748.

[67] Martin-Zanca, D.; Oskam, R.; Mitra, G.; Copeland, T. & Barbacid, M. (1989). Molecular and biochemical characterisation of the human Trk oncogene. *Molecular and Cellular Biology*, 9, 24-33.

[68] Greco, A.; Villa, R. & Pierotti, M. A. (1996). Genomic organization of the human NTRK1 gene. *Oncogene*, 13, 2463-2466.

[69] Weier, H-U. G.; Rhein, A. P.; Shadravan, F.; Collins, C. & Polikoff, D. (1995). Rapid physical mapping of the human protoncogene (NTRK1) to human chromsome 1q21-22 by P1 clone selection, fluorescence in situ hybridisation (FISH), and computer-assisted microscopy. *Genomics*, 26, 390-393.

[70] Valent, A.; Danglot, G. & Bernheim, A. (1997). Mapping of the tyrosine kinase receptors trkA (NTRK1), trkB (NTRK2) and trkC (NTRK3) to human chromosomes 1q22, 9q22 and 15q25 by fluorescence in situ hybridization. *Europrean Journal of human genetics*, 5, 102-104.

[71] Dubus, P.; Parrens, M.; El-Mokhtari, Y.; Ferrer, J.; Groppi, A. & Merlio, J. P. (2000). Identification of novel TrkA variants with deletions in the leucine-rich motifs of the extracellular domain. *Journal of Neuroimmunology*, 107, 42-49.

[72] Barker, P. A.; Lomen-Hoerth, C.; Gensch, E. M.; Meakin, S. O.; Glass, D. J. & Shooter, E. M. (1993). Tissue specific alternative splicing generates two isoforms of the TrkA receptor. *Journal of Biological Chemistry*, 268, 15150-15157.

[73] Tacconelli, A., Farina, A. R.; Cappabianca, L.; DeSantis, G.; Tessitore, A.; Vetuschi, A.; Sferra, R.; Rucci, N.; Argenti, B.; Screpanti, I.; Gulino, A. & Mackay, A. R. (2004). TrkA alternative splicing: A regulated tumor-promting switch in human neuroblastoma. *Cancer Cell*, 6, 347-360.

[74] Windisch, J. M.; Marksteiner, R. & Schneider, R. (1995). Nerve growth factor binding site on TrkA mapped to a single 24-amino acid rich leucine motif. *Journal of Biological Chemistry*, 270, 28133-28136.

[75] Ninkina, N.; Grashchuck, M.; Buchman, V. L. & Davies, A. M. (1997). TrkB variants with deletions in the leucine-rich motifs of the extracellular domain. *Journal of Biological Chemistry*, 272, 13019-13025.

[76] Clary, D. O.; & Reichardt, L. F. (1994). An alternative splice form of the nerve growth factor receptor confers an enhanced response to neurotrophin 3. *Proceedings of the National Academy of Science. USA*, 91, 11133-11137.

[77] Tacconelli, A., Farina, A. R.; Cappabianca, L.; Cea, G.; Panella, S.; Chioda, A.; Gallo, R.; Cinque, B.; Sferra, R.; Vetuschi, A.; Campese, A. F.; Screpanti, I.; Gulino, A. & Mackay, A. R. (2007). TrkAIII expression in the thymus. *Journal of Neuroimmunology*, 183, 151-161.

[78] Farina, A. R.; Tacconelli, A.; Cappabianca, L.; Cea, G.; Chioda, A.; Romanelli, A.; Pensato, S.; Pedone, C.; Gulino, A. & Mackay, A. R. (2009). The neuroblastoma tumour-suppressor TrkAI and its oncogenic alternative TrkAIII splice variant exhibit geldanamycin-sensitive interactions with Hsp90 in human neuroblastoma cells. *Oncogene*, 28, 4075-4094.

[79] Farina, A. R.; Tacconelli, A.; Cappabianca, L.; Cea, G.; Pannella, S.; Chioda, A.; Romanelli, A.; Pedone, C.; Gulino, A. & Mackay, A. R. (2009). The TrkAIII splice variant targets the centrosome and promotes genetic instability. *Molecular and Cellular Biology*, 29, 4812-4830.

[80] Berkemeier, L. R.; Winslow, J. W.; Kaplan, D. R.; Nikolics, K.; Goeddel, D. V. & Rosenthal, A. (1991). Neurotrophin-5: a novel neurotrophic factor that activates Trk and TrkB. *Neuron*, 7, 857-866.

[81] Glass, D. J.; Nye, S. H.; Hantzopoulos, P.; Macchi, M. J.; Squinto, S. P.; Goldfarb, M. & Yancopoulos, G. D. (1991). TrkB mediates BDNF/NT-3-dependent survival and proliferation in fibroblasts lacking low affinity NGF receptor. *Cell*, 66, 405-413.

[82] Squinto, S. P.; Stitt, T. N.; Aldrich, T. H.; Davis, S.; Bianco, S. M.; Radziejewski, C.; Glass, D. J.; Masiakowski, P.; Furth, M. E.; Venezuela, D. M.; Distefano, P. S. & Yan-

copoulos, G. D. (1991). trkB encodes a functional receptor for brain-derived neurotrophic factor and neurotrophin-3 but not nerve growth factor. *Cell*, 65, 885-893.

[83] Soilov, P.; Castren, E. & Stamm, S. (2002). Analysis of the human TrkB gene genomic
organization reveals novel TrkB isoforms, unusual gene length, and splicing mechanism. *Biochemical and Biophysical Research Communications*, 290, 1054-1065.

[84] Eide, F. F.; Vining, E. R.; Eide, B. L.; Zang, K.; Wang, X. Y. & Reichardt, L. F. (1996).
Naturally occurring truncated TrkB receptors have dominant inhibitory effects on
brain-derived neurotrophic factor signalling. *Journal of Neuroscience*, 16, 3123-3129.

[85] Luberg, K.; Wong, J.; Weickert, C. S. & Timmusk, T. (2010). Human TrkB gene: novel
alternative transcripts, protein isoforms and expression pattern in the prefrontal cerebral cortex during postnatal development. *Journal of Neurochemistry*, 113, 952- 964.

[86] Fenner, B. M. (2012). Truncated TrkB: Beyond a dominant negative receptor. *Cytokine
& Growth factor Reviews*, 23, 15-24.

[87] Middlemas, D. S.; Kihl, B. K.; Zhou, J. F et al., (1999). Brain-derived neurotrophic factor promotes survival and hemoprotection of human neuroblastoma cells. *Journal of
Biological Chemistry*, 274, 16451-16460.

[88] Lamballe, F.; Klein, R. & Barbacid, M. (1991). trkC, a new member of the trk family of
tyrosine protein kinases, is a receptor for neutotrophin-3. *Cell*, 66, 967-979.

[89] Lamballe, F.; Tapley, P. & Barbacid, M. (1993). trkC encodes multiple neurotrophin-3
receptors with distinct biological properties and biological activities. *EMBO Journal*,
12, 3083-3094.

[90] Tsoulfas, P.; Soppet, D.; Escandon, E.; Tessarollo, L.; Mendoza-Ramirez, J. L.; Rosenthal, A.; Nikolics, K. & Parada, L. F. (1993). The rat TrkC locus encodes multiple neurogenic receptors that exhibit differential response to neurotrophin-3 in PC-12 cells.
Neuron, 10, 975-990.

[91] Valenzuela, D. M.; Maisonpierre, P. C.; Glass, D. J.; Rojas, E.; Nunez, L.; Kong, Y.;
Stitt, Ip, N. Y. & Yancopoulos, G. D. (1993). Alternative forms of rat TrkC with different functional capabilities. *Neuron*, 10, 963-974.

[92] Menn, B.; Timsit, S.; Calothy, G. & Lamballe, F. (1998). Differential expression of trkC
catalytic and noncatalytic isoforms suggests that they act independently or in association. *Journal of Comparative Neurology*, 410, 47-64.

[93] Tsoulfas, P.; Stephens, R. M.; Kaplan, D. R. & Parada, L. F. (1996). trkC isoforms with
insert in the kinase domain show impaired signalling responses. *Journal of Biological
Chemistry*, 271, 5691-5697.

[94] Liepenish, E.; Llag, L. L.; Otting, G. & Ibanez, C. F. (1997). NMR structure of the
death domain of the p75 neurotrophin receptor. *EMBO Journal*, 16, 4999-5005.

[95] Yano, H. & Chao, M. V. (2000). Neurotrophin receptor structure and function. *Pharmaceutica acta Helvetiae*, 74, 253-260.

[96] Wartiovaara, K.; Paavola, P.; Suvanto, P.; Paulin, L.; Saarma, M.; Peltonen, L. & Sariola, H. (1997). Exclusion of the p75 neurotrophin receptor gene as a candidate gene for Meckel syndrome. *Clinical Dysmorphology*, 6, 213-217.

[97] Von Shack, D.; Casademunt, E.; Schweigreiter, R.; Meyer, M.; Bibel, M. & Dechant, G. (2001). Complete ablation of the neurotrophin receptor p75NTR causes defects both in the nervous and vascular system. *Nature Neuroscience*, 4, 977-978.

[98] Nykjaer, A.; Lee, R.; Teng, K. K.; Jansen, P.; Madsen, P.; Nielsen, M. S.; Jacobsen, C.; Kliemannel, M.; Schwarz, E.; Willnow, T. E.; Hempstead, B. & Petersen, C. M. (2004). Sortilin is essential for proNGF-induced neuronal cell death. *Nature*, 427, 843-847.

[99] Zampieri, N. & Chao, M. V. (2004). Structural biology. The p75 NGF receptor exposed. *Science*, 304, 833-834.

[100] Harel, L.; Costa, B. & Fainzilber, M. (2010). On the death Trk. *Developmental Neurobiology*, 70, 298-303.

[101] Teng, H. K.; Teng, K. K.; Lee, R.; Wright, S.; Tevar, S.; Almeida, R. D.; Kermani, P.; Torkin, R.; Chen, Z. Y.; Lee, F. S.; Kraemer, R. T.; Nykjaer, A. & Hempstead, B. L. (2005). ProBDNF induces neuronal apoptosis via activation of a receptor complex of p75NTR and Sortilin. *Journal of Neuroscience*, 25, 5455-5463.

[102] Yano, H.; Torkin, R.; Martin, L. A.; Chao, M. V. & Teng, K. K. (2009). Proneurotrophin-3 is a neuronal apoptotic ligand: evidence for retrograde-directed cell killing. Journal of Neuroscience, 29, 14790-14802.

[103] Petersen, C. M.; Nielsen, M. S.; Nykjaer, A.; Jacobsen, L.; Tommerup, N.; Rasmussen, H. H.; Roigarard, H.; Gliemann, J.; Madsen, P. & Moestrup, S. K. (1997). Molecular identification of a novel candidate sorting receptor purified from human brain by receptor-associated protein affinity chromatography. *Journal of Biological Chemistry*, 272, 3599-3605.

[104] Vincent, J-P.; Mazella, J. & Kitabgi, P. (1999). Neurotensin and neurotensin receptors. *Trends in Pharmacological Sciences*, 20, 302-309.

[105] Schweigreiter, R. (2006). The dual nature of neurotrophins. *Bioessays*, 28, 583-594.

[106] Schneider, R. & Schweiger, M. (1991). A novel modular mosaic of cell adhesion morifs in the extracellular domains of the neurogenic trk and trkB tyrosine kinase receptors. *Oncogene*, 6, 1807-1811.

[107] Holden, P. H.; Asopa, V.; Robertson, A. G.; Clarke, A. R.; Tyler, S.; Bennett, G. S.; Brain, S. D.; Wilcock, G. K.; Allen, S. J.; Smith, S. K. & Dawbarn, D. (1997). Immunoglobulin-like domains define the nerve growth factor binding site of the trkA receptor. *Nature Biotechnology*, 15, 668-672.

[108] Perez, P.; Coll, P. M.; Hempstead, B. L.; Martin-Zanca, D. & Chao, M. V. (1995). NGF binding to the trk tyrosine kinase receptor requires the extracellular immunoglobulin-like domains. *Molecular and Cellular Neuroscience*, 6, 97-105.

[109] Urfer, R.; Tsoulfas, P.; O'Connell, L. & Presta, L. G. (1997). Specificity determinants in neurotrophin-3 and design of nerve growth factor-based trkC agonists by changing central beta strand bundle residues to their neurotrophin-3 analogs. *Biochemistry*, 36, 4775-4781.

[110] Arevalo, J. C.; Conde, B.; Hemstead, B. I.; Chao, M. V.; Martin-Zanca, D. & Perez, P. (2000). TrkA immunoglobulin-like ligand binding domains inhibit spontaneous activation of the receptor. *Molecular and Cellular Biology*, 20, 5908-5916.

[111] Peng, X.; Green, L. A.; Kaplan, D. R. & Stephens, R. M. (1995). Deletion of a conserved juxtamembrane sequence in Trk abolishes NGF-promoted neuritogenesis. *Neuron*, 15, 395-406.

[112] Monshipouri, M.; Jiang, H. & Lazarovici, P. (2000). NGF stimulation of erk phosphorylation is impaired by a point mutation in the transmembrane domain of the trkA receptor. *Journal of Molecular Neuroscience*, 14, 69-76.

[113] Kaplan, D. R.; Martin-Zanca, D. & Prada, L. F. (1991). Tyrosine phosphorylation and tyrosine kinase activity of the trk proto-oncogene product induced by NGF. *Nature*, 350, 358-360.

[114] Wiesman, C.; Muller, Y. A. & de Vos, A. M. (2000). Ligand binding sites in Ig-like domains of receptor tyrosine kinases. *Journal of Molecular Medicine*, 78, 247-260.

[115] Arevalo, J. C.; Conde, B.; Hemstead, B. I.; Chao, M. V.; Martin-Zanca, D. & Perez, P. (2001). A novel mutation within the extracellular domain of TrkA causes constitutive receptor activation. *Oncogene*, 20, 1229-1234.

[116] Benedetti, M.; Levi, A. & Chao, M. V. (1993). Differential expression of nerve growth factors leads to altered binding affinity and neurotrophin responsiveness. *Proceeding of the National Academy of Science. USA*, 90, 7859-7863.

[117] Mahadeo, D.; Kaplan, L.; Chao, M. V. & Hempstead, B. L. (1994). High affinity nerve growth factor binding displays a faster rate of association than p140trk binding implications for multi-subunit polypeptide receptors. *Journal of Biological Chemistry*, 269, 6884-6891.

[118] Esposito, D.; Patel, P.; Stephens, R. M.; Perez, P.; Chao, M. V.; Kaplan, D. R. & Hempstead, B. L. (2001). The cytoplasmic and transmembrane domains of the p75 and trkA receptors regulate high affinity binding to nerve growth factor. *Journal of Biological Chemistry*, 276, 32687-32695.

[119] Bibel, H.; Hoppe, E. & Barde, Y-A. (1999). Biochemical and functional interactions between the neurotrophin receptors trk and p75NTR. *EMBO Journal*, 18, 616-622.

[120] Mischel, P. S.; Smith, S. G.; Vining, E. R.; Valletta, J. S.; Mobley, W. C. & Reichardt, L. F. (2001). The extracellular domain of p75NTR is necessary to inhibit neurotrophin-3 signaling through TrkA. *Journal of Biological Chemistry*, 276, 11292-11301.

[121] Murray, S. S.; Perez, P.; Lee, R.; Hempstead, B. L. & Chao, M. V. (2004). A novel p75 neurotrophin receptor-related protein, NRH2, regulates nerve growth factor binding to the TrkA receptor. *Journal of Neuroscience*, 24, 2742-2749.

[122] Pratcha, G. & Ibanez, C. F. (2002). Lipid rafts and the control of neurotrophic factor signaling in the nervous system: variations on a theme. *Current Opinions in Neurobiology*, 12, 542-549.

[123] Marsh, H. N.; Dubreuil, C. I.; Quevedo, C.; Lee, A.; Majdan, M.; Walsh, G. S.; Hausdorff, S.; Said, F. A.; Zoueva, O.; Kozlowski, M.; Siminovitch, K.; Neel, B. G.; Miller, F. D. & Kaplan, D. R. (2003). SHP-1 negatively regulates neuronal survival by functioning as a TrkA phosphatase. *Journal of Cell Biology*, 163, 999-1010.

[124] Watson, F. L.; Porcionatto, M. A.; Bhattacharyya, A.; Stiles, C. & Segal, R. C. (1999). TrkA glycosylation regulates localisation and activity. *Journal of Neurobiology*, 39, 323-336.

[125] Ostman, A. & Bohmer, F. D. (2001). Regulation of receptor tyrosine kinase signalling by protein tyrosine phosphatases. *Trends in Cell Biology*, 11, 258-266.

[126] Sastry, S. K. & Elferink, L. A. (2011). Checks and balances: interplay of RTKs and PTPs in cancer progression. *Biochemical Pharmacology* http://dx.doi.org/10.1016/j.bcp.2011.06.016.

[127] Kaplan, D. R. & Stephens, R. M. (1994). Neurotrophin signal transduction by the trk receptor. *Journal of Neurobiology*, 25, 1404-1417.

[128] Green, L. A. & Kaplan, R. M. (1995). Early events in neurotrophin signaling via Trk and p75 receptors. *Current Opinions in Neurobiology*, 5, 579-587.

[129] Hallberg, B.; Ashcroft, M.; Loeb, D. M. & Kaplan, R. M. (1998). Nerve factor induced stimulation of Ras requires Trk interaction with Shc but does not involve phosphoinositol 3-OH kinase. *Oncogene*, 17, 691-697.

[130] Meakin, S. O.; MacDonald, J. I. S.; Gryz, E. A.; Kubu, C. J. & Verdi, J. M. (1999). The signalling adapter FRS-2 competes with Shc for binding to the nerve growth factor receptor TrkA. A model discriminating between proliferation and differentiation. *Journal of Biological Chemistry*, 274, 9861-9870.

[131] Cunningham, M. E.; Stephens, R. M.; Kaplan, D. R. & Greene, L. A. (1997). Autophosphorylation of activation loop tyrosines regulates signaling by the Trk nerve growth factor receptor. *Journal of Biological Chemistry*, 272, 10957-10967.

[132] Obermeier, A.; Haltre, H.; Weismuller, K. H.; Jung, G.; Schlessinger, J. & Ullrich, A. (1993). Tyrosine 785 is a major determinant of Trk-substrate interaction. *EMBO Journal*, 12, 933-941.

[133] Obermeier, A.; Bradshaw, R. A.; Seedorf, K.; Choidas, A.; Schlessinger, J. & Ullrich, A. (1994). Neuronal differentiation signals are controlled by nerve growth factor receptor/Trk binding sites for Shc and PLCγ. *EMBO Journal*, 13, 1585-1590.

[134] Segal, R. A. & Greenberg, M. E. (1996). Intracellular signalling pathways activated by neurotrophic factors. *Annual Reviews in Neuroscience*, 19, 463-489.

[135] Yao, R. & Cooper, G. M. (1995). Requirement for phosphoinositol-3 kinase in the prevention of apoptosis by nerve growth factor. *Science*, 267, 2003-2005.

[136] MacDonald, J. I.; Gryz, E. A.; Kubu, C. J.; Verdi, J. M. & Meakin, S. O. (2000). Direct binding of the signalling adapter protein Grb2 to the activation loop tyrosines on the nerve growth factor receptor tyrosine kinase, TrkA. *Journal of Biological Chemistry*, 275, 18225-18233.

[137] Hagag, N.; Halegoua, S. & Viola, M. (1986). Inhibition of growth factor induced differentiation of PC12 cells by microinjection of antibody to ras p21. *Nature*, 319, 680-682.

[138] Hampstead, B. L.; Martin-Zanca, D.; Kaplan, D. R.; Parada, L. F. & Chao, M. V. (1991). High affinity NGF binding requires coexpression of the trk proto-oncogene and low affinity NGF receptor. *Nature*, 350, 678-683.

[139] Majdan, M.; Walsh, G. S.; Aloyz, R. & Miller, F. D. (2001). TrkA mediates developmental sympathetic neuron survival by silencing an ongoing p75NTR-mediated death signal. *Journal of Cell Biology*, 155, 1275-1285.

[140] Zaccaro, M. C.; Ivanisevic, L.; Perez, P.; Meakin, S. O. & Saragovi, H. U. (2002). P75 coreceptors regulate ligand dependent and ligand independent Trk receptor activation, in part by altering trk docking subdomains. *Journal of Biological Chemistry*, 276, 31023-31029.

[141] Nykjaer, N.; Willnow, T. E.; & Munk-Peterson, C. (2005). P75NTR-liver or let die. *Current Opinions in Neurobiology*, 15, 40-57.

[142] York, R. D.; Yao, H.; Dillon, T.; Ellig, C. L.; Eckert, S. P.; McCleskey, E. W. & Stork, P. J. (1998). Rap1 mediates sustained MAP kinase activation induced by nerve growth factor. *Nature*, 392, 622-626.

[143] Wu, C.; Lai, C. F. & Mobley, W. C. (2001). Nerve growth factor activates persistent Rap1 signaling in endosomes. *Journal of Neuroscience*, 21, 5406-5416.

[144] Minichiello, L.; Casagrande, F.; Tatche, R. S.; Stucky, C. L.; Postigo, A.; Lewin, G. R.; Davies, A. M. & Klein, R. (1998). Point mutation in trkB causes loss of NT-4-dependent neurons without major effect on diverse BDNF responses. *Neuron*, 21, 335-345.

[145] Postigo, A.; Calella, A. M.; Fritzsch, B.; Knipper, M.; Katz, D.; Eilers, A.; Schimmang, T.; Lewin, G. R.; Klein, K. & Minichiello, L. (2002). Distinct requirements for TrkB and TrkC signalling in target innervation by sensory neurons. *Genes and Development*, 16, 633-645.

[146] Kong, H.; Boulter, J.; Weber, J. L.;lai, C. & Chao, M. V. (2001). An evolutionaily conserved transmembrane protein that is a novel downstream target of neurotrophin and aphrin receptors. *Journal of Neuroscience*, 21, 176-185.

[147] Arevalo, J. C.; Yano, H.; Teng, K. K. & Chao, M. V. (2004). A unique pathway for sustained neurotrophin signalling through an akyrin-rich membrane-soanning protein. *EMBO Journal*, 23, 2358-2368.

[148] Ginty, D. D.; Bonni, A. & Greeberg, M. E. (1994). Nerve growth factor activates a Ras-dependent protein kinase that stimulates c-fos transcription via phosphorylation of CREB. *Cell*, 77, 713-725.

[149] Xing, J.; Ginty, D. D. & Greenberg, M. E. (1998). Coupling of the RAS-MAPK pathway to gene activation by RSK2, a growth factor-regulated CREB kinase. *Science*, 273, 959-963.

[150] Deak, M.; Clifton, A. D.; Lucocq, L. M. & Alessi, D. R. (1998). Mitogen- and stress-activated protein kinase-1 (MSK1) is directly activated by MAPK and SAPK2/p38, and may mediate activation of CREB. *EMBO Journal*, 17, 4426-4441.

[151] Atwal, J. K.; Massie, B.; Miller, F. D. & Kaplan, D. R. (2000). The TrkB-Shc site signals neuronal survival and local axon growth via MEK and PI3-kinase. *Neuron*, 27, 265-277.

[152] Ecinas, M.; Iglesias, M.; Llecha, N. & Comella, J. X. (1999). Extracellular-regulated kinases and phosphoinositol 3-kinase are involved in brain-derived growth factor-mediated survival and neuritogenesis of the neuroblastoma cell line SH-SY5Y. *Journal of Neurochemistry*, 73, 1409-1421.

[153] Florez, A. I.; Mallon, B. S.; Matsui, T.; Ogawa, W.; Rosenzweig, A.; Okamoto, T. & Macklin, W. B. (2000). Akt-mediated survival of oligodendrocytes induced by neuro-regulins. *Journal of Neuroscience*, 20, 7622-7630.

[154] Wooten, M. W.; Vandenplas, M. L.; Seibenhener, M. L.; Geetha, T. & Diaz-Meco, M. T. (2001). Nerve growth factor stimulates tyrosine phosphorylation and activation of the atypical protein kinase C's via a src kinase pathway. *Molecular and Cellular Biology*, 21, 8414-8427.

[155] Corbit, K. C.; Foster, D. A. & Rosner, M. R. (1999). Protein kinase Cdelta mediates neurogenic but not mitogenic activation of mitogen-activated protein kinase in neuronal cells. *Molecular and Cellular Biology*, 19, 4209-4218.

[156] Simpson, A. M.; Iyer, R.; Mangino, J. L.; Minturn, J. E.; Zhao, H.; Kolla, V. & Brodeur, G. M. (2012). TrkA3 isoform expression upregulates stem cell markers and correlates

with worse outcome in neuroblastomas (NBs). *Proceedings of the Advances in Neuroblastoma Research (2012)* (Meeting Abstract POT055), p 164.

[157] Moises, T.; Dreieir, A.; Flohr, S.; Esser, M.; Brauers, E.; Reiss, K.; Merken, D.; Weis, J. & Kruttgen, A. (2007). Tracking TrkA's trafficking: NGF receptor trafficking controls NGF receptor signalling. *Molecular Neurobiology*, 35, 151-159.

[158] Howe, C. L. & Mobley, W. C. (2004). Signaling endosome hypothesis: a cellular mechanism for long distance communication. *Journal of Neurobiology*, 58, 207-216. 2004

[159] Valdez, G.; Akmentin, W.; Philippidou, P.; Kuruvilla, R.; Ginty, D. D. & Halegoua, S. (2005). Pincher-mediated macroendocytosis underlies retrograde signalling by neurotrophin receptors. *Journal of Neuroscience*, 25, 5236-5247.

[160] Rajagopal, R.; Chen, Z. Y.; Lee, F. S. & Chao, M. V. (2004). Transactivation of Trk neurotrophin receptors by G-protein-coupled receptor ligands occurs on intracellular membranes. *Journal of Neuroscience*, 24, 6650-6658.

[161] Shi, G. X.; Jin, L. & Andres, D. A. (2010). Src-dependent TrkA transactivation is required for pituitary adenylate cyclase- activating polypeptide 38-mediated Rit activation and neuronal differentiation. *Molecular Biology of the Cell*, 21, 1597-1608.

[162] He, X. L. & Garcia, K. C. (2004). Structure of nerve growth factor complexed with the shared neurotrophin receptor p75. *Science*, 304, 870-875.

[163] Huang, E. J. & Reichardt, L. F. (2003). Trk receptors: roles in neuronal signal transduction. *Annual Reviews in Biochemistry*, 72, 609-642.

[164] Kuruvilla, R.; Zweifel, L. S.; Glebova, N. O.; Lonze, B. E.; Valdez, G.; Ye, H. & Ginty, D. D. (2004). A neurotrophin signaling cascade coordinates sympathetic neuron development through differential control of TrkA trafficking and retrograde signaling. *Cell* 118, 243-255.

[165] Epa, W. R.; Markovska, K. & Barrett, G. L. (2004). The p75 neurotrophin receptor enhances TrkA signaling by binding to Shc and augmenting its phosphorylation. *Journal of Neurochemistry*, 89, 344-353.

[166] Hannila, S. S.; Lawreance, G. M.; Ross, G. M. & Kawaja, M. D. (2004). TrkA and mitogen-activated protein kinase phosphorylation are enhanced in sympathetic neurons lacking functional p75 neurotrophin receptor expression. *European Journal of Neuroscience*, 19, 2903-2908.

[167] Lad, S. P.; Peterson, D. A.; Bradshaw, R. A. & Neet, K. E. (2003). Individual and combined effects of TrkA and p75NTR nerve growth factor receptors. A role for high affinity receptor sites. *Journal of Biological Chemistry*, 278, 24808-24817.

[168] Paul, C. E.; Vereker, E.; Dickson, K. M. & Barker, P. A. (2004). A pro-apoptotic fragment of the p75 neurotrophin receptor is expressed in p75NTR exon IV null mice. *Journal of Neuroscience,* 24, 1917-1923.

[169] Gentry, J. J.; Barker, P. A. & Carter, B. D. (2004). The p75 neurotrophin receptor: multiple interactors and numerous functions. *Progress in Brain Research,* 146, 25-39.

[170] Miller, F. D. & Kaplan, D. R. (2001). Neurotrophin signalling pathways regulating neuronal apoptosis. *Cellular and Molecular Life Sciences,* 58, 7879-7887.

[171] Bhakar, A. L.; Howell, J. L.; Paul, C. E.; Salehi, A. H.; Becker, E. B.; Said, F.; Bonni, A. & Barker, P. A. (2003). Apoptosis induced by p75NTR overexpression requires jun kinase-dependent phosphorylation of Bad. *Journal of Neuroscience,* 23, 11373-11381.

[172] Okuno, S.; Saito, A.; Hayashi, T. & Chan, P.H. (2004). The c-Jun N-terminal protein kinase signaling pathway mediates bax activation and subsequent neuronal apoptosis through interaction with bim after transient focal cerebral ischemia. *Journal of Neuroscience,* 24, 7879-7887.

[173] Barker, P. A. (2004). P75NTR is positively promiscuous: novel partners and new insights. *Neuron,* 42, 529-533.

[174] Becker, E. B. E.; Howell, J.; Kodama, Y.; Barker, P. A. & Bonni, A. (2004). Characterisation of the c-Jun N-terminal kinase-BimEL signaling pathway in neuronal apoptosis. *Journal of Neuroscience,* 24, 8762-8770.

[175] Casademunt, E.; Carter, B. D.; Benzel, I.; Frade, J. M.; Dechant, G. & Barde, Y-A. (1999). The zinc finger protein NRIF interacts with the neurotrophin receptor p75(NTR) and participates in programmed cell death. *EMBO Journal,* 18, 6050-6061.

[176] Salehi, A. H.; Roux, P. P.; Kubu, C. J.; Zeindler, C.; Bhakar, A.; Tannis, L. L.; Verdi, J. M. & Barker, P. A. (2000). RAGE, a novel MAGE protein, interacts with the p75 neurotrophin receptor and facilitates nerve growth factor-dependent apoptosis. *Neuron,* 27. 279-288.

[177] Park, J. A.; Lee, J. Y.; Sato, T. A. & Koh, J. Y. (2000). Co-induction of p75NTR and p75NTR-associated death executor in neurons after zinc exposure in cortical culture or transient ischemia in the rat. *Journal of Neuroscience,* 20, 9069-9103.

[178] Chittka, A.; Arevalo, J. C.; Rodriguez-Guzman, M.; Perez, P.; Chao, M. V. & Sendtner, M. (2004). The p75NTR-interacting protein SC1 inhibits cell cycle progression by transcriptional repression of cyclin E. *Journal of Cell Biology,* 164, 985-996.

[179] Arevalo, J. C. & Wu, S. H. (2006). Neurotrophin signalling: many exciting surprises. *Cell Mol Life Sci* 63, 1523-1537.

[180] Yamashito, H.; Avraham, S.; Jiang, S.; Dikic, I. & Avram, H. (1999). The Csk homologous kinase associates with TrkA receptors and is involved in neurite outgrowth of PC12 cells. *Journal of Biological Chemistry,* 274, 15059-15065.

[181] Frade, J. M. (2005). Nuclear translocation of the p75 neurotrophin receptor cytoplas-
       mic domain in response to neurotrophin binding. *Journal of Neuroscience*, 25,
       1407-1411.

[182] Datta, S. R.; Dudek, H.; Tao, X.; Masters, S.; Fu, H.; Gotoh, Y. & Greenberg, M. E.
       (1997). Akt phosphorylation of BAD couples survival signals to the cell-intrinsic
       death machinary. *Cell*, 91, 231-241.

[183] Orike, M.; Middleton, G.; Borthwick, E.; Buchman, V. Cowen, T. & Davies, A. M.
       (2001). Role of PI-3 kinase, Akt and Bcl-2-related proteins in sustaining the survival
       of neurotrophic factor-dependent adult sympathetic neurons. *Journal of Cell Biology*,
       154, 995-1005.

[184] Brunet, A.; Bonni, A.; Zigmond, A. J.; Lin, M. Z.; Juo, P.; Hu, L. S.; Anderson, M. J.;
       Arden, K. C.; Blenis, J. & Greenberg, M. E. (1999). Akt promotes cell survaival by
       phosphorylating and inhibiting a Forkhead transcription factor. *Cell*, 96, 857-868.

[185] Wyttenbach, A. & Tolkovsky, A. M. (2006). The BH3-only protein Puma is both nec-
       essary and sufficient for neuronal apoptosis induced by DNA damage in sympathet-
       ic neurons. *Journal of Neurochemistry*, 96, 1213-11226.

[186] Putcha, G. V.; Moulder, K. L.; Golden, J. P.; Bouillet, P.; Adams, J. A.; Strasser, A. &
       Johnson, E. M. (2001). Induction of BIM, a proapoptotic BH3-only BCL-2 family
       member, is critical for neuronal apoptosis. *Neuron*, 29, 615-628.

[187] Gilley, J.; Coffer, P. J. & Ham, J. (2003). FOXO transcription factors directly activate
       bim gene expression and promote apoptosis in sympathetic neurons. *Journal of Cell
       Biology*, 162, 613-622.

[188] Whitfield, J.; Neame, S. J.; Parquet, L.; Bernard, O. & Ham, J. (2001). Dominant-nega-
       tive c-Jun promotes neuronal survival by reducing BIM expression and inhibiting
       mitochondrial cytochrome c release. *Neuron*, 29, 629-643.

[189] Du, K. & Mintiminy, M. (1998). CREB is a regulatory target for the protein kinase
       Akt/PKB. *Journal of Biological Chemistry*, 273, 32377-32379.

[190] Riccio, A.; Ahn, S.; Davenport, C. M.; Blendy, J. A. & Ginty, D. D. (1999). Mediation
       by a CREB family transcription factor of NGF-dependent survival of sympathetic
       neurons. *Science*, 286, 2358-2361.

[191] Tauszig-Delamasure, S.; Yu, L-Y.; Cabrera, J. R.; Bouzas-Rodriguez, J.; Mermet-Bouv-
       ier, C.; Giux, C.; Bordeux, M-C.; Arumae, U. & Mehlen, P. (2007). The TrkC receptor
       induces apoptosis when the dependence receptor meets the neurotrophin paradigm.
       Proceedings of the National Acadamy of Sciences, USA, 104, 13361-13366.

[192] Nikoletopoulou, V.; Lickert, H.; Frade, J. M.; Rencurel, C.; Giallonardo, P.; Zhang, L.;
       Bibel, M. & Barde, Y-A. (2010). Neurotrophin receptors TrkA and TrkC cause neuro-
       nal death whereas TrkB does not. *Nature*, 467, 59-64.

[193] Bernd, P. (2008). The role of neurotrophins during early development. *Gene Expression*, 14, 241-250.

[194] Kahane, N. & Kalcheim, C. (1994). Expression of trkC receptor mRNA during development of the avian nervous system. *Journal of Neurobiology*, 25, 571-584.

[195] Chalazonitis, A.; Pham, T. D.; Rothman, T. P.; DiStefano, P. S.; Bothwell, M.; Blair-Flynn, J.; Tassarollo, L. & Gershon, M. D. (2001). Neurotrophin-3 is required for the survival-differentiation of subsets of developing enteric neurons. *Journal of neuroscience*, 21, 5620-5636.

[196] Ernfors, P.; Kucera, J.; Lee, K. F.; Loring, J. & Jaenisch, R. (1995). Studies on the physiological role of brain-derived neurotrophic factor and neurotrophin-3 in knockout mice. *International Journal of Developmental Biology*, 39, 799-807.

[197] Farinas, I.; Jones, K. R.; Backus, C.; Wang, X. Y. & Reichardt, L. F. (1994). Severe sensory and sympathetic deficits in mice lacking neurotrophin-3. *Nature*, 369, 658-661.

[198] Yao, L.; Zhang, D. & Bernd, P. (1994). The onset of neurotrophin and trk mRNA expression in early embryonic tissue of the quail. *Developmental Biology*, 165, 727-730.

[199] Zhang, D.; Yao, L. & Bernd, P. (1994). Expression of trk and neurotrophin mRNA in dorsal root and sympathetic ganglia of the quail during development. *Journal of Neurobiology*, 25, 1517-1532.

[200] Henion, P. D.; Garner, A. S.; Large, T. H. & Weston, J. A. (1995). trkC-mediated NT-3 signaling is required for the early development of a subpopulation of neurogenic neural crest cells. *Developmental Biology*,172, 602-613.

[201] Kalcheim, C.; Carmeli, C. & Rosenthal, A. (1992). Neurotrophin-3 is a mitogen for cultured neural crest cells. *Proceeding of the National Acadeny of Science. USA*, 89, 1661-1665.

[202] Maisonpierre, P. C.; Belluscio, L.; Friedman, B.; Alderson, R. F.; Wiegand, S. J.; Furth, M. E.; Lindsay, R. M. & Yancopoulos, G. D. (1990). NT-3, BDNF, and NGF in the developing rat nervous system: parallel as well as reciprocal petterns of expression. *Neuron*, 5, 501-509.

[203] Ernfors, P.; Merlio, J. P. & Persson, H. (1992). Cells expressing mRNA for neurotrophins and their receptors during embryonic rat development. *European Journal of Neuroscience*, 4, 1140-1158.

[204] Verdi, J. M.; Groves, A. K.; Farinas, I.; Jones, K.; Marchionni, M. A.; Reichardt, L. F. & Anderson, D. J. (1996). A reciprocal cell-cell interaction mediated by NT-3 and neuregulins controls the early survival and development of sympathetic neuroblasts. *Neuron*, 16, 515-527.

[205] DiCicco-Bloem, E.; Friedman, W. J. & Black, I. B. (1993). NT-3 stimulates sympathetic neuroblast proliferation by promoting precursor survival. *Neuron*, 11, 1101-1111.

[206] Levi-Montalcini, R. (1987). The nerve growth factor: thirty-five years later. *EMBO Journal*, 6, 1145-1154.

[207] Verdi, J. M. & Anderson, D. J. (1994). Neurotrophins regulate sequential changes in neurotrophin receptor expression by sympathetic neuroblasts. *Neuron*, 13, 1359-1372.

[208] Wetmore, C. & Olson, L. (1995). Neuronal and non neuronal expression of neurotrophins and their receptors in sensory and sympathetic ganglia suggest new intercellular trophic interactions. *Journal of Comparative Neurology*, 353, 143-159.

[209] Rosenthal, A.; Goeddel, D. V.; Nguyen, T.; Lewis, M.; Shih, A.; Laramee, G. R.; Nikolics, K. & Winslow, J. W. (1990). Primary structure and biological activity of a novel human neurotrophic factor. *Neuron*, 4, 767-773.

[210] Reichardt , L. F. (2006). Neurotrophin-regulated signalling pathways. *Philosophical Transactions of the Royal Society of London. Series B, Biological Sciences*, 361, 1545-1564.

[211] ElShamy, W. M.; Linnarsson, S.; Lee, K. F.; Jaenisch, R. & Enfors, P. (1996a). Prenatal and postnatal requirements of NT-3 for sympathetic neuroblast survival and innervation of specific targets. . *Development*, 122, 491-500.

[212] ElShamy, W. M. & Enfors, P. (1996b). A local action of neurotrophin-3 prevents death of proliferating sensory neuron precusor cells. *Neuron*, 16, 963-972.

[213] Schecterson, L. C. & Bothwell, M. (1992). Novel roles for neurotrophins are suggested by BDNF and NT-3 mRNA expression in developing neurons. *Neuron*, 9, 449-463.

[214] Zhou, X-F. & Rush, R. A. (1996). Functional roles for neurotrophin-3 in the developing and mature sympathetic nervous system. *Molecular Neurobiology*, 13, 185-197.

[215] Francis, N.; Farinas, I.; Brennan, C.; Rivas-Plata, K.; Backus, C.; Reichardt, L. & Landis, S. (1999). NT-3, like NGF, is required for survival of sympathetic neurons, but not their precursors. *Developmental Biology*, 210, 411-427.

[216] Davies, A. M. (1994). The role of neurotrophins in the developing nervous system. *Journal of Neurobiology*, 25, 1134-1148.

[217] Ockel, M.; von Schack, D.; Schropel, A.; Dechant, G.; Lewin, G. R. & Barde, Y-A. (1996). Roles of neurotrophin-3 during early development of the peripheral nervous system. *Philosophical Transactions of the Royal Society: Biological Science*, 351, 383-387.

[218] Rush, R. A.; Chie, E.; Liu, D.; Tafreshi, A.; Zettler, C. & Zhou, X. F. (1997). Neurotrophic factors are required by mature sympathetic neurons for survival, transmission and connectivity. *Clinical and Experimental Pharmacology and Physiology*, 24, 549-555.

[219] Schecterson, L. C. & Bothwell, M. (2009). Neurotrophin receptors: old friends with new partners. *Developmental Neurobiology*, 70, 332-338.

[220] Scarisbrick, I. A.; Jones, E. G. & Isackson, P. J. (1993). Coexpression of mRNAs for NGF, BDNF, and NT-3 in the cardiovascular system of pre- and postnatal rats. *Journal of Neuroscience*, 13, 875-893.

[221] Hamberger, V. & Levi-Montalcini, R. (1949). Proliferation, differentiation and degeneration in the spinal ganglia of the chick embry under normal and experimental conditions. *Journal of Experimental Zoology*, 111, 457-501.

[222] Saltis, J. & Rush, R. A. (1995). Effects of nerve growth factor on sympathetic neuron development in normal and limbless chick embryos. *International Journal of Developmental Neuroscience*, 13, 577-584.

[223] Lee, K. F.; Davies, A. M. & Jaenisch, R. (1994). P75-deficient embryonic dorsal root sensory and neonatal sympathetic neurons display a decreased sensitivity to NGF. *Development*, 120, 1027-1033.

[224] Birren, S.; Lo, L. & Anderson, D. J. (1993). Sympathetic neuroblasts undergo a developmental switch in trophic dependence. *Development* ,119, 597-610.

[225] Straub, J. A.; Saulnier Sholler, G. L. & Nishi, R. (2007). Embryonic sympathoblasts transiently express TrkB in vivo and proliferate in response to brian-derived neurotrophic factor in vitro. *BMC Developmental Biology*, 7, 1-13.

[226] Elkabes, S.; Dreyfus, C. F.; Schaar, D. G. & Black, I. B. (1994). Embryonic sensory development: local expression of neurotrophin-3 and target expression of nerve growth factor. *Journal of Comparative Neurology*, 341, 204-213.

[227] Pizzuti, A.; Borsani, G.; Falini, A.; Sidoli, A.; Baralle, F. E.; Scarlato, G. & Silani, V. (1990). Detection of beta-nerve growth factor mRNA in the human fetal brain. *Brain Research*, 518, 337-341.

[228] Quartu, M.; Geic, M. & Del Flacco, M. (1997). Neurotrophin-like immunoreactivity in the human trigeminal ganglion. *Neuroreports*, 8, 3611-3617.

[229] Schober, A.; Wolf, N.; Huber, K.; Hertel, R.; Krieglstein, K.; Minichiello, L.; Kahane, N.; Widenfalk, J.; Kalcheim, C.; Olsen, L.; Klein, R.; Lewin, G. R. & Unsicker, K. (1998). TrkB and neurotrophin-4 are important for development and maintenance of sympathetic preganglion neurons innervating the adrenal medulla. *Journal of Neuroscience*, 18, 7272-7284.

[230] Schober, A.; Minichiello, L.; Keller, M.; Huber, K.; Layer, P. G.; Roig-Lopez, J. L.; Garcia-Arraras, J. E.; Klein, R. & Unsicker, K. (1997). Reduced acetylcholinesterase (AChE) activity in adrenal medulla and loss of sympathetic preganglionic neurons in TrkA-deficient, but not TrkB-deficient, mice. *Journal of Neuroscience*, 17, 891-903.

[231] Snider, W. D. (1994). Functions of the neurotrophins during nervous system development: what the knockouts are teaching us. *Cell*, 77, 627-638.

[232] Bode, K.; Hofmann, H. D.; Muller, T. H.; Otten, U.; Schmidt, R. & Unsicker, K. (1986). Effects of pre- and postnatal administration of antibodies to nerve growth factor on

the morphological and biochemical behaviour of the rat adrenal medulla: a reinvestigation. *Brain Research*, 392, 139-150.

[233] Shibayama, E. & Koizima, H. (1996). Cellular localisation of the Trk neurotrophin receptor family in human non-neural tissues. *American Journal of Pathology*, 148, 1807-1818.

[234] Lillien, L. E. & Claude, P. (1985). Nerve growth factor is a mitogen for cultured chromaffin cells. *Nature*, 317, 632-634.

[235] Aloe L.; Alleva, E.; Bohm, A. & Levi-Montalcino, R. (1986). Aggressive behaviour induces release of nerve growth factor from mouse salivary glands. *Proceedings of the National Acadamy of Sciences USA*, 83, 6184-6187.

[236] Otten, U.; Schwab, M.; Gangnon, C. & Thoenen, H. (1977). Selective induction of tyrosine hydroxylase and beta-hydroxylase by nerve growth factor: comparison between adrenal medulla and sympathetic ganglia of adult and newborn rats. *Brain Research*, 133, 291-303.

[237] Yamamoto, M. & Iseki, S. (2003). Co-expression of NGF and its high-affinity receptor trkA in the rat Carotic body chief cells. *Acta Histochem Cytochem* 36, 377-383.

[238] Suter-Crazzolara, C.; Lachmund, A.; Arab, S. F. & Unsicker, K. (1996). Expression of neurotrophins and their receptors in the developing and adult rat adrenal gland. *Molecular Brain Research*, 43, 351-355.

[239] Unsicker, K. & Kriegelstein, K. (1996). Growth factors in chromaffin cells. *Progress in Neurobiology*, 48, 307-324.

[240] Unsicker, K.; Huber, K.; Schutz, G. & Kalcheim, C. (2005). The chromaffin cell and its development. *Neurochemistry Research*, 30, 921-925.

[241] Doupe, A. J.; Landis, S. C. & Patterson, P. H. (1985). Environmental factors in the development of neural crest derivatives: glucocorticoids, growth factors, and chromaffin cell plasticity. *Journal of Neuroscience*, 5, 2119-2142.

[242] Wyatt, S. & Davies, A. M. (1995). Regulation of nerve growth factor receptor gene expression in sympathetic neurons during development. *Journal of Cell Biology*, 130, 1435-1446.

[243] Jungbluth, S.; Koentges, G. & Lumsden, A. (1997). Coordination of early neural tube development by BDNF/trkB. *Development*, 124, 1877-1885.

[244] Pinon, L. G.; Minichiello, L.; Klein, R. & Davies, A. M. (1996). Timing of neuronal death in trkA, trkB and trkC mutant embryos reveals developmental changes in sensory neuron dependence on Trk signalling. *Development*, 122, 3255-3261.

[245] Dixon, J. E. & McKinnon, D. (1994). Expression of trk gene family of neurotrophin receptors in prevertebral sympathetic ganglia. *Brain Research Developmental Brain Research*, 77, 177-182.

[246] Causing, C. G.; Gloster, A.; Aloyz, R.; Bamj, S. X.; Chang, E.; Fawcett, J.; Kuchel, G. & Miller, F. D. (1997). Synaptic innervation density is regulated by neuron-derived BDNF. *Neuron*, 257-267.

[247] Timmusk, T.; Belluardo, N.; Metsis, M. & Persson, H. (1993). Widespread and developmentally regulated expression of neurotrophin-4 mRNA in rat brain and peripheral tissues. *European Journal of Neuroscience*, 5, 605-613.

[248] Kondo, Y.; Saruta, J.; To, M.; Shiiki, N.; Sato, C. & Tsukinoki, K. (2010). Expression and role of the BDNF receptor-TrkB in rat adrenal gland under acute immobilisation stress. *Acta Histochemica Cytochemica*, 43, 139-147.

[249] Morrison, S. J.; White, P. M.; Zock, C.; & Anderson, D. J. (1999). Prospective identification, isolation by flow cytometry, and in vivo self-renewal of multipotent mammalian neural crest stem cells. *Cell*, 96, 737-749.

[250] Boiko, A, D.; Razorenova, O. V.; van de Rijn, M.; Swetter, S. M.; Johnson, D. L.; Ly, D. P.; Butler, P. D.; Yang, G. P.; Joshua, B.; Kaplan, M. J.; Longaker, M. T. & Weissman, I. L. (2010). Human melanoma initiating cells express neural crest nerve growth factor receptor CD-271. *Nature*, 466, 133-137.

[251] Baker, D. L.; Molenaar, W. M.; Trojanowski, J. Q.; Evans, A. E.; Ross, A. H.; Rorke, L. B.; Packer, R. J.; Lee, V. M-Y. & Pleasure, D. (1991). Nerve growth factor receptor expression in peripheral and central neuroectodermal tumors, other pediatric brain tumors and during development of the adrenal gland. *American Journal of Patholology*, 139, 115-122.

[252] Garin-Chesa, P.; Rettig, W.; Thomson, T. M.; Old, L. J. & Melamed, M. R. (1988). Immunohistochemical analysis of nerve growth factor receptor expression in normal and malignant human tissues. *Journal of Histochemistry and Cytochemistry*, 36, 383-389.

[253] Barrett, G. L.; Georgiou, A.; Ried, K.; Bartlett, P. F. & Leung, D. (1998). Rescue of dorsal root sensory neurons by nerve growth factor and neurotrophin-3, but not brain-derived neurotrophic factor or neurotrophin-4, is dependent on the level of the p75 neurotrophin receptor. *Neuroscience*, 85, 1321-1328.

[254] Bamji, S. X.; Majdan, M.; Pozniak, C. D.; Belliveau, D. J.; Aloyz, R.; Kohn, J.; Causing, C. G. & Miller, F. D. (1998). The p75 neurotrophin receptor mediates neuronal apoptosis and is essential for naturally occurring sympathetic neuron death. *Journal of Cell Biology*, 140, 911-923.

[255] Ibanez, C. F. & Simi, A. (2012). P75 neurotrophin receptor signalling in nervous system injury and degeneration: paradox and opportunity. *Trends in Neuroscience*, 35, 431-440

[256] Lorentz, C. U.; Woodward, W. R.; Tharp, K. & Habecker, B. A. (2011). Altered norepinephrine content and ventricular function in p75NTR-/- mice after myocardial infarction. *Autonomic Neuroscience*, 164, 13-19.

[257] Nakagawara, A.; Arima, M.; Azar, C. G.; Scavards, N. J. & Brodeur, G. M. (1992). In-
       verse relationship between trk expression and N-myc amplification in human neuro-
       blastomas. *Cancer Research*, 52, 1364-1368.

[258] Nakagawara, A.; Arima-Nakagawara, M.; Scavarda, N. J.; Azar, C. G.; Cantor, A. B.
       & Brodeur, G. M. (1993). Association between high levels of expression of the trk
       gene and favourable outcome in human neuroblastoma. *New England Journal of Medi-
       cine*, 328, 847-854.

[259] Kogner, P.; Barbany, G.; Dominici, C.; Castello, C.; Raschella, G. & Persson, H. (1993).
       Coexpression of messenger RNA for TRK protooncogene and low affinity nerve
       growth factor receptor in neuroblastoma with favourable prognosis. *Cancer Research*,
       53, 2044-2050.

[260] Cheung, N. –K. V.; Kushner, B. H.; LaQuaglia, M. P.; Kramer, K.; Ambros, P.; Am-
       bros, I.; Ladanyi, M.; Eddy, J.; Bonilla, M.-A. & Gerald, W. (1997). Survival from non-
       stage 4 neuroblastoma without cytotoxic therapy: an analysis of clinical and
       biological markers. *European Journal of Cancer*, 33, 2117-2120.

[261] Combaret, V.; Gross, N.; Lasset, C.; Balmas, K.; Bouvier, R.; Frappaz, D.; Beretta-
       Brognara, C.; Philip, T.; Favrot, M. C. & Coll, J-L. (1997). Clinical relevance of trkA
       expression on neuroblastoma: camparison with Nmyc amplification and CD44 ex-
       pression. *British Journal of Cancer* , 75, 1151-1155.

[262] Matsunaga, T.; Shirasawa, H.; Enomoto, H.; Yoshida, H.; Iwai, J.; Tanabe, M.; Kawa-
       mura, K.; Etoh, T. & Ohnuma, N. (1998). Neuronal Src and Trk A protoncogene ex-
       pression in neuroblastomas and patient prognosis. *International Journal of Cancer
       (Predictive Oncology)*, 79, 226-231.

[263] Matsunaga, T.; Shirasawa, H.; Hishiki, T.; Yoshida, H.; Kouchi, K.; Ohtsuka, Y.; Ka-
       wamura, K.; Etoh, T. & Ohnuma, N. (2000). Enhanced expression of N-myc messen-
       ger RNA in neuroblastoma found by mass screening. *Clinical Cancer Research*, 6,
       3199-3204.

[264] Suzuki, T.; Bogenmann, E.; Shimada, H.; Stram, D. & Seeger, R. C. (1993b) Lack of
       high-affinity nerve growth factor receptors in aggressive neuroblastomas. *Journal of
       the National Cancer Institute*, 85, 377-384.

[265] Terui, E.; Matsunaga, T. ; Yoshida, , H.; Kouchi, K.; Kuroda, H.; Hishiki, T.; Saito, T.;
       Yamada, S-I.; Shirasawa, H. & Ohnuma, N. (2005). Shc family expression in neuro-
       blastoma: high expression of Shc C is associated with a poor prognosis in advanced
       neuroblastoma. *Clinical Cancer Research*, 11, 3280-3287.

[266] Warnat, P.; Oberthuer, A.; Fischer, M.; Westermann, F.; Eils, R. & Brors, B. (2007).
       Cross-study analysis of gene expression data for intermediate neuroblastoma identi-
       fies two biological subtypes. *BMC Cancer*, 7, 89-100.

[267] Tajiri, T.; Higashi, M.; Souzaki, R.; Tatsuta, K.; Kinoshita, Y. & Taguchi, T. (2007). Classification of neuroblastomas based on an analysis of the expression of genes related to prognosis. *Journal of Pediatric Surgery*, 42, 2046-2049.

[268] Weinreb, I.; Goldstein, D.; Irish, J. & Perez-Ordonez, B. (2009). Expression patterns of Trk-A, Trk-B, GRP78, and p75NRT in olfactory neuroblastoma. *Hum Pathol* 40, 1330-1335.

[269] Light, J. E.; Koyama, H.; Minturn, J. E.; Ho, R.; Simpson, A. M.; Iyer, R.; Mangino, J. L.; Kolla, V.; London, W. B. & Brodeur, G. M. (2012). Clinical significance of NTRK family gene expression in neuroblastomas. *Pediatric Blood Cancer*, 59, 226-232.

[270] Shimada, H.; Nakagawara, A.; Peters, J.; Wang, H.; Wakamatsu, P- K.; Lukens, J. N.; Matthay, K. K.; Siegel, S. E. & Seeger, R. C. (2004). TrkA expression in peripheral neuroblastic tumours. *Cancer*, 101, 1873-1881.

[271] Cheng, A. J.; Cheng, N. C.; Ford, J.; Smith, J.; Murray, J. E.; Flemming, C.; Lastowska, M.; Jackson, M. S.; Hackett, C. S.; Weiss, W. A.; Marshall, G. M.; Kees, U. R.; Murray, D. N. & Haber, M. (2007). Cell lines from MycN transgenic murine tumours reflect molecular and biological characteristics of human neuroblastoma. *European Journal of Cancer*, 43, 1467-1475.

[272] Cohn, S. L.; Look, T. A.; Joshi, V. V.; Holbrook, T.; Salwern, H.; Chagnovich, D.; Chesler, L.; Rowe, S. T.; Valentine, M. B.; Komuro, H.; Castleberry, R. P.; Bpwman, L. C.; Rao, P. V.; Seeger, R. C. & Brodeur, G. M. (1995). Lack of correlation of N-myc gene amplification with prognosis in localised neuroblastoma: a pediatric oncology group study. *Cancer Research*, 55, 721-726.

[273] Comstock, J. M.; Willmore-Payne, C.; Holden, J. A. & Coffin, C. M. (2009). Composite pheochromocytoma: a clinicopathologic and molecular comparison with ordinary pheochromocytoma and neuroblastoma. *American Journal of Clinical Phology*,132, 69-73.

[274] Iraci, N.; Diolati, D.; Papa, A. et al., (2011). A SP1/MIZ1/MYCN repression complex recruits HDAC1 at the TrkA and p75NTR promoters and effects neuroblastoma malignancy by inhibiting the cell response to NGF. *Cancer Research*, 71, 404-412.

[275] Lau, D. T.; Hesson, L. B.; Norris, M. D.; Marshall, G. M.; Haber, M. & Ashton, L. J. (2012). Prognostic significance of promoter DNA methylation in patients with childhood neuroblastoma. *Clinical Cancer Research*, 18, 5690-5700.

[276] De Preter, K.; Vandesompele, J.; Heimann, P.; Yigit, N.; Beckman, S.; Schramm, A.; Eggert, A.; Stallings, R. L.; Benoit, Y.; Renard, M.; De Paepe, A.; Laureys, G.; Pahlman, S. & Speleman, F. (2006). Human fetal neuroblasts and neuroblastoma transcriptome analysis confirms neuroblast origin and highlights neuroblastoma candidate genes. *Genome Biology*, 7 (R84) 3-17.

[277] Lucarelli, E.; Kaplan, D. & Thiele, C. J. (1995). Selective regulation of TrkA and TrkB receptors by retinoic acid and interferon-γ in human neuroblastoma cells. *Journal of Biological Chemistry*, 270, 24725-24731.

[278] Chang, B. B.; Persengiev, S. P.; de Diego, J. G.; Sacristan, M. P.; Martin-Zanca, D. & Kilpatrick, D. L. (1998). Proximal promoter sequences mediate cell specific and elevated expression of favourable prognosis marker TrkA in human neuroblastoma cells. *Journal of Biological Chemistry*, 273, 39-44.

[279] Condello, S.; Caccamo, D.; Curro, M.; Ferlazzo, N.; Parisi, G. & Ientile R. (2008). Transglutaminase and NF-kB interplay during NGF-induced differentiation in neuroblastoma cells. *Brain Research*, 1207, 1-8.

[280] Azar, C. G.; Scavarda, N. J.; Nakagawara, A. & Brodeur, G. M. (1994). Expression and function of the nerve growth gactor receptor (TRK-A) in human neuroblastoma cell lines. *Progress in Clinical and Biological Research*, 385, 169-175.

[281] Matsushima H & Bogenmann, E. (1993). Expression of TrkA cDNA in neuroblastomas mediates differentiation in vitro and in vivo. *Molecular and Cellular Biology*, 13, 7447-7456.

[282] Hartman, D. S. & Hertel, C. (1994). Nerve growth factor-induced differentiation in neuroblastoma cells expressing trkA but lacking p75NTR. *Journal of Neurochemistry*, 63, 1261-1270.

[283] Poluha, W.; Poluha, D. K. & Ross, A. H. (1995). TrkA neurogenic receptor regulates differentiation of neuroblastoma cells. *Oncogene*, 10, 185-189.

[284] Gryz, A. A. & Meakin, S. O. (2003). Acidic substitution of the activation loop tyrosines in TrkA supports nerve growth factor-dependent, but not nerve growth factor-independent differentiation and cell cycle arrest in the human neuroblastoma cell line, SY5Y. *Oncogene*, 22, 8774-8785.

[285] Kim, C. J.; Matsuo, T.; Lee, K-H. & Thiele, C. J. (1999). Up-regulation of insulin-like growth factor-II expression is a feature of TrkA but not TrkB activation in SH-SY5Y neuroblastoma cells. *American Journal of Pathology*, 155, 1661-1670.

[286] Peterson, S. & Bogemann, E. (2004). The RET and TrkA pathways collaborate to regulate neuroblastoma differentiation. *Oncogene*, 23, 213-215.

[287] Tsuruda, A.; Suzuki, S.; Maekawa, T. & Oka, S. (2004). Constitutively active Src facilitates NGF-induced phosphorylation of TrkA and causes enhancement of MAPK signalling in SK-N-MC cells. *FEBS Letters*, 560, 215-220.

[288] Fagerstrom, S.; Pahlman, S. Gestblom, C. & Nanberg, E. (1996). Protein kinase C-ε is implicated in neurite outgrowth in differentiating neuroblastoma cells. *Cell Growth & Differentiation*, 7, 775-785.

[289] Eggert, A.; Ikegaki, N.; Liu, X-G.; Chou, T. T.; Lee, M. V. & Brodeur, G. M. (2000). Molecular dissection of TrkA signal transduction pathways leading to differentiation in human neuroblastoma cells. *Oncogene*, 19, 2043-2051.

[290] Olsson, A-K. & Nanberg, E. (2001). A functional role for ERK in gene induction, but not in neurite outgrowth in differentiating neuroblastoma cells. *Experimental Cell Research*, 265, 21-30.

[291] Eggert, A.; Grotzer, M. A.; Ikegaki, N.; Liu, X-G.; Evans, A. E. & Brodeur, G. M. (2000). Expression of neurotrophin receptor TrkA inhibits angiogenesis in neuroblastoma. *Medical and Pediatric Oncology*, 35, 569-572.

[292] Eggert, A.; Grotzer, M. A.; Ikegaki, N.; Liu, X. G.; Evans, A. E. & Brodeur, G. M. (2002). Expression of the neurotrophin receptor TrkA down-regulates expression and function of angiogenic stimulators in SH-SY5Y neuroblastoma cells. *Cancer Research*, 62, 1802-1808.

[293] Schulte, J. H.; Kuhfittig-Kulle, S.; Klein-Hitpass, L.; Schramm, A.; Baird, D. S. F.; Pfeiffer, P. & Eggert, A. (2008). Expression of the TrkA and TrkB receptor tyrosine kinase alters the double-strand break (DSB) repair capacity of SY5Y neuroblastoma cells. *DNA Repair*, 7, 1757-1764.

[294] Matsumoto, K.; Wada, R. K. & Yamashiro, J. M. (1995). Expression of brain derived neurotrophic factor and p145TrkB affects survival, differentiation, and invasiveness of human neuroblastoma cells. *Cancer Research*, 55, 1798-1806.

[295] Lavoie, J-F.; LeSauteur, L.; Kohn, J.; Wong, J.; Furtoss, O.; Thiele, C. J.; Miller, F. D. & Kaplan, D. R. (2005). TrkA induces apoptosis of neuroblastoma cells and does so via a p53-dependent mechanism. *Journal of Biological Chemistry*, 280, 29199-29207.

[296] Harel, L.; Costa, B.; Tcherpakov, M.; Zapatka, M.; Oberthuer, A.; Hansford, L. M.; Vojvodic, M.; Levy, Z.; Chen, Z-Y.; Lee, F. S.; Avigad, S.; Yaniv, I.; Shi, L.; Eils, R.; Fischer, M.; Brors, B.; Kaplan, D. R. & Fainzilber, M. (2009). CCM2 mediates death signaling by the TrkA receptor tyrosine kinase. *Neuron*, 63, 585-591.

[297] Jung, E. J. & Kim, D. R. (2008). Apoptotic death in TrkA-overexpressing cells: kinetic regulation of ERK phosphorylation and caspase-7 activation. *Molecular Cells*, 26, 12-17.

[298] Kogner, P.; Barbany, G.; Bjork, O.; castello, C.; Donfrancesco, A.; Falkmer, U. G.; Hedborg, F.; Kouvidou, H.; Persson, H.; Raschella et al., (1994). Trk mRNA and low affinity nerve growth factor receptor mRNA expression and triploid DNA content in favourable neuroblastoma tumors. *Progress in Clinical and Biological Research*, 385, 137-145.

[299] Schulte, J. H.; Pentek, F.; Hartmann, W.; Schramm, A.; Friedrichs, N.; Ora, I.; Koster, J.; Versteeg, R.; Kirfel, J.; Buettner, R. & Eggert, A. (2009). The low affinity neurotrophin receptor, p75, is upregulated in ganglioneuroblastoma/ ganglioneuroma and re-

duces tumorigenicity of neuroblastoma in vivo. *International Journal of Cancer*, 124, 2488-2494.

[300] Bogemann, E. (1996). A metastatic neuroblastoma model in SCID mice. *International Journal of Cancer*, 67, 379-385.

[301] Morandi, F.; Scaruffi, P.; Gallo, F.; Stigliani, S.; Moretti, S.; Bonassi, S.; Gambini, C.; Mazzocco, K.; Fardin, P.; Haupt, R.; Arcamone, G.; Pistoia, V.; Tonini, G. P. & Corrias, M. V. (2012). Bone marrow infiltrating human neuroblastoma cells express high levels of calprotectin and HLA-G- proteins. *PloS ONE*, 7, e2pp22

[302] Lipska, B. S.; Drozynska, E.; Scaruffi, P.; Tonini, G. P.; Izycka-Swieszewska, E.; Zietkiewicz, S.; Balcerska, A.; Perek, D.; Chybicka, A.; Biernat, W. & Limon, J. (2009). C. 1810C>T polymorphism of NTRK1 gene is associated with reduced survival in neuroblastoma patients. *BMC Cancer*, 9, 436-444.

[303] Cao, F.; Liu, X.; Zhang, L.; Wang, Y. & Zhang, N. (2010). Expression of TrkA splice isoforms in neuroblastoma and its clinical significance. *Chinese Journal of Clinical Oncology*, 37, 1282-1285.

[304] Minturn, J. E.; Evans, A. E.; Villablanca, J. G.; Yanik, G. A.; Park, J. R.; Shusterman, S.; Groshen, S.; Hellriegel, E. T.; Bensen-Kennedy, D.; Matthay, K. K.; Brodeur, G. M. & Maris, J. M. (2011). Phase I trial of laustaurtinib for children with refractory neuroblastoma: a new approaches to neuroblastoma therapy consortium study. *Cancer Chemotherapy and Pharmacology*, 68, 1057-1065.

[305] Schramm, A.; Vandesompele, J.; Schulte, J. H.; Dreesman, S.; Kaderali, L.; Brors, B.; Eils, R.; Speleman, F. & Eggert, A. (2007). Translating expression profiling into a clinically feasible test to predict neuroblastoma outcome. *Clinical Cancer Research*, 13, 1459-1465.

[306] Guo, X.; Chen, Q-R.; Song, Y. K.; Wei, J. S. & Khan, J. (2011). Exon array analysis reveals neuroblastoma tumors have distinct alternative splicing patterns according to stage and MYCN amplification status. *BMC Medical Genomics*, 4, 35-50.

[307] Hishiki, T.; Saito, T.; Terui, K.; Sato, Y.; Takenouchi, A.; Yahata, E.; Ono, S.; Nakagawara, A.; Kamijo, T.; Nakamura, Y.; Matsunga, T. & Yoshida, H. (2010). Reevaluation of trkA expression as a biological marker of neuroblastoma by high-sensitivity expression analysis – a study of 106 primary neuroblastomas treated in a single study. *Journal of Pediatric Surgery*, 45, 2293-2298.

[308] Farina, A. R.; Cappabianca, L.; Ruggeri, P.; Di Ianni, N.; Ragone, M.; Merolla, S.; Gulino, A. & Mackay, A. R. (2012). Alternative TrkA Splicing and neuroblastoma. In: *Neuroblastoma-Present and Future* (Ed. Hiroyuki Shimada) Intech, Rijeka Croatia, pp111-136.

[309] Brodeur, G. M.; Nakagawara, A.; Yamashiro, D. J.; Ikegaki, N.; Liu, X. G.; Azar, C. G.; Lee, C. P. & Evans, A. E. (1997). Expression of TrkA, TrkB and TrkC in human neuro-blastomas. *Journal of Neurooncology*, 31, 49-55.

[310] Brodeur, G. M; Minturn, J. E.; Ho, R.; Simpson, A. M.; Iyer, R.; Varela, C. R.; Light, J. E.; Kolla, V. & Evans A. E. (2009). Trk expression and inhibition in neuroblastomas. *Clinical Cancer Research*, 15, 3244-3256.

[311] Nakagawara, A.; Azar, C. G.; Scavarda, N. J. & Brodeur, G. M. (1994). Expression and function of Trk-B and BDNF in human neuroblastomas. *Molecular and Cellular Biology*, 14, 759-767.

[312] Aoyama, M.; Sai, K.; Shishikura, T.; Kawamoto, T.; Miyachi, T.; Yokoi, T.; Togari, H.; Wada, Y.; Kato, T. & Nakagawara, A. (2001). Human neuroblastomas with unfavour-able biologies express high levels of brain-derived neurotrophic factor mRNA and a variety of its variants. *Cancer Letters*, 164, 51-60.

[313] Baj, G. & Tongiorgi, E. (2008). BDNF splice variants from the second promoter cluster support cell survival of differentiated neuroblastoma upon cytotoxic stress. *Journal of Cell Science*, 122, 36-43.

[314] Bouzas-Rodrigues, J.; Cabrera, J. R.; Delloye-Bourgeois, C.; Ichim, G.; Delcros, J-G.; Raquin, M-A.; Rousseau, R.; Combaret, V.; Bénard, J.; Tauszig-Delamasure, S. & Mehlen, P. Neurotrophin-3 production promotes human neuroblastoma cell survival by inhibiting TrkC-induced apoptosis. *Journal of Clinical Investigation*, 120, 850-858.

[315] Stemple, D. L. & Anderson, D. J. (1992). Isolation of a stem cell for neurons and glia from the mammalian neural crest. *Cell*, 71, 973-985.

[316] Biagiotti, T.; D'Amico, M.; Marzi, I.; Di Gennaro, P.; Arcangeli, A.; Wanke, E. & Oli-votto, M. (2006). Cell renewing in neuroblastoma: electrophysiological and immuno-cytochemical characterization of stem cells and derivatives. *Stem Cells*, 24, 443-453.

[317] Marzi, I.; D'Amico, M. ; Biagiotti, T.; Giunti, S.; Carbone, M. V.; Fredducci, D.; Wanke, E. & Olivotto, M. (2007). Purging of the neuroblastoma stem cell component and tumor regression on exposure to hypoxia or cytotoxic treatment. *Cancer Research*, 67, 2402-2407.

[318] Islam, O.; Loo, T. X. & Heese, K. (2009). Brain-derived neurotrophic factor (BDNF) has proliferative effects on neural stem cells through the truncated Trk-B receptor, MAP kinase, Akt, and STAT-3 signaling pathways. *Current Neurovascular Reseach*, 6, 42-53.

[319] Fanburg-Smith, J. C. & Miettinen, M. (2001). Low-affinity nerve growth factor recep-tor (p75) in Dermatofibrosarcoma Protuberans and other neural tumors: A study of 1,150 tumors and fetal and adult normal tissues. *Human Pathology*, 32, 976-983.

[320] Perosio, P. M. & Brooks, J. J. (1988). Expression of nerve growth factor receptor in paraffin-embedded soft tissue tumors. *American Journal of Pathology*, 132, 152-160.

[321] Kimura, N.; Nakamura, M.; Kimura, I. & Nagura, H. (1996). Tissue localisation of nerve growth factor receptors: TrkA and low-affinity nerve growth factor receptor in neuroblastoma, pheochromocytoma, and retinoblastoma. *Endocrine Pathology, 7,* 281-289.

[322] Ho, R.; Minturn, J. E.; Simpson, A. M.; Iyer, R.; Light, J. E.; Evans, A. E. & Brodeur, G. M. (2011). The effect of P75 on Trk receptors in neuroblastoma. *Cancer Letters, 305,* 76-85.

[323] Zhao, S. P. (2003). Co-expression of TrkA and p75 neurotrophin receptor in extracranial olfactory neuroblastoma cells. *Humnan Yi Ke Da Xue Xue Bao, 28,* 50-52.

[324] Matsushima, H. & Bogenmann, E. (1994). NGF induces terminal differentiation in trkA expressing neuroblastoma cells in vitro and in vivo. *Progress in Clinical and Biological Research, 385,* 177-183.

[325] Ehrehard, P.B.; Ganter, U.; Schmutz, B.; Bauer, J. & Otten, U. (1993). Expression of low affinity nerve growth factor receptor and TrkB messenger RNA in human SH-SY5Y neuroblastoma cells. *FEBS letters, 330,* 287-292.

[326] Roux, P. P.; Bhakar, A. L.; Kennedy, T. E. & Barker, P. A. (2001). The p75 neurotrophin receptor activates Akt (protein kinase B) through a phosphoinositol 3-kinase-dependent pathway. *Journal of Biologcal Chemistry, 276,* 23097-23104.

[327] Levrerrier, Y.; Thomas, J.; Mathieu, A. L.; Low, W.; Blanquier, B. & Marvel, J. (1999). Role of PI-3kinase in Bcl-X induction and apoptosis inhibition mediated by IL-3 or IGF in Baf-3 cells. *Cell Death & Differentiation, 6,* 290-296.

[328] Gargano, N.; Levi, A. & Alema, S. (1997). Modulation of nerve growth factor internalisation by direct interaction between p75 and trkA receptors. *Journal of Neuroscience Research, 50,* 1-12.

[329] Wehrman, T.; He, X.; Raab, B.; Dukipatti, A.; Blau, H. & Garcia, K. C. (2007). Structural and mechanistic insights into nerve growth factor interactions with the TrkA and p75 receptors. *Neuron, 53,* 25-38.

[330] Makkerth, J. P.; Ceni, C.; Auld, D. S.; Vaillancourt, F.; Dorval, G. & Barker, P. A. (2005). P75 neurotrophin receptor reduces ligand-induced Trk receptor ubiquination and delays Trk receptor internalisation and degradation. *EMBO Reports, 6,* 936-941.

[331] Zhang, C.; Helmsing, S.; Zagrebelsky, M.; Schirrmann, T.; Marschall, A. L. J.; Schungel, M.; Korte, M.; Hust, M. & Dubel, S. (2012). Suppression of p75 neurotrophin receptor surface expression with itraantibodies influences Bcl-X mRNA expression and neurite outgrowth in PC12 cells. *PloS ONE, 7,* e30684.

[332] Ito, H.; Nomoto, H. & Furukawa, S. (2003). Growth arrest of PC12 cells by nerve growth factor is dependent on the phosphoinositol 3-kinase pathway via p75 neurotrophin receptor. *Journal of Neuroscience, 72,* 211-217.

[333] Chen, J. & Zhe, X. (2003). Cotransfection of TrkA and p75(NTR) in neuroblastoma cell line (IMR32) promotes differentiation and apoptosis of tumor cells. *Chinese Medical Journal*, 116, 906-912.

[334] Yan, C.; Liang, Y.; Nylander, K. D.; Wong, J.; Rudavsky, R. M.; Saragovi, H. U. & Schor, N. F. (2002). P75-Nerve growth factor as an antiapoptotic complex: Independence versus cooperativity in protection from enediyne chemotherapeutic agents. *Molecular Pharmacology*, 61, 710-719.

[335] Holub, J. L.; Qui, Y. Y.; Chu, F. & Madonna, M. B. (2011). The role of nerve growth factor in caspase-dependent apoptosis in human BE(2)C neuroblastoma. *Journal of Pediatric Surgery*, 46, 1191-1196.

[336] Bunone, G.; Mariotti, A.; Compagni, A.; Morandi, E. & Della Valle, G. (1997). Induction of apoptosis by p75 neurotrophin receptor in human neuroblastoma cells. *Oncogene*, 14,1463-1470.

[337] Eggert, A.; Sieverts, H.; Ikegaki, X-G. & Brodeur, G. M. (2000). P75 mediated apoptosis in neuroblastoma cells is inhibited by expression of TrkA. *Medical and Pediatric Oncology*, 35, 573-576.

[338] Giraud, S.; Lautrette, B.; Bessette, B.; Decourt, C.; Mathonnet, M. & Jauberteau, M. O. (2005). Modulation of Fas-induced apoptosis by p75 neurotrophin receptor in a human neuroblastoma cell line. *Apoptosis*, 10, 1271-1283.

[339] Bai, Y.; Qiang, Li.; Yang, J.; Zhou.; X.; Yin, X. & Zhao, D. (2008). P75NTR activation of NF-kB is involved in prP106- 126-induced apoptosis in mouse neuroblastoma cells. *Neuroscience Research*, 62, 9-14.

[340] Rogers, M-L.; Beare, A.; Zola, H. & Rush, R. A. (2008). CD-271 (P75 neurotrophin receptor). *Journal of Biological Regulation & Homeostatic Agents*, 22, 1-6.

[341] Kuwako, K-I.; Taniura, H. & Yoshikawa, K. (2004). Necdin-related MAGE proteins differentially interact with the E2F1 transcription factor and the p75 neurotrophin receptor. *Journal of Biological Chemistry*, 279, 1703-1712.

[342] Kenchappa, R. S.; Zampieri, N.; Chao, M. V.; Barker, P. A.; Teng, H. K.; Hempstead, B. L. & Carter, B. D. (2006). A ligand-dependent cleavage of P75 neurotrophin receptor is necessary for NRIF nuclear translocation and apoptosis in sympathetic neurons. *Neuron*, 50, 219-232.

[343] Christiansen, H.; Christiansen, N. M.; Wagner F et al., (1990). Neuroblastoma-inverse relationship between expression of N-Myc and NGF-R. *Oncogene*, 5, 437-440.

[344] Wang, C.; Liu, Z.; Woo, C-W.; Li, Z.; Wang, L.; Wei, J. S.; Marquez, V. E.; Bates, S. E.; Jin, Q.; Khan, J.; Ge, K. and Thiele, C. J. (2011). EZH2 mediates epigenetic silencing of neuroblastoma suppressor genes CASZ1, CLU, RUNX3, and NGFR. *Cancer Research*, 72, 315-324.

[345]   Cortazzo, M. H.; Kassis, E. S.; Sproul, K. A. & Schor, N. F. (1996). Nerve growth fac-
        tor (NGF)-mediated protection of neural crest cells from antimitotic agent-induced
        apoptosis: the role of low-affinity NGF receptor. *Journal of Neuroscience*, 16, 3895-3899.

[346]   Panicker, J.; Li, Z.; McMahon, C.; Sizer, C.; Steadman, K.; Piekarz, R.; Bates, S. E. &
        Thiele, C. J. (2010). Romidepsin (FK228/depsipeptide) controls growth and induces
        apoptosis in neuroblastoma tumor cells. *Cell Cycle*, 9, 1830-1838.

[347]   Borrello, M. G.; Bongarzone, I.; Pierotti, M. A.; Luksch, R.; Gasparini, M.; Collini, P.;
        Pilotti, S.; Rizzetti, M. G.; Mondellini, P.; De Bernardi, B.; Di Martino, D.; Garaventa,
        A.; Brisigotti, M. & Tonini, G. P. (1993). Trk and ret proto-oncogene expression in hu-
        man neuroblastoma specimens: high frequency of trk expression in non-advanced
        stages. *International Journal of Cancer*, 54, 540-545.

[348]   Edsjo, A.; Lavinius, E.; Nilsson, H.; Hoehner, J. C.; Simonsson, P.; Culp, L. A.; Mar-
        tinsson, T.; Larsson, C.; Pahlman, S. (2003). Expression of trkB in human neuroblasto-
        ma in relation to MycN expression and retinoic acid treatment. *Laboratory
        Investigation*, 83, 813-823.

[349]   Fung, W.; Hasan, M. Y.; Loh, A. H.; Chua, J. H.; Yong, M. H.; Knight, L.; Hwang, W.
        S.; Chan, M. Y.; Seow, W. T.; Jacobsen, A. S. & Chui, C. H. (2011). Gene expression of
        Trk neurotrophin receptors in advanced stage neuroblastomas in Singapore - a pilot
        study. *Pediatric Hematology and Oncology*, 28, 571-578.

[350]   Zhang, J.; Zhend, Y.; Wang, Y. & Tong, H. (2010). The studies on the correlation for
        gene expression of tyrosine-kinase receptors and vascular endothelial growth factor
        in human neuroblastomas. *Journal of Pediatric Hematology and Oncology*, 32, 180-184.

[351]   Pastor, R.; Bernal, J. & Rodriguez-Pena, A. (1994). Unliganded c-erbA/thyroid hor-
        mone receptor induces trkB expression in neuroblastoma cells. *Oncogene*, 1081-1089.

[352]   Martens, L. K.; Kirschner, K. M.; Warnecke, C. & Scholz, H. (2007). Hypoxia-induci-
        ble factor-1 (HIF-1) is a transcriptional activator of the TrkB neurotrophin receptor
        gene. *Journal of Biological Chemistry*, 282, 14379-14388.

[353]   Hoehner, J. C.; Olsen, L.; Sandstedt, B.; Kaplan, D. R. & Pahlman, S. (1995). Associa-
        tion of neurotrophin receptor expression and differentiation in human neuroblasto-
        ma. *American Journal of Pathology*, 147, 102-113.

[354]   Lucarelli, E.; Kaplan, D. & Thiele, C. J. (1997). Activation of trk-A but not trk-B signal
        transduction pathway inhibits growth of neuroblastoma cells. *European Journal of
        Cancer*, 33, 2068-2070.

[355]   Kaplan, D. R.; Matsumoto, K.; Lucarelli, E. & Thiele, C. J. (1993). Induction of TrkB by
        retinoic acid mediates biologic responsiveness to BDNF and differentiation of human
        neuroblastoma cells. *Neuron*, 11, 321-331.

[356] Esposito, C. L.; D'Alessio, A.; de Franciscis, V. & Cerchia, L. (2008). A cross-talk be-tween TrkB and Ret tyrosine kinases receptors mediates neuroblastoma cells differ-entiation. *PloS ONE*,3(2):e1643.doi:10.1371/journal.pone. 001643

[357] Shirohira, H.; Kitaoka, A.; Enjoji, M.; Uno, T. & Nakashima, M. (2012). AM80 induces neuronal differentiation via increased tropomyosin-related kinase B expression in human neuroblastoma SH-SY5Y cell line. *Biomedical Research*, 33, 291-297.

[358] Middlemas, D. S.; Kihl, B. K.; Zhou, J. & Zhu, X. (1999). Brain-derived neurotrophic factor promotes survival and chemoprotection of human neuroblastoma cells. *Journal of Biological Chemistry*, 274, 16451-16460.

[359] Scala, S.; Wosikowski, K.; Giannakakou, P.; Valle, P.; Biedler, J.; Spengler, B. A.; Lu-carelli, E.; Bates, S. E. & Thiele, C. J. (1996). Brain-derived neurotrophic factor pro-tects neuroblastoma cells from vinblastine toxicity. *Cancer Research*, 56, 3737-3742.

[360] Ho, R.; Eggert, A.; Hishiki, T.; Minturn, J. E.; Ikegaki, N.; Foster, P.; Camoratto, A. M.; Evans, A. E. & Brodeur, G. M. (2002). Resistance to chemotherapy mediated by TrkB in neuroblastoma. *Cancer Research*, 62, 6462-6466.

[361] Jaboin, J.; Kim, C. J.; Kaplan, D. R. & Thiele, C. J. (2002). Brain-derived neurotrophic factor activation of TrkB protects neuroblastoma cells from chemotherapy-induced apoptosis via phosphatidylinositol 3'-kinase pathway. *Cancer Research*, 62, 6756-6763.

[362] Jaboin, J.; Hong, A.; Kim, C. J. & Thiele, C. J. (2003). Cisplatin-induced cytotoxicity is blocked by brain-derived neurotrophic factor activation of TrkB signal transduction path in neuroblastoma. *Cancer Letters*, 193, 109-114.

[363] Li, Z. & Thiele, C. J. (2007). Targeting Akt to increase the sensitivity of neuroblastoma to chemotherapy: lessons learned from the brain derived neurotrophic factor/TrkB signal transduction pathway. *Expert Opinions in Therapeutic Targets*, 11, 1611-1621.

[364] Hecht, M.; Schulte, J. H.; Eggert, A.; Wilting, J. & Schweigerer, L. (2005). The neuro-trophin receptor TrkB cooperates with c-Met in enhancing neuroblastoma invasive-ness. *Carcinogenesis*, 26, 2105-2115.

[365] Cimmino, F.; Schulte, J. H.; Zollo, M.; Koster, J.; Versteeg, R.; Iolascon, A.; Eggert, A. & Schramm, A. (2009). Galectin-1 is a major effector of Trk-B-mediated neuroblasto-ma aggressiveness. *Oncogene*, 28, 2015-2023.

[366] Nakamura, K.; Martin, K. C.; Jackson, J. K.; Beppu, K.; Woo, C-W. & Thiele, C. J. (2006). Brain-derived neurotrophic factor activation of TrkB induces vascular endo-thelial growth factor expression via hypoxia-inducible factor-1a in neuroblastoma cells. *Cancer Research*, 66, 4249-4255.

[367] Geiger, T. R. & Peeper, D. S. (2005). The neurotrophic receptor TrkB in anoikis and metastasis: a perspective. *Cancer Research*, 65, 7033-7036.

[368] Haapsalo, A.; Saarelainen, T.; Moshynakov, M.; Arumae, U.; Kiema, T. R.; Saarma, M.; Wong, G. & Castrén, E. (1999). Expression of the naturally occurring truncated

trkB neurotrophin receptor induces outgrowth of filopodia and processes in neuro-blastoma cells. *Oncogene*, 18, 1285-1296.

[369] Olivieri, G.; Otten, U.; Meier, F.; Baysang, G.; Dimitriades-Schmutz, B.; Muller-Spahn, F. & Savaskan, E. (2003). β-Amyloid modulates tyrosine kinase B receptor ex-pression in SHSY5Y neuroblastoma cells: influence of the antioxidant melatonin. *Neuroscience*, 120, 659-665.

[370] Ryden, M.; Sehgal, R.; Dominici, C.; Schilling, F. H.; Ibanez, C. F. & Kogner, P. (1996). Expression of mRNA for the neurotrophin receptor TrkC in neuroblastomas with fa-vourable tumour stage and good prognosis. *British Journal of Cancer* ,74, 773-779.

[371] Yamashiro, D. J.; Liu, X-G.; Lee, C. P.; Nakagawara, A.; Ikegaki, N.; McGregor, L. M.; Baylin, S. B. & Brodeur, G. M. (1997). Expression and function of Trk-C in favourable human neuroblastomas. *European Journal of Cancer* 33, 2054-2057.

[372] Svensson, T.; Ryden, M.; Schilling, F. H.; Dominici, C.; Sehgal, R.; Ibanez, C. F. & Kogner, P. (1997). Coexpression of mRNA for the full-length neurotrophin receptor Trk-C and trk-A in favourable neuroblastoma. *European Journal of Cancer*, 33, 2058-2063.

[373] Menn, B.; Timsit, S.; Represa, A.; Mateos, S.; Calothy, G. & Lamballe, F. (2000). Spa-tiotemporal expression of noncatalytic TrkC NC2 isoform during early and late CNS neurogenesis: a comparative study with TrkC catalytic and p75NTR receptors. *Euro-pean Journal of Neuroscience*, 12, 3211-3223.

[374] Edsjo, A.; Hallberg, B.; Fagerstrom, S.; Larsson, C.; Axelson, H. & Pahlman, S. (2001). Differences in the early and late responses between neurotrophin-stimulated TrkA and TrkC transfected SH-SY5Y neuroblastoma cells. *Cell Growth & Differentiation*, 12, 39-50.

[375] Bassili, M.; Birman, E.; Schor, N. F. & Saragovi, U. H. (2010). Differential roles of Trk and p75 neurotrophin receptors in tumorigenesis and chemoresistance ex vivo and in vivo. *Cancer Chemother Pharmacol* 65, 1047-1056.

[376] Nara, K.; Kasafuka, T.; Yoneda, A.; Oue, T.; Sangkhathat, S. & Fukuzawa, M. (2007). Silencing MYCN by RNA interference induces growth inhibition, apoptotic activity and cell differentiation in a neuroblastoma cell line with MYCN amplification. *Inter-national Journal of Oncology*, 30, 1189-1196.

[377] Laneve, P.; Di Marcotullio, L.; Gioia, U.; Fiori, M. E.; Ferretti, E.; Gulino, A.; Bozzoni, I. & Caffarelli, E. (2007). The interplay between microRNAs and the neurotrophin re-ceptor tropomyosin-related kinase C controls proliferation of human neuroblastoma cells. *Proceedings of the National Academy of Science. USA.* 104, 7957-7962.

[378] Guidi, M.; Muinos-Gimeno, M.; Kagerbauer, B.; Martl, E.; Estivilli, X. & Espinosa-Parrilla, Y. (2010). Overexpression of miR-128 specifically inhibits the truncated iso-

form of NTRK3 and upregulates BCL2 in SH-SY5Y neuroblastoma cells. *BMC Molecular Biology,* 11, 95.

[379] Thress, K.; Macintyre, T.; Wang, H.; Whitston, D.; Liu, Z. Y.; Hoffmann, E.; Wang, T.; Brown, J. L.; Webster, K.; Omer, C.; Zage, P. E.; Zeng, L. & Zweidler-McKay, P. A. (2009). Identification and preclinical characterisation of AZ-23, a novel, selective, and orally bioavailable inhibitor of the Trk kinase pathway. *Molecular Cancer Therapeutics,* 8, 1818-1827.

[380] Zage, P. E.; Graham, T. C.; Zeng, L.; Fang, W.; Pien, C.; Thress, K.; Omer, C.; Brown, J. L. & Zweidler-McKay, P. A. (2011). The selective Trk inhibitor AZ623 inhibits brain-derived neurotrophic factor-mediated neuroblastoma cell proliferation and signalling and is synergistic with topotecan. *Cancer,* 117, 1321-1329.

[381] Iyer, R.; Varela, C. R.; Minturn, J. E.; Ho, R.; Simpson, A. M.; Light, J. E.; Evans, A. E.; Zhao, H.; Thress, K.; Brown, J. L. & Brodeur, G. M. (2012). AZ64 inhibits TrkB and enhances the efficacy of chemotherapy and local radiation in neuroblastoma xenografts. *Cancer Chemotherapy and Pharmacology,* 10.1007/s00280-012-1879-x

[382] Evans, A. E.; Kisselbach, K. D.; Yamashiro, D. J.; Ikegaki, N.; Camoratto, A. M.; Dionne, C. A. & Brodeur, G. M. (1999). Antitumor activity of CEP-751 (KT-6587) on human neuroblastoma and medulloblastoma xenografts. *Clinical Cancer Research,* 5, 3594-3602.

[383] Evans, A. E.; Kisselbach, K. D.; Liu, X.; Eggert, A.; Ikegaki, N.; Camoratto, A. M.; Dionne, C. A. & Brodeur, G. M. (2001). Effect of CEP-751 (KT-6587) on neuroblastoma xenografts expressing trkB. *Medical Pediatric Oncology,* 36, 181-184.

[384] Iyer, R.; Evans, A. E.; Qi, X.; Ho, R.; Minturn, J. E.; Zhao, H.; Balamuth, N.; Maris, J. M. & Brodeur, G. M. (2010). Lestaurtinib enhances the antitumour efficacy of chemotherapy in murine xenograft models of neuroblastoma. *Clinical Cancer Research,* 16, 1478-1485.

[385] Minturn, J. E.; Evans, A. E.; Villablanca, J. G.; Yanik, G. A.; Park, J. R.; Shusterman, S.; Groshen, S.; Hellriegel, E. T.; Bensen-Kennedy, D.; Matthay, K. K.; Brodeur, G. M. & Maris, J. M. (2011). Phase I trial of laustaurtinib for children with refractory neuroblastoma: a new approaches to neuroblastoma therapy consortium study. *Cancer Chemotherapy and Pharmacology,* 68, 1057-1065.

[386] Norris, R. E.; Minturn, J. E.; Brodeur, G. M.; Maris, J. M. & Adamson, P. C. (2011). Preclinical evaluation of lesaurtinib (CEP-701) in combination with retinoids from neuroblastoma. *Cancer Chemotherapy and Pharmacology,* 68, 1469-1475.

[387] Saulnier Sholler, G. L.; Brard, L.; Straub, J. A.; Dorf, L.; Illeyne, S.; Koto, K.; Kalkunte, S.; Bosenberg, M.; Ashikaga, T. & Nishi, R. (2009). Nifurtimox induces apoptosis of neuroblastoma cells in vitro and in vivo. *Journal of Pediatric Hematology and Oncology,* 31, 187-193.

[388] Yamaguchi, Y.; Tabata, K.; Asami, S.; Miyake, M. & Suzuki, T. (2007). A novel cyclophane compound, CPPy, facilitates NGF-induced TrkA signal transduction and induces cell differentiation in neuroblastoma. *Biological and Pharmacological Bullitin*, 30, 638-643.

[389] Ikegaki, N.; Gotoh, T.; Kung, B.; Riceberg, J. S.; Kim, D. Y.; Zhao, H.; Rappaport, E. F.; Hicks, S. L.; Seeger, R. C. & Tang, X. X. (2007). De novo identification of MIZ-1 (ZBTB1) encoding MYC-interacting zinc finger protein as a new favourable neuroblastoma gene. *Clinical Cancer Research*, 13, 6001-6009.

[390] Wang, C.; Liu, Z.; Woo, C. W.; Li, Z.; Wang, L.; Wei, J. S.; Marquez, V. E.; Bates, S. E.; Jin, Q.; Khan, J.; Ge, K. & Thiele, C. J. (2012). EZH2 mediates epigenetic silencing of neuroblastoma suppressor genes CASZ1, CLU, RUNX3, and NGFR. *Cancer Research*, 72, 315-324.

[391] Tang, X. X.; Robinson, M. E.; Riceberg, J. S.; Kim, D. Y.; Kung, B.; Titus, T. B.; Hayashi, S.; Flake, A. W.; Carpentieri, D. & Ikegaki, N. (2005). Favorable neuroblastoma genes and molecular therapeutics of neuroblastoma. *Clinical Cancer Research*, 10, 5837-5844.

Chapter 4

Close Neighbours on Chromosome 2 the ALK and MYCN Genes. Implications for Targeted Therapeutics in Neuroblastoma

Fergal C. Kelleher

Additional information is available at the end of the chapter

1. Introduction

Neuroblastoma is a neural crest-derived embryonal malignancy of the postganglionic sympathetic division of the peripheral autonomic nervous system. It is the most frequent extra cranial solid malignancy of childhood and the most common cancer in children less than one year of age. It accounts for 7% of childhood cancers and 15% of all childhood cancer deaths. It most commonly occurs sporadically but familial cases can also occur with one subdivision attributable to germline mutation of the PHOX2B gene and another due to germline ALK gene mutations [1,2,3,4]. Recurring chromosomal aberrations are detected in this disease and three major genomic subdivisions represent greater than 80% of cases; i.e. hyperdiploid neuroblastoma; near diplod neuroblastoma that has 17q gain and 11q deletions; and MYCN amplified neuroblastoma with 17q gain and 1p deletion [5,6,7,8]. A whole-genome analysis and assessment of structural defects in 87 primary neuroblastomas found few recurrent amino-acid changing mutations, with ALK mutations in 6%, but identified local shredding of chromosomes (chromothripsis) in 18% of high stage neuroblastomas. High stage tumours that did not have amplifications of MYCN had recurrent structural alterations in genes involved in cone stabilisation and neuritogenesis [9]. Indeed in this study tumours with a genomic signature involving defective genes responsible for neuritogenesis or growth cone guidance were mostly aggressive high-stage tumours.

Activating mutations of the anaplastic lymphoma kinase (ALK) genes and amplification of the MYCN oncogene can occur in neuroblastoma. The ALK gene resides on chromosome 2p23 centromeric to the MYCN locus on chromosome 2q24. Approximately 2-3% of cases of neuroblastomas have amplification of ALK and these occur almost invariably concomitant with amplification of MYCN [10]. However, amplification of the ALK gene without concomitant MYCN gene amplification can occur, for example a particularly informative case of a neuroblastoma with a high level amplicon involving and solely limited to the ALK gene was described by French investigators in 2008 in one of the landmark papers that established the importance of ALK in neuroblastoma [11]. Activating ALK mutations are found in 80% of familial cases and 6-11% of sporadic cases. It is considered that once the expression of wild type ALK exceeds a certain threshold it can have oncogenic activity[10]. Twenty percent of all cases of neuroblastomas have amplification of MYCN which is associated with a worse prognosis and can be used to stratify treatment. This chapter appraises the current knowledge and potential therapeutic implications arising from ALK and MYCN abnormalities in neuroblastoma. In a concluding reflection the chromosomal proximity and interaction of these genes as well as the potential for therapeutic advancement in neuroblastoma is discussed.

2. The anaplastic lymphoma kinase gene in neuroblastoma

2.1. The ALK gene

The anaplastic lymphoma kinase gene is a 200kDa member of the insulin receptor super family. It is an orphan tyrosine kinase receptor and has homology with the MET oncogene and the neurotrophin receptor. It is normally expressed by the developing nervous system and at a much lower level in the nervous system of adults [12]. In mouse embryo studies *Alk* transcripts were detected in the central nervous system (CNS) and peripheral nervous system. E15 embryos had expression in the Gasserian ganglion of the trigeminal nerve (cell bodies of V_1, V_2 and sensory component V_3) as well as the superior cervical ganglion, posterior root ganglia of the spinal cord and the myenteric plexus of the enteric nervous system. In the 1 week old mouse *Alk* transcripts are clustered in particular neuronal regions in the CNS such as the mesencephalon, thalamic nuclei which act as relay stations for nerve impulses and olfactory bulb, mitral cells and tufted cells that receive primary afferents from olfactory epithelial neurones. Relatively high levels of *Alk* transcripts were present in the superior colliculus, which is the centre of visual sensation and the red nucleus, a crucial part of the rubrospinal tract which regulates the contraction of flexor muscles [13]. Lower levels were detected in the hypothalamus, inferior colliculus, subiculum, cerebral cortex and cerebellum (Purkinje's cells and Golgi cells). Interestingly one patient in a phase 1 study of an ALK inhibitor in children with relapsed/refractory ALK-driven tumors (57 evaluated for toxicity) developed grade 3 dizziness [14]. It remains speculative as to whether it is possible to attribute it to cerebellar Alk expression based on the finding of low level *Alk* expression in the murine cerebellum.

The anaplastic lymphoma kinase gene has a restricted pattern of expression in adults in that it is expressed in testis, small intestine and brain but is not expressed in normal lymphoid tissue. It has been shown to be important in the pathogenesis of ALK positive anaplastic large cell lymphoma, inflammatory myofibroblastic tumours and adenocarcinoma of the lung (NSCLC) [15]. Its importance in cancer was first described in 1994 in anaplastic large cell lymphoma where a translocation (2; 5) (p23; q35) fuses NPM a non-ribosomal nucleolar phosphoprotein with ALK in 50-75% of cases [16]. The most frequent abnormality involving ALK in non-small cell lung cancer is an inversion of a segment of chromosome 2 creating a chimeric fusion gene involving ALK and the Echinoderm microtubule-associated protein; ALK-EML4 [17]. In inflammatory myofibroblastic tumours, tropomyosin TMP3 or TMP4 create fusion oncoproteins with ALK. Clonal rearrangements at chromosome 2p23 occur in 50% of these tumours [18]. More recently ALK protein expression has been seen in rhabdo-myosarcomas with 81% of cases of the alveolar subtype having strong cytoplasmic staining for ALK compared to 31% of cases of the embryonal subtype. These subtypes have gene copy number gain of 88% and 52% respectively. In the embyonal subgroup ALK aberrations were associated with disease progression and outcome [19].

The ALK receptor is a dependence receptor and in the absence of ligand enhances apoptosis by autologous cleavage by caspase [12]. Therefore ALK belongs to the subcategory of onco-genes in which inappropriate expression in a cellular context or in the absence of ligand can induce apoptosis. This is considered to be a mechanism to abrogate frequent tumour formation if oncogenes become deregulated. Myc is also considered to be an established comparator gene in this respect. Additionally in the visual system of Drosophila ALK in the presence of a ligand appears essential for axonal guidance. It is known that perturbations of the visual system, in particular in the first 5 years of life can cause amblyopia [20, 21]. Also, in an expanded cohort study of 82 adults with ALK positive NSCLC treated with crizotinib, mild visual disturbances were reported by 41% of patients. These were most frequently described as trails of light following moving objects particularly seen with changes in ambient lighting usually improv-ing with duration of time receiving treatment [22]. It may be the case that the aforementioned finding of *Alk* transcripts in the superior colliculus of the 1 week old mouse is relevant as the superior colliculus is important for saccadic and smooth pursuit eye movements. Though not described to date in patients with neuroblastoma treated with ALK inhibitors, given the age demographics of patients with neuroblastoma it is the author's contention that clinicians conducting ongoing trials need to be cognisant of the theoretical potential to damage the developing neuroanatomical visual system with resulting amblyopa. The visual system includes the optic nerves, optic chiasma and optic tracts; the lateral geniculate body a swelling beneath the posterior projection of the pulvinar of the thalamus and the geniculoclcarine tract which originates within the lateral geniculate body and terminates at the calcarine sulcus of the medial surface of the cerebral hemisphere. Evaluation of the regional ALK status of this system is a subject for further research.

2.2. ALK in neuroblastoma

Neuroblastoma is considered to be a malignancy derived from the embryonic neural crest. Evidence of neuroblastoma being derived from neural crest progenitor cells are (i) neuroblas-toma primary sites are anatomically consistent with arising from the sympatho-adrenergic lineage of neural crest differentiation (ii) The gene expression patterns of neuroblastomas and neural crest progenitor cells are similar [23] (iii) In situ neuroblastomas occur in the adrenal glands of 1/200 newborns with most spontaneously regressing later in life and there is a histological similarity to residual nests of sympathogonia [24].

A small proportion of cases of neuroblastoma display autosomal dominant Mendelian inheritance patterns and a familial history of neuroblastoma is elicited in 1-2% of cases [25, 26, 27]. There is a standardized incidence ratio of 9.7 for disease occurrence in siblings of index cases [28]. Previously it had been recognized that neuroblastoma can arise in the context of concurrent neurocristopathies related to abnormal development of neural-crest derived tissues such as concomitant Hirschsprung's disease or central congenital hypoventilation syndrome. Nonsense and missense mutations of the homeobox gene PHOX2B were shown to predispose to this abnormality of the sympathoadrenal lineage [4, 29, 30].

In October 2008 four articles were published in the journal *Nature* that established the importance of aberrations in ALK as a feature of some neuroblastomas [11,31,32,33]. Mossé and colleagues of Children's Hospital Philadelphia found that ALK is a major neuroblastoma predisposition gene with germline ALK mutations accounting for most cases of familial neuroblastoma [31]. Using a whole-genome scan of neuroblastoma pedigrees (8 unrelated families) a significant linkage signal at 2p23-24 was identified. Re-sequencing 194 high risk neuroblastomas found somatically acquired ALK mutations in 12.4% of cases. Most mutations mapped to the kinase domain of ALK and caused constitutive phosphorylation. Cell line studies also showed that knockdown of ALK mRNA caused growth inhibition suggesting that therapeutics targeting ALK may have clinical efficacy in neuroblastoma.

In another study lead by investigators at Dana Farber Cancer Institute, Boston mutations of ALK were found in 8% of primary neuroblastomas [32]. A genome wide study of primary neuroblastomas identified amplification of the ALK gene. Analysis of 94 tumours with amplification of MYCN found 14 (15%) with concomitant ALK amplification. This was not identified in 51 tumors without MYCN amplification. DNA resequencing of the ALK open reading frame identified in primary neuroblastomas found 5 non-synonymous sequence variations in the ALK tyrosine kinase domain in 7 of 93 samples (8%). The most frequent mutation which was in 4.3% (4) of the 93 cases was a cytosine to adenine alteration in exon 23 causing a phenylalanine to leucine substitution in codon 1174 (F1174L). This mutation was also found in 3 different neuroblastoma cell lines. Three of the mutations were somatic and 2 were germline. Interestingly 4 of the 5 identified mutations involved residues which correspond to those that are affected by activating EGFR gene mutation. The ALK 1174 residue correlated with V769 in EGFR and ERBB2 [34]. A F1245C ALK mutation correlated with the L833V mutation in EGFR, which is a gefitinib resistant mutation in NSCLC. The R1275Q mutation is positioned adjacent to the homologous position of L858R in EGFR, the most common mutation of EGFR in NSCLC [35, 36]. ALK cDNA encoding either the F1174L or the R1275Q variants transformed interleukin-3 dependent murine hematopoietic Ba/F3 cell lines to cytokine independent cell growth. Furthermore these autonomously growing cells were sensitive to the ALK inhibitor TAE684. Additionally 2 human neuroblastoma cell lines were sensitive to TAE684. It has been observed by Mossé and colleagues that there are disorder involving oncogenes such as RET in medullary thyroid cancer arising in the context of multiple endocrine neoplasia type 2 and MET in papillary carcinoma of the kidney that are analogous to the sequential 'two hit model' of Knudson. Knudsons' was first used to describe retinoblastoma arising from aberrations of a tumor suppressor gene. In the oncogene 'two hit' model the second hit is a somatically acquired duplicate of the mutant allele or mutant gene amplification [37]. In neuroblastoma oncogenic activation of ALK can occur by mutation of the tyrosine kinase domain and for example with respect to a 'second hit' in the Dana Farber led study, ALK gene amplification was found in 15% of 94 tumours with MYCN amplification.

French investigators assessed ALK copy number variation by comparative genomic hybridization in 592 cases of neuroblastomas [11]. Within this group 26 cases (4.4%) had in excess of a twofold copy number increase of ALK and a further 135 cases (22.8%) had lower level gains. The level of expression of ALK is strongly correlated with copy number [38]. Within the genomic analysis a subcategory without MYCN amplification was assessed using 100K single nucleotide polymorphism arrays. A notable case within this cohort was an instance of neuroblastoma with a high level amplicon involving and solely limited to the ALK gene. Also a series of 28 cell lines and 115 tumor samples found 16 ALK mutations grouped into 2 main hotspots. The F1174L mutation was seen in one primary tumor but was more frequent in cell lines suggesting that this particular mutation confers an in vitro growth advantage. Cell lines are usually over-represented by metastatic tumors with a greater propagating potential and this finding may be vicarious evidence of the F1174L mutation being correlated with a poorer clinical outcome. Finally a Japanese study identified 8 novel missense mutations in the ALK gene in 13 out of 215 cases of neuroblastoma (6.1%) and 8 of 33 (33%) neuroblastoma cell lines. The mutated kinases could transform NIH3T3 fibroblasts and form tumors in nude mice [33].

These four studies were a landmark advance in the field, however later a European group of international collaborators performed a meta-analysis of 709 neuroblastomas (254 new cases and 455 previously published) to comprehensively described the correlation of ALK mutation type and frequency with clinical and genomic factors. They also assessed the prognostic significance of ALK copy number and expression [39]. Mutations in ALK were detected in 6.9% of cases with a mutation frequency of ALK of 5.7% in favorable (International neuroblastoma Staging System INSS 1, 2 and 4s) cases and 7.5% in unfavorable tumors (INSS 2 and 4). There was no statistical difference with respect to mutation frequency between the favorable and unfavorable groups (P=0.087). Mutation hot spots R1275Q (49%) and F1174L (34.7%) were observed within the mutated cases. However the F1174L mutations occurred in a greater proportion of the MYCN amplified cases (P=0.0001) and the concurrence of a F1174L mutation in a MYCN amplified neuroblastoma was found to confer an especially poor prognosis. It was described that there was a skewed ALK mutation spectrum within the MYCN amplified cohort with over-representation of the F1174L mutation. F1174 mutated ALK was present in 1.3% of single copy MYCN tumors compared with 6.1% of MYCN amplified tumors. To consider it another way, within the 17 cases of F1174 ALK mutated neuroblastoma 58.8% had amplification of MYCN compared to a rate of 21.6% in cases of neuroblastoma with wild type ALK. There also was no difference in the frequency for MYCN amplification between the R1275Q cases and wild type ALK. The skewed distribution of F1174L mutations being overrepresented in MYCN amplified cases of neuroblastoma was also confirm in 27 neuroblastoma cell lines most of which were MYCN amplified. Five had the F1174L mutation with only one case of R1275Q mutant neuroblastoma found. F1174 mutated neuroblastoma compared to the R1275Q mutant variant had a greater transforming ability with a higher amount of auto phosphory-lation. Gain in Chr. 2p that included ALK (91.8%) also was correlated with poor survival.

2.3. Possible new treatments for neuroblastoma that target ALK

Crizotinib is an orally bio-available small molecule that inhibits the tyrosine kinase activity of ALK and c-Met which is approved by the U.S. Food and Drug administration for the treatment of cases of NSCLC that have rearrangements of the ALK gene. Crizotinib competes with adenosine triphosphate to bind to the ALK tyrosine kinase. The two most common ALK mutations in neuroblastoma are F1174L and R1275Q and both mutations promote autophos-phorylation of the ALK tyrosine kinase region. F1174 mutated ALK in particular is a more lethal variant. Using neuroblastoma cell lines and xenograft models it has been shown that different ALK mutations can affect both kinase activity and inhibitor sensitivity [40]. Both F1174L and R1275Q ALK mutations cause amino acid substitutions in the intracellular tyrosine kinase domain of the ALK receptor and constitutively activate the ALK tyrosine kinase domain. Neuroblastoma cell lines and xenograft mouse models that expressed R1275Q-ALK are sensitive to crizotinib. By comparison F1174L mutated ALK cell lines were relatively resistant to crizotinib. The $K_{m, ATP}$ for F1174L of ~0.127Mm was approximately 2.3 times lower than the $K_{m, ATP}$ of 0.326 for the R1275Q mutant ALK variant. The F1174L mutation combines the characteristics of an activating gene mutation and a resistance mutation, increasing k_{cat} and maintaining a wild type like $K_{m, ATP}$. The derived overall inference of these findings is that comparative crizotinib resistance of the F1174L mutant ALK is due to greater ATP binding affinity and it is hoped that the resistance may be overcome by increasing the doses of crizotinib or using ALK inhibitors with increased affinity to the ALK tyrosine kinase domain.

The U.S. National Cancer Institute is sponsoring a phase I/II study of crizotinib in children with relapsed or refractory solid tumors and anaplastic large cell lymphoma. The phase I study was presented at the American Society of Clinical Oncology Annual Meeting in Chicago, June 2012 (Protocol IDs: COG-ADVL0912, ADVL0912, NCT00939770) by Yael Mossé; abstract 9500 [14]. The study enrolled 70 patients with confirmed ALK fusion proteins, mutations or amplification with 57 fully evaluable for toxicity. This was a heterogeneous study population with respect to cancer type and included other cancers in addition to neuroblastoma. Six different dose levels of crizotinib were evaluated using the rolling-six design and dosing was bid on 28 day cycles without interruption. The recommended phase II dose that emerged was 280mg/m²/dose. Seven of eight (88%) of patients with anaplastic large cell lymphoma had a complete response (2 differing dose levels). 27 patients in the trial had neuroblastomas. Within the cohort of neuroblastoma cases with a known ALK mutation (n=8), one patient had a complete response and 2 had stable disease. Of the 19 patients with neuroblastoma and an unknown ALK status, 1 had a complete response and 6 had prolonged stable disease.

With respect to toxicity there were two grade 5 cases of haemorrhage within the central nervous system in patients with neuroblastoma and the protocol was updated to exclude patients with a previous history of central nervous system involvement. Other toxicities observed within the study and not necessarily within the neuroblastoma subgroup were grade 4 transaminitis (n=1), grade 4 neutropenia (n=1) and grade 3 dizziness (n=1). A discussant at the meeting

Thomas Gross of The Ohio State University Nationwide Children's Hospital referenced some Crizotinib toxicities observed in adults with NSCLC including gastrointestinal complaints, transient vision disorders, self-limited lower testosterone levels and rare renal cysts. He felt that these toxicities necessitated further investigation in the paediatric population. Regarding efficacy he noted that there can be variability in oncogenic partners with ALK within chimeric fusion genes in differing disease types that may partly account for the rates of complete responses seen in different malignancies. He also observed that some responses were seen in ALK negative cases in the phase 1 trial. Phase II data on the efficacy and toxicity of Crizotinib in neurblastoma will be required.

3. The MYCN gene in neuroblastoma

3.1. The MYCN family

MYC is a pleotropic evolutionary conserved family of basic helix-loop-helix leucine zipper transcription factors, comprising c-Myc, L-Myc and N-Myc [41, 42]. These transcription factors regulate the expression of ~15% of all genes [43, 44]. MYC proteins have numerous roles in malignancy with roles of special importance in neuroblastoma being that of driving cellular proliferation and angiogenesis while concurrently inhibiting apoptosis and maintaining the neoplastic 'stem cell' compartment. MYCN is amplified in ~20% of cases of neuroblastoma and amplification of MYCN is independently correlated with a higher disease stage and a poor clinical outcome. It is amplified in 40% of cases with a high risk phenotype. It has been contended that targeting Myc is a therapeutically attractive strategy to treat cancer but difficulties persist. These include (i) Myc exerts effects by protein-protein and protein-DNA interactions. Small molecule inhibitors have not usually been effective in this context. (ii) Most Myc aberrations in malignancies are not due to intrinsic abnormalities of Myc but rather due to 'upstream' aberrant oncogenic signals causing it's induction (iii) Myc is required for stem cell compartment maintenance and proliferation in normal tissues with a theoretical concern of serious bystander tissue toxicities [45] (iv) Analysis of the role of c-Myc and N-Myc in cancer is difficult to assess in tissues as embryonic lethality is conferred by germline deletion of these genes. Much of the data on the consequences of inhibiting Myc is derived from conditional knockouts of the c-Myc gene using Cre mediated recombination which can be very variable and unpredictable in the extent of c-myc deletion in the cells targeted (iv) Conditional knockout models are irreversible and therefore not good representative models of transient inhibition of Myc conferred by inhibitor medications.

One particularly important experimental example of Myc inhibition was in an adenocarcinoma of lung murine model [45]. Omomyc is a competitive inhibitor of Myc-dependent gene transcription by preventing the binding of Myc to its consensus E-box CACGTG DNA elements thereby preventing Myc binding to its obligate dimerization partner Max. This prevents the transactivation of its target genes. Omomyc may also augment Myc-dependent trans repression [46, 47]. The LSL-Kras^{G12D} murine model of NSCLC has irreversible activation of oncogenic KRas^{G12D} driven by the *kras* promoter when it inhales adenovirus expressing Cre recombinase.

This causes multifocal lung tumours to occur within 18 weeks. Shut down of Myc transactivation using transgenic Omomyc expression caused profound tumour reduction within 3 days and mice become overtly tumour free after 28 days [45]. Reassuringly murine tissue integrity was maintained with no major unexpected toxicities emerging. Considering neuroblastoma, treatments directed at MYCN are particularly appealing as genetic mouse models with MYCN targeted to neural crest tissue develop tumours which are similar to neuroblastomas [48].

3.2. MYCN in neuroblastoma

Double minutes and homogeneously staining regions are the cytogenetic hallmarks of genomic amplification in malignancies. Neuroblastoma karyotyes frequently have these cytogenetic markers and MYCN amplifications are often found [49]. Tumours that have an aggressive phenotype frequently have amplification of the MYCN oncogene and amplification of MYCN is correlated with the extent of disease at diagnosis [50]. Correlative International Neuroblastoma Staging System (INSS) stage at diagnosis and the respective frequency of MYCN amplification described by data from the Children's Oncology Group Statistical Office are; Stage 1, 3%; Stage 2a/2b, 4%; Stage 3, 25%; Stage 4, 32% and Stage 4s, 8% (Wendy, London; John, Maris, Principles and Practice of Paediatric Oncology, page 890). Amplification of MYCN is normally detected by interphase FISH with a usual increase in copy number of 50 to 400 copies in neuroblastomas and a cut off of 4 times the normal copy number being the definition of MYCN amplification by many pathologists. Other genes can be co-amplified with MYCN [51, 52]. Also comparative genomic hybridisation of tumours arising in a transgenic mouse model that overexpresses MYCN in neuroectodermal cells, found losses and gains of at least seven chromosomal regions. These were syntenic with comparable abnormalities detected in human neuroblastomas [52].

NVP-BEZ235 a dual inhibitor of the phosphatidylinositol 3-kinase (PI3K)/mammalian target of rapamycin (mTOR) pathway decreases levels of MYCN protein and suppresses tumour proliferation and angiogenesis in neuroblastomas [53]. This partly arises because MYCN in tumour cells contributes to paracrine signalling between tumour cells and endothelial cells. It has previously been shown that blocking PI3K/mTOR causes destabilisation of MYCN protein with reduced VEGF secretion and inhibition of progression of neuroblastomas in murine models [54]. A study published in *Science Translational Medicine* in 2012 by Chanthery and colleagues provided new information as to the separate 'intrinsic' and 'paracrine' including 'anti-angiogenic' mediated anti-tumour effects of inhibiting PI3K/mTOR signalling in neuroblastomas using NVP-BEZ235. Improved survival was seen in two mouse models, the first a xenograft tumour derived from a patient (MYCN-amplified human orthoptic xenograft) and the second a MYCN dependent transgenic model (transgenic for TH-MYCN; that recapitulates a MYCN amplified tumour arising in an autochthonous site) in which MYCN causes spontaneous tumour formation in mice. In both models there were reductions in tumour growth without tumour regression. This was attributed to a reduction in proliferation of neuroblasts and decreased tumour vascular density. PI3K inhibition caused de-repression of GSK3β with consequential Thr58 phosphorylation and destabilisation of MYCN with a remarkable reduction in MYCN levels in tumours treated with NVP-BEZ235.

To establish tumour cell autonomous effects of NVP-BEZ235 on MYCN degradation, HUWE1 knockdown tumour cells (deficient in PI3K/mTOR-mediated MYCN proteolysis; a Thr58 mutant MYCN) were used to establish orthoptic xenograft models. It was demonstrated that HUWE1 were resistant to the anti-angiogenic effects of NVP-BEZ235 showing that MYCN was a critical target in vivo and part of the anti-angiogenic effect is a consequence of the transcription regulatory function of MYCN. It is possible that NVP-BEZ235 may emerge as a new therapeutic choice for the treatment of neuroblastoma.

4. ALK and MYCN

4.1. ALK and MYC co-operating neighbours

ALK and MYCN are the only established oncogenes in neuroblastoma [55, 56]. ALK mutations occur at an equal frequency in both low and high risk neuroblastomas and within all genomic subtypes which is suggestive that mutations within the ALK gene are not the only molecular aberrations that drives oncogenesis in this disease [57]. ALKF1174L mutated neuroblastomas are more common within the high risk neublastoma category [10]. In neuroblastoma cell line studies overexpression of wild type or mutated ALK stimulates the transcription of MYCN and the concurrent expression of MYCN and activated ALK increases the in vitro transformation of NIH3T3 cells [58].

A series of experiments on pathogenic cooperation between ALK and MYCN were conducted using a transgenic zebrafish model of neuroblastoma in which MYCN induced tumour arose from a subpopulation of neuroblasts which migrate to the interrenal gland, the zebrafish equivalent of the adrenal medulla (50% of neuroblastomas in humans arise in the adrenal medulla) [59]. Sympathoadrenal precursors in the interrenal gland co-express the cholaminergic enzymes tyrosine hydroxylase and dopamine-β-hydroxylase as well as neuronal specific Hu proteins. In this model the dopamine-β-hydroxylase promoter was used to drive EGFR-MYCN expression. Using this experimental model it was found that 17.3% of MYCN induced zebrafish develop neuroblastomas. Transgenic zebrafish that expressed wild type ALK or that expressed F1174L mutant ALK did not develop neuroblastomas. Activated ALK accelerate the onset of neuroblastoma and increased the penetrance of MYCN-induced neuroblastoma with a 3 fold increase for fish co-expressing both MYCN and ALK F1174L compared to wild type or F1174L mutant ALK fish. The mechanism as to how neuroblastomas arise within the zebrafish model was also investigated. MYCN overexpressing transgenic fish has an increased number of Hu+ neuroblasts that fail to differentiate resulting in increased cell number with reduced numbers of chromaffin cells compared to controls at 3-5 weeks post fertilization (wpf). An apoptotic response significantly reduced the number of these Hu+ cells at the 5-7 wpf interval. In the presence of a cooperating activated ALK there is continuous accumulation of Hu+ neuroblasts with failure of differentiation but there is decreased apoptosis of high penetrance and transformed neuroblastoma. Overall it has been inferred that ALK mutant F1174L attenuates the sequential apoptotic response in MYCN transformed Hu+

neuroblasts constituting the 'second' hit when considering it as an oncogenic equivalent of the Knudson 'two hit' model.

Another study found that ALK regulates the initiation of MYCN transcription in neuroblastoma [58]. ALK (including wild type ALK and mutated variants) stimulated the transcription of MYCN mRNA by affecting the MYCN promoter in neuronal and neuroblastoma cell lines. Similarly the transcription of MYCN can be abrogated by using ALK inhibitors such as crizotinib or NVP-TAE684. A series of experiments found that ALK^{F1174L} or ALK^{R1275Q} mediated a marked transformation of NIH3T3 cells but MYCN alone or wild type ALK failed to initiate cellular transformation. Co-transfection of ALK^{1174L} concurrent with MYCN caused a 3 fold increase in transformation compared to activated ALK^{F1174L} alone. Results consistent with this finding were seen when ALK^{R1275Q} was expressed with MYCN. It was consistently noted that ALK^{F1175L} has a greater transforming potential than ALK^{R1275Q} [60]. Overall it appears that ALK drives the initiation of MYCN transcription. Concomitant expression of a constitutively active mutant ALK variant causes increased transformation and MYCN protein levels compared with expression of ALK^{F1174L}, ALK^{R1275Q} or MYCN alone. Trials of ALK inhibitors alone in neuroblastoma may not succeed as dysregulation of MYC is the main 'oncogenic driver' in the disease and initiation of MYCN transcription can occur by ways other than by the mutation or amplification of ALK.

5. Recent therapeutic advances in neuroblastoma and the promise of targeted therapies changing the treatment paradigm

The treatment of neuroblastoma varies according to risk group stratification and prognosis. Therefore prognosis needs to be considered first prior to contextualizing recent therapeutic advances.

5.1. Prognosis

Phenotypic and prognostic variation occurs in neuroblastoma as some clinical phenotypes spontaneously regress while other patients have rapidly progressive high risk disease in which despite intensive myeloablative chemotherapy relapses are common and almost invariably fatal [61,62]. Neuroblastoma prognosis can be subdivided into low risk, intermediate risk, high risk, and stage 4S disease [63]. The U.S. National Cancer Institute also has listed different subdivisions of neuroblastoma. Firstly neuroblastomas can be subdivided into three biologically discrete types of tumor. These categories can be used to sub-stratify patient prognosis but do not have treatment implications [64,65].

Type 1: Hyperdiploid, expression of TrkA neurotropin receptor. Tends to spontaneously regress.

Type 2: Expression of TrkB neurotropin receptor and its ligand. Additional copy of chromosome 17q, loss of heterozygosity 14q or 11q. Genome unstable.

Type 3: Gain chromosome 17q, loss of chromosome 1p, MYCN amplification.

There also is a risk assignment system in North America that has been used clinically by the Children's Oncology Group in studies such as COG-9641 and COG-A3961 [66, 67]. It has categories of low, intermediate and high-risk based on INSS stage, age, and tumor biology. Tumor biology characteristics considered are International Neuroblastoma Pathologic Classification (INPC), MYCN status and tumor DNA index. The INPC system involves the evaluation of pre-treatment tissue for the amount of stromal development, the mitosis-karyorrhexis index and the degree of neuroblastic maturation [68,69,70,71]. Stage 4S disease though included in these studiers is a particular case.

5.1.1. Treatment advances in high risk neuroblastoma in the ' ALK Era'

In 2009 long term outcomes of 379 patients with high risk neuroblastoma (CCG-3891) all of whom received the same induction treatment (5 cycles' cisplatin, doxorubicin, etoposide and cyclophosphamide plus surgery and received radiotherapy for residual local and metastatic disease) was reported [72]. Subsequent to induction patients were randomly assigned to consolidation with myeloablative chemotherapy, total body irradiation, and autologous purged bone marrow transplantation versus 3 cycles of intensive chemotherapy (cisplatin, etoposide, doxorubicin and ifosfamide). Of the participants that completed consolidation without disease progression, they were randomly assigned to no further therapy or 6 cycles of 13-cis retinoic acid (160mg/m^2/d in 2 divided doses for 14 days every 28 days). Myeloablative therapy and autologous hematopoietic rescue had a significantly better 5 year event free (~30% versus ~19%) and overall survival compared with non-myeloablative chemotherapy. 13 cis-retinoic acid after consolidation independently lead to significantly improved overall survival. 5 year overall survival from time of second random assignment for patients who underwent both sequential randomisations is documented in table 1.

Treatment randomly assigned to	5-year overall survival
ABMT / 13-cis retinoic acid	59%+/-8%
ABMY / no 13-cis retinoic acid	41%+/-7%
Continuing chemotherapy / 13-cis retinoic acid	38%+/-7%
Chemotherapy / no 13-cis retinoic acid	36%+/-7%

Table 1. please add caption

In 2010 a new treatment advance was reported in high risk neuroblastoma involving ch14.18 a chimeric human-murine anti-GD2 monoclonal antibody that targets GD2 a disialoganglio-side tumour associated antigen [73]. Patients that had a response to induction therapy and stem-cell transplantation were treated with immunotherapy (six cycles of isotretinoin and five concomitant cycles of ch14.18 in combination with alternating GM-CSF and interleukin-2). This regimen was found to be better than standard treatment (six cycles of isotretinoin) with a 2 year event free survival rate of 66% compared to 46% respectively, P=0.02.

High risk disease has a generic treatment paradigm of intensive chemotherapy to induce remission followed by surgery, radiotherapy and myeloablative chemotherapy. A presentation at the 2011 ASCO Annual meeting changed the treatment standard for high risk disease. The HR-NLB1 trial was a comparator trial between two high dose myeloablative chemotherapeutic regimens in high risk neuroblastoma. 563 children with stage IV disease (high risk distant metastatic disease or local disease; median age 3 years) received busulphan and myelphalan (281 patients) or a 3 drug chemotherapeutic combination of carboplatin, etoposide and melphalan (CEM; 282 patients). The 3 year event free survival was 49% versus 33% respectively. The 3 year overall survival was 60% versus 48% again favouring busulphan-melphalan over CEM. Busulphan-melphalan also had a lower rate of relapse 47% versus 60% [74].

5.1.2. Intermediate risk neuroblastoma advances in the 'ALK Era'

A phase 3 non randomized trial of newly diagnosed intermediate risk neuroblastoma without MYCN amplification was performed on 479 patients (323 patients had favourable biology tumours; 141 patients had tumours with unfavourable biology) [75]. Patients with favourable histopathology and hyperdiploidly received 4 cycles of chemotherapy (carboplatin, etoposide, cyclophosphamide and doxorubicin, administered at 3-week intervals) and patients with unfavourable features or an incomplete response received 8 cycles. The 3 year overall survival rate was ~ 96% with an overall survival rate of 98% for patients with favourable biology tumour and 93% for patients with unfavourable biology neuroblastomas. Using this biologic based risk assignment high rates of survival were preserved in intermediate risk disease with reduced doses and duration of chemotherapy compared to historic controls (e.g. Children's Oncology Group trial CCG-3881; overall survival INSS stage 4s, 92%; stage 4, 93%; stage 3, 100%)[76,77,78]. Recent years have seen advancements in high risk neuroblastoma involving myleoablative conditioning regimens, 13-cis retinoic acid and immunotherapeutic. However in intermediate risk disease the evolution of treatment involves preservation of treatment efficacy using a biologically defined stratification approach with a reduction in the patient exposure to chemotherapy.

5.1.3. What of ALK and MYC and targeted treatments?

MYC gene transcription can be diminished by targeting BET bromodomainds using small molecular inhibitors of the BET family of chromatin adaptors [79]. Inhibition of BET bromo-domain-promoter interactions with reduced MYC mRNA transcription and translation of MYC protein caused G1 cycle arrest with apoptosis in a diverse number of lymphoma and leukaemia cells. There was dysregulation of the MYC transcriptome including reactivation of the tumour suppressor p21. Treating xenograft models of Burkitt's lymphoma or acute myeloid leukaemia with a BET inhibitor demonstrated significant anti-tumour activity. Activation of the c-MYC gene is the *sine qua non* of Burkitt's lymphoma with the c-MYC locus at Chr. 8q24 involved in t (8;14)(q24;q32) epidemic Burkitt's lymphoma and other abnormalities involving the MYC gene in sporadic cases including a different t(8;14) translocation and point mutation of exon 2 of c-MYC. In neuroblastoma cell lines with MYCN amplification high dose transient treatment with (+)-JQ1 (a small molecule enantiomer BET bromodomaine inhibitor) caused transcriptional repression of MYCN.

Zhu and colleagues in the zebrafish model of neuroblastoma show that ALK F1174L attenuates MYCN induced apoptosis [59]. Given the previous experience with targeted therapeutics in other disease types and the emergence of drug resistance it has been contended that responses to crizotinib are unlikely to be durable [57]. As ALK and MYCN have collaborative roles with MYCN being the primary oncogenic driver it may be the case that some of the initial optimism pertaining to Crizotinib in neuroblastoma may not be fulfilled and that dual targeting of ALK and MYCN once technically feasible may revolutionise the outcome for many patients with neuroblastoma. In a fascinating caveat it is notable that in MYCN single-copy cases of neuroblastoma, increased MYCN mRNA and protein levels are paradoxically associated with a more favourable clinical phenotype. Gene expression profiling of 251 primary neuroblastomas identified a core set of MYCN/c-MYC target genes with a successive gradual increase in that target gene signature in localized non-amplified cases to stage 4s-non amplified followed by stage 4-non-amplified and finally MYCN amplified cases. High expression of the MYCN/c-MYC gene signature identified patients with poor overall survival independent of some of the usual clinico-pathologic variables such as age at diagnosis (> or equal 1.5 years; stage 4 versus stages 1,2,3, and 4s and amplified MYCN) [80]. It is apparent that MYCN's role in the quite heterogenous disease neuroblastoma is complex and the development of targeted therapeutics in neuroblastoma needs to appreciate these complexities. Of course treatments that target MYCN remain therapeutic lacunae to be filled. A final ancillary comment on ALK and MYC. German investigators have designed and performed experiments using JoMa1 which is a multipotent neural crest progenitor cell line that is kept in an undifferentiated but viable state by a tamoxifen activated c-Myc transgene (c-MycER^T) [81]. Expression of ALKF1174L in primary neuroblastomas caused in vitro growth of these cells independent of c-MycER^T activity and the in vivo growth of neuroblastoma like tumours. Tumorigenicity was further enhanced by serial transplantation and remained susceptible to NBT-272 a MYC inhibitor. Therefore it appears that targeting ALK alone may result in regression of neuroblastoma with the potential to further augment tumour regression by inhibition of MYC. Maybe new hope for children with neuroblastoma does not fully rely on neighbourly gene relations!

6. Conclusion

The improvement in outcome in neuroblastoma treatment in recent decades is a tremendous success however outcomes for high risk disease have changed little. The importance of the ALK gene in this disease and an established ALK inhibitor already being used in other types of cancer offers new hope for improving outcomes. Therapeutic targeting of Myc is a long aspired for hope in the wider field of oncology which may be realised. Chromosomal proximity of genes such as topoisomerase II and Her-2 in breast cancer has been a topical subject but aside from the concept of co-amplification of genes as in the breast cancer 'topo II-Her2' paradigm ALK and Myc interact in many nuanced and therapeutically exploitable ways with the prospect of many advances still to come.

Author details

Fergal C. Kelleher

Peter MacCallum Cancer Centre, Melbourne, Victoria, Australia

References

[1] Maris JM, Hogarty MD, Bagatell R, Cohn SL. Neuroblastoma. Lancet. 2007 Jun 23;369(9579):2106-20.

[2] Brodeur GM. Neuroblastoma: biological insights into a clinical enigma.Nat Rev Cancer. 2003 Mar;3(3):203-16.

[3] Tonini GP, Longo L, Coco S, Perri P. Familial neuroblastoma: a complex heritable disease. Cancer Lett. 2003 Jul 18;197(1-2):41-5.

[4] Trochet D, Bourdeaut F, Janoueix-Lerosey I, Deville A, de Pontual L, Schleiermacher G, Coze C, Philip N, Frébourg T, Munnich A, Lyonnet S, Delattre O, Amiel J. Germline mutations of the paired-like homeobox 2B (PHOX2B) gene in neuroblastoma. Am J Hum Genet. 2004 Apr;74(4):761-4.

[5] Vandesompele J, Baudis M, De Preter K, Van Roy N, Ambros P, Bown N, Brinkschmidt C, Christiansen H, Combaret V, Lastowska M, Nicholson J, O'Meara A, Plantaz D, Stallings R, Brichard B, Van den Broecke C, De Bie S, De Paepe A, Laureys G, Speleman F. Unequivocal delineation of clinicogenetic subgroups and development of a new model for improved outcome prediction in neuroblastoma. J Clin Oncol. 2005 Apr 1;23(10):2280-99.

[6] Michels E, Vandesompele J, De Preter K, Hoebeeck J, Vermeulen J, Schramm A, Molenaar JJ, Menten B, Marques B, Stallings RL, Combaret V, Devalck C, De Paepe A, Versteeg R, Eggert A, Laureys G, Van Roy N, Speleman F. ArrayCGH-based classification of neuroblastoma into genomic subgroups. Genes Chromosomes Cancer. 2007 Dec;46(12):1098-108.

[7] Janoueix-Lerosey I, Schleiermacher G, Michels E, Mosseri V, Ribeiro A, Lequin D, Vermeulen J, Couturier J, Peuchmaur M, Valent A, Plantaz D, Rubie H, Valteau-Couanet D, Thomas C, Combaret V, Rousseau R, Eggert A, Michon J, Speleman F, Delattre O. Overall genomic pattern is a predictor of outcome in neuroblastoma. J Clin Oncol. 2009 Mar 1;27(7):1026-33. Epub 2009 Jan 26.

[8] Brodeur GM. Molecular basis for heterogeneity in human neuroblastomas. Eur J Cancer. 1995;31A(4):505-10.

[9] Molenaar JJ, Koster J, Zwijnenburg DA, van Sluis P, Valentijn LJ, van der Ploeg I, Hamdi M, van Nes J, Westerman BA, van Arkel J, Ebus ME, Haneveld F, Lakeman A,

Schild L, Molenaar P, Stroeken P, van Noesel MM, Ora I, Santo EE, Caron HN, Westerhout EM, Versteeg R. Sequencing of neuroblastoma identifies chromothripsis and defects in neuritogenesis genes. Nature. 2012 Feb 22;483(7391):589-93.

[10]   Azarova AM, Gautam G, George RE. Emerging importance of ALK in neuroblastoma. Semin Cancer Biol. 2011 Oct;21(4):267-75. Epub 2011 Sep 16.

[11]   Janoueix-Lerosey I, Lequin D, Brugières L, Ribeiro A, de Pontual L, Combaret V, Raynal V, Puisieux A, Schleiermacher G, Pierron G, Valteau-Couanet D, Frebourg T, Michon J, Lyonnet S, Amiel J, Delattre O. Somatic and germline activating mutations of the ALK kinase receptor in neuroblastoma. Nature. 2008 Oct 16;455(7215):967-70.

[12]   Mourali J, Bénard A, Lourenço FC, Monnet C, Greenland C, Moog-Lutz C, Racaud-Sultan C, Gonzalez-Dunia D, Vigny M, Mehlen P, Delsol G, Allouche M. Anaplastic lymphoma kinase is a dependence receptor whose proapoptotic functions are activated by caspase cleavage. Mol Cell Biol. 2006 Aug;26(16):6209-22.

[13]   Iwahara T, Fujimoto J, Wen D, Cupples R, Bucay N, Arakawa T, Mori S, Ratzkin B, Yamamoto T. Molecular characterization of ALK, a receptor tyrosine kinase expressed specifically in the nervous system. Oncogene. 1997 Jan 30;14(4):439-49.

[14]   Mosse YP, Balis FM, Lim MS, Laliberte J, Voss SD, Fox E, Bagatell R, Weigel B, Adamson PC, Ingle AM, Ahern CH, Blaney S; The Children's Hospital of Philadelphia, Philadelphia, PA; C S Mott Children's Hospital, Ann Arbor, MI; Children's Hospital of Boston, Boston, MA; Children's Hospital of Philadelphia, Philadelphia, PA; University of Minnesota, Minneapolis, MN; Children's Oncology Group, Arcadia, CA; Baylor College of Medicine, Houston, TX; Texas Children's Cancer Center, Houston, TX. Efficacy of crizotinib in children with relapsed/refractory ALK-driven tumors including anaplastic large cell lymphoma and neuroblastoma: A Children's Oncology Group phase I consortium study. Abstract No: 9500; J Clin Oncol 30, 2012 (suppl; abstr 9500).

[15]   Kelleher FC, McDermott R. The emerging pathogenic and therapeutic importance of the anaplastic lymphoma kinase gene. Eur J Cancer. 2010 Sep;46(13):2357-68. Epub 2010 May 5.

[16]   Morris SW, Kirstein MN, Valentine MB, Dittmer KG, Shapiro DN, Saltman DL, Look AT. Fusion of a kinase gene, ALK, to a nucleolar protein gene, NPM, in non-Hodgkin's lymphoma. Science. 1994 Mar 4;263(5151):1281-4.

[17]   Soda M, Choi YL, Enomoto M, Takada S, Yamashita Y, Ishikawa S, Fujiwara S, Watanabe H, Kurashina K, Hatanaka H, Bando M, Ohno S, Ishikawa Y, Aburatani H, Niki T, Sohara Y, Sugiyama Y, Mano H. Identification of the transforming EML4-ALK fusion gene in non-small-cell lung cancer. Nature. 2007 Aug 2;448(7153):561-6.

[18]   Griffin CA, Hawkins AL, Dvorak C, Henkle C, Ellingham T, Perlman EJ. Recurrent involvement of 2p23 in inflammatory myofibroblastic tumors. Cancer Res. 1999 Jun 15;59(12):2776-80.

[19] van Gaal JC, Flucke UE, Roeffen MH, de Bont ES, Sleijfer S, Mavinkurve-Groothuis AM, Suurmeijer AJ, van der Graaf WT, Versleijen-Jonkers YM. Anaplastic lymphoma kinase aberrations in rhabdomyosarcoma: clinical and prognostic implications. J Clin Oncol. 2012 Jan 20;30(3):308-15.

[20] Donahue SP. Clinical practice. Pediatric strabismus. N Engl J Med. 2007 Mar 8;356(10):1040-7.

[21] Keech RV, Kutschke PJ. Upper age limit for the development of amblyopia. J Pediatr Ophthalmol Strabismus. 1995 Mar-Apr;32(2):89-93.

[22] Kwak EL, Bang YJ, Camidge DR, Shaw AT, Solomon B, Maki RG, Ou SH, Dezube BJ, Jänne PA, Costa DB, Varella-Garcia M, Kim WH, Lynch TJ, Fidias P, Stubbs H, Engelman JA, Sequist LV, Tan W, Gandhi L, Mino-Kenudson M, Wei GC, Shreeve SM, Ratain MJ, Settleman J, Christensen JG, Haber DA, Wilner K, Salgia R, Shapiro GI, Clark JW, Iafrate AJ. Anaplastic lymphoma kinase inhibition in non-small-cell lung cancer. N Engl J Med. 2010 Oct 28;363(18):1693-703.

[23] De Preter K, Vandesompele J, Heimann P, Yigit N, Beckman S, Schramm A, Eggert A, Stallings RL, Benoit Y, Renard M, De Paepe A, Laureys G, Påhlman S, Speleman F. Human fetal neuroblast and neuroblastoma transcriptome analysis confirms neuroblast origin and highlights neuroblastoma candidate genes. Genome Biol. 2006;7(9):R84.

[24] Beckwith JB, Perrin EV. In situ neuroblastomas; A contribution to the natural history of neural crest tumors. Am J Pathol. 1963 Dec;43:1089-104.

[25] Knudson AG Jr, Strong LC. Mutation and cancer: neuroblastoma and pheochromocytoma. Am J Hum Genet. 1972 Sep; 24(5):514-32.

[26] Kushner BH, Gilbert F, Helson L. Familial neuroblastoma. Case reports, literature review, and etiologic considerations. Cancer. 1986 May 1;57(9):1887-93.

[27] Maris JM, Kyemba SM, Rebbeck TR, White PS, Sulman EP, Jensen SJ, Allen C, Biegel JA, Brodeur GM. Molecular genetic analysis of familial neuroblastoma. Eur J Cancer. 1997 Oct;33(12):1923-8.

[28] Friedman DL, Kadan-Lottick NS, Whitton J, Mertens AC, Yasui Y, Liu Y, Meadows AT, Robison LL, Strong LC. Increased risk of cancer among siblings of long-term childhood cancer survivors: a report from the childhood cancer survivor study. Cancer Epidemiol Biomarkers Prev. 2005 Aug;14(8):1922-7.

[29] Amiel J, Laudier B, Attié-Bitach T, Trang H, de Pontual L, Gener B, Trochet D, Etchevers H, Ray P, Simonneau M, Vekemans M, Munnich A, Gaultier C, Lyonnet S. Polyalanine expansion and frameshift mutations of the paired-like homeobox gene PHOX2B in congenital central hypoventilation syndrome. Nat Genet. 2003 Apr; 33(4):459-61. Epub 2003 Mar 17.

[30] Mossé YP, Laudenslager M, Khazi D, Carlisle AJ, Winter CL, Rappaport E, Maris JM.
      Germline PHOX2B mutation in hereditary neuroblastoma. Am J Hum Genet. 2004
      Oct;75(4):727-30.

[31] Mossé YP, Laudenslager M, Longo L, Cole KA, Wood A, Attiyeh EF, Laquaglia MJ,
      Sennett R, Lynch JE, Perri P, Laureys G, Speleman F, Kim C, Hou C, Hakonarson H,
      Torkamani A, Schork NJ, Brodeur GM, Tonini GP, Rappaport E, Devoto M, Maris
      JM. Identification of ALK as a major familial neuroblastoma predisposition gene. Na-
      ture. 2008 Oct 16;455(7215):930-5. Epub 2008 Aug 24.

[32] George RE, Sanda T, Hanna M, Fröhling S, Luther W 2nd, Zhang J, Ahn Y, Zhou W,
      London WB, McGrady P, Xue L, Zozulya S, Gregor VE, Webb TR, Gray NS, Gilliland
      DG, Diller L, Greulich H, Morris SW, Meyerson M, Look AT. Activating mutations in
      ALK provide a therapeutic target in neuroblastoma. Nature. 2008 Oct 16;455(7215):
      975-8.

[33] Chen Y, Takita J, Choi YL, Kato M, Ohira M, Sanada M, Wang L, Soda M, Kikuchi A,
      Igarashi T, Nakagawara A, Hayashi Y, Mano H, Ogawa S. Oncogenic mutations of
      ALK kinase in neuroblastoma. Nature. 2008 Oct 16;455(7215):971-4.

[34] Greulich H, Chen TH, Feng W, Jänne PA, Alvarez JV, Zappaterra M, Bulmer SE,
      Frank DA, Hahn WC, Sellers WR, Meyerson M. Oncogenic transformation by inhibi-
      tor-sensitive and -resistant EGFR mutants. PLoS Med. 2005 Nov;2(11):e313. Epub
      2005 Oct 4.

[35] Lynch TJ, Bell DW, Sordella R, Gurubhagavatula S, Okimoto RA, Brannigan BW,
      Harris PL, Haserlat SM, Supko JG, Haluska FG, Louis DN, Christiani DC, Settleman
      J, Haber DA. Activating mutations in the epidermal growth factor receptor underly-
      ing responsiveness of non-small-cell lung cancer to gefitinib. N Engl J Med. 2004 May
      20;350(21):2129-39. Epub 2004 Apr 29.

[36] Paez JG, Jänne PA, Lee JC, Tracy S, Greulich H, Gabriel S, Herman P, Kaye FJ, Linde-
      man N, Boggon TJ, Naoki K, Sasaki H, Fujii Y, Eck MJ, Sellers WR, Johnson BE,
      Meyerson M. EGFR mutations in lung cancer: correlation with clinical response to
      gefitinib therapy. Science. 2004 Jun 4;304(5676):1497-500. Epub 2004 Apr 29.

[37] Vogelstein B, Kinzler KW. Cancer genes and the pathways they control. Nat Med.
      2004 Aug;10(8):789-99.

[38] Fix A, Lucchesi C, Ribeiro A, Lequin D, Pierron G, Schleiermacher G, Delattre O, Ja-
      noueix-Lerosey I. Characterization of amplicons in neuroblastoma: high-resolution
      mapping using DNA microarrays, relationship with outcome, and identification of
      overexpressed genes. Genes Chromosomes Cancer. 2008 Oct;47(10):819-34.

[39] De Brouwer S, De Preter K, Kumps C, Zabrocki P, Porcu M, Westerhout EM, Lake-
      man A, Vandesompele J, Hoebeeck J, Van Maerken T, De Paepe A, Laureys G,
      Schulte JH, Schramm A, Van Den Broecke C, Vermeulen J, Van Roy N, Beiske K, Re-
      nard M, Noguera R, Delattre O, Janoueix-Lerosey I, Kogner P, Martinsson T, Naka-

gawara A, Ohira M, Caron H, Eggert A, Cools J, Versteeg R, Speleman F. Meta-analysis of neuroblastomas reveals a skewed ALK mutation spectrum in tumors with MYCN amplification. Clin Cancer Res. 2010 Sep 1;16(17):4353-62. Epub 2010 Aug 18.

[40] Bresler SC, Wood AC, Haglund EA, Courtright J, Belcastro LT, Plegaria JS, Cole K, Toporovskaya Y, Zhao H, Carpenter EL, Christensen JG, Maris JM, Lemmon MA, Mossé YP. Differential inhibitor sensitivity of anaplastic lymphoma kinase variants found in neuroblastoma. Sci Transl Med. 2011 Nov 9;3(108):108ra114.

[41] Oster SK, Ho CS, Soucie EL, Penn LZ. The myc oncogene: MarvelouslY Complex. Adv Cancer Res. 2002;84:81-154.

[42] Soucek L, Evan GI. The ups and downs of Myc biology. Curr Opin Genet Dev. 2010 Feb;20(1):91-5.

[43] Fernandez PC, Frank SR, Wang L, Schroeder M, Liu S, Greene J, Cocito A, Amati B. Genomic targets of the human c-Myc protein. Genes Dev. 2003 May 1;17(9):1115-29. Epub 2003 Apr 14.

[44] O'Connell BC, Cheung AF, Simkevich CP, Tam W, Ren X, Mateyak MK, Sedivy JM. A large scale genetic analysis of c-Myc-regulated gene expression patterns. J Biol Chem. 2003 Apr 4;278(14):12563-73. Epub 2003 Jan 14.

[45] Soucek L, Whitfield J, Martins CP, Finch AJ, Murphy DJ, Sodir NM, Karnezis AN, Swigart LB, Nasi S, Evan GI. Modelling Myc inhibition as a cancer therapy. Nature. 2008 Oct 2;455(7213):679-83.

[46] Soucek L, Helmer-Citterich M, Sacco A, Jucker R, Cesareni G, Nasi S. Design and properties of a Myc derivative that efficiently homodimerizes. Oncogene. 1998 Nov 12;17(19):2463-72.

[47] Soucek L, Jucker R, Panacchia L, Ricordy R, Tatò F, Nasi S. Omomyc, a potential Myc dominant negative, enhances Myc-induced apoptosis.Cancer Res. 2002 Jun 15;62(12): 3507-10.

[48] Weiss WA, Aldape K, Mohapatra G, Feuerstein BG, Bishop JM. Targeted expression of MYCN causes neuroblastoma in transgenic mice. EMBO J. 1997 Jun 2;16(11): 2985-95.

[49] Schwab M, Alitalo K, Klempnauer KH, Varmus HE, Bishop JM, Gilbert F, Brodeur G, Goldstein M, Trent J. Amplified DNA with limited homology to myc cellular onco-gene is shared by human neuroblastoma cell lines and a neuroblastoma tumour. Na-ture. 1983 Sep 15-21;305(5931):245-8.

[50] Maris JM, Weiss MJ, Mosse Y, Hii G, Guo C, White PS, Hogarty MD, Mirensky T, Brodeur GM, Rebbeck TR, Urbanek M, Shusterman S. Evidence for a hereditary neu-roblastoma predisposition locus at chromosome 16p12-13. Cancer Res. 2002 Nov 15;62(22):6651-8.

[51] Reiter JL, Brodeur GM. High-resolution mapping of a 130-kb core region of the MYCN amplicon in neuroblastomas. Genomics. 1996 Feb 15;32(1):97-103.

[52] Reiter JL, Brodeur GM. MYCN is the only highly expressed gene from the core amplified domain in human neuroblastomas. Genes Chromosomes Cancer. 1998 Oct; 23(2):134-40.

[53] Chanthery YH, Gustafson WC, Itsara M, Persson A, Hackett CS, Grimmer M, Charron E, Yakovenko S, Kim G, Matthay KK, Weiss WA. Paracrine signaling through MYCN enhances tumor-vascular interactions in neuroblastoma. Sci Transl Med. 2012 Jan 4;4(115):115ra3.

[54] Chesler L, Schlieve C, Goldenberg DD, Kenney A, Kim G, McMillan A, Matthay KK, Rowitch D, Weiss WA. Inhibition of phosphatidylinositol 3-kinase destabilizes Mycn protein and blocks malignant progression in neuroblastoma. Cancer Res. 2006 Aug 15;66(16):8139-46.

[55] Hogarty MD, Maris JM. PI3King on MYCN to improve neuroblastoma therapeutics. Cancer Cell. 2012 Feb 14;21(2):145-7.

[56] Brodeur GM, Seeger RC, Schwab M, Varmus HE, Bishop JM. Amplification of N-myc in untreated human neuroblastomas correlates with advanced disease stage. Science. 1984 Jun 8;224(4653):1121-4.

[57] Liu Z, Thiele CJ. ALK and MYCN: when two oncogenes are better than one. Cancer Cell. 2012 Mar 20;21(3):325-6.

[58] Schönherr C, Ruuth K, Kamaraj S, Wang CL, Yang HL, Combaret V, Djos A, Martinsson T, Christensen JG, Palmer RH, Hallberg B. Anaplastic Lymphoma Kinase (ALK) regulates initiation of transcription of MYCN in neuroblastoma cells.Oncogene. 2012 Jan 30.

[59] Zhu S, Lee JS, Guo F, Shin J, Perez-Atayde AR, Kutok JL, Rodig SJ, Neuberg DS, Helman D, Feng H, Stewart RA, Wang W, George RE, Kanki JP, Look AT. Activated ALK collaborates with MYCN in neuroblastoma pathogenesis. Cancer Cell. 2012 Mar 20;21(3):362-73.

[60] Schönherr C, Ruuth K, Yamazaki Y, Eriksson T, Christensen J, Palmer RH, Hallberg B. Activating ALK mutations found in neuroblastoma are inhibited by Crizotinib and NVP-TAE684. Biochem J. 2011 Dec 15;440(3):405-13.

[61] Matthay KK, Villablanca JG, Seeger RC, Stram DO, Harris RE, Ramsay NK, Swift P, Shimada H, Black CT, Brodeur GM, Gerbing RB, Reynolds CP. Treatment of high-risk neuroblastoma with intensive chemotherapy, radiotherapy, autologous bone marrow transplantation, and 13-cis-retinoic acid. Children's Cancer Group. N Engl J Med. 1999 Oct 14;341(16):1165-73.

[62] George RE, Li S, Medeiros-Nancarrow C, Neuberg D, Marcus K, Shamberger RC, Pulsipher M, Grupp SA, Diller L. High-risk neuroblastoma treated with tandem au-

tologous peripheral-blood stem cell-supported transplantation: long-term survival update. J Clin Oncol. 2006 Jun 20;24(18):2891-6.

[63] Maris JM. Recent advances in neuroblastoma. N Engl J Med. 2010 Jun 10; 362(23): 2202-11.

[64] Maris JM, Matthay KK. Molecular biology of neuroblastoma. J Clin Oncol. 1999 Jul; 17(7):2264-79.

[65] Lastowska M, Cullinane C, Variend S, Cotterill S, Bown N, O'Neill S, Mazzocco K, Roberts P, Nicholson J, Ellershaw C, Pearson AD, Jackson MS; United Kingdom Children Cancer Study Group and the United Kingdom Cancer Cytogenetics Group. Comprehensive genetic and histopathologic study reveals three types of neuroblastoma tumors. J Clin Oncol. 2001 Jun 15;19(12):3080-90.

[66] Kushner BH, Cheung NK.Treatment reduction for neuroblastoma. Pediatr Blood Cancer. 2004 Nov;43(6):619-21

[67] Kushner BH, Kramer K, LaQuaglia MP, Modak S, Cheung NK. Liver involvement in neuroblastoma: the Memorial Sloan-Kettering Experience supports treatment reduction in young patients. Pediatr Blood Cancer. 2006 Mar;46(3):278-84.

[68] Shimada H, Ambros IM, Dehner LP, Hata J, Joshi VV, Roald B, Stram DO, Gerbing RB, Lukens JN, Matthay KK, Castleberry RP. The International Neuroblastoma Pathology Classification (the Shimada system). Cancer. 1999 Jul 15;86(2):364-72.

[69] Shimada H, Umehara S, Monobe Y, Hachitanda Y, Nakagawa A, Goto S, Gerbing RB, Stram DO, Lukens JN, Matthay KK. International neuroblastoma pathology classification for prognostic evaluation of patients with peripheral neuroblastic tumors: a report from the Children's Cancer Group. Cancer. 2001 Nov 1;92(9):2451-61.

[70] Goto S, Umehara S, Gerbing RB, Stram DO, Brodeur GM, Seeger RC, Lukens JN, Matthay KK, Shimada H. Histopathology (International Neuroblastoma Pathology Classification) and MYCN status in patients with peripheral neuroblastic tumors: a report from the Children's Cancer Group. Cancer. 2001 Nov 15;92(10):2699-708.

[71] Peuchmaur M, d'Amore ES, Joshi VV, Hata J, Roald B, Dehner LP, Gerbing RB, Stram DO, Lukens JN, Matthay KK, Shimada H. Revision of the International Neuroblastoma Pathology Classification: confirmation of favorable and unfavorable prognostic subsets in ganglioneuroblastoma, nodular. Cancer. 2003 Nov 15;98(10):2274-81.

[72] Matthay KK, Reynolds CP, Seeger RC, Shimada H, Adkins ES, Haas-Kogan D, Gerbing RB, London WB, Villablanca JG. Long-term results for children with high-risk neuroblastoma treated on a randomized trial of myeloablative therapy followed by 13-cis-retinoic acid: a children's oncology group study. J Clin Oncol. 2009 Mar 1;27(7): 1007-13. Epub 2009 Jan 26.

[73] Yu AL, Gilman AL, Ozkaynak MF, London WB, Kreissman SG, Chen HX, Smith M, Anderson B, Villablanca JG, Matthay KK, Shimada H, Grupp SA, Seeger R, Reynolds

CP, Buxton A, Reisfeld RA, Gillies SD, Cohn SL, Maris JM, Sondel PM; Children's Oncology Group. Anti-GD2 antibody with GM-CSF, interleukin-2, and isotretinoin for neuroblastoma. N Engl J Med. 2010 Sep 30;363(14):1324-34.

[74] Ladenstein RL, et al.: Busulphan-melphalan as a myeloablative therapy (MAT) for high-risk neuroblastoma: Results from the HR-NBL1/SIOPEN trial. Presented at the 47th Annual Meeting of the American Society of Clinical Oncology: June 2011; Chicago, IL.

[75] Baker DL, Schmidt ML, Cohn SL, Maris JM, London WB, Buxton A, Stram D, Castleberry RP, Shimada H, Sandler A, Shamberger RC, Look AT, Reynolds CP, Seeger RC, Matthay KK; Children's Oncology Group. Outcome after reduced chemotherapy for intermediate-risk neuroblastoma. N Engl J Med. 2010 Sep 30;363(14):1313-23.

[76] Nickerson HJ, Matthay KK, Seeger RC, Brodeur GM, Shimada H, Perez C, Atkinson JB, Selch M, Gerbing RB, Stram DO, Lukens J. Favorable biology and outcome of stage IV-S neuroblastoma with supportive care or minimal therapy: a Children's Cancer Group study. J Clin Oncol. 2000 Feb;18(3):477-86.

[77] Schmidt ML, Lukens JN, Seeger RC, Brodeur GM, Shimada H, Gerbing RB, Stram DO, Perez C, Haase GM, Matthay KK. Biologic factors determine prognosis in infants with stage IV neuroblastoma: A prospective Children's Cancer Group study. J Clin Oncol. 2000 Mar;18(6):1260-8.

[78] Matthay KK, Perez C, Seeger RC, Brodeur GM, Shimada H, Atkinson JB, Black CT, Gerbing R, Haase GM, Stram DO, Swift P, Lukens JN. Successful treatment of stage III neuroblastoma based on prospective biologic staging: a Children's Cancer Group study. J Clin Oncol. 1998 Apr;16(4):1256-64.

[79] Mertz JA, Conery AR, Bryant BM, Sandy P, Balasubramanian S, Mele DA, Bergeron L, Sims RJ 3rd. Targeting MYC dependence in cancer by inhibiting BET bromodomains. Proc Natl Acad Sci U S A. 2011 Oct 4;108(40):16669-74. Epub 2011 Sep 26.

[80] Westermann F, Muth D, Benner A, Bauer T, Henrich KO, Oberthuer A, Brors B, Beissbarth T, Vandesompele J, Pattyn F, Hero B, König R, Fischer M, Schwab M. Distinct transcriptional MYCN/c-MYC activities are associated with spontaneous regression or malignant progression in neuroblastomas. Genome Biol. 2008 Oct 13;9(10):R150.

[81] Schulte JH, Lindner S, Bohrer A, Maurer J, De Preter K, Lefever S, Heukamp L, Schulte S, Molenaar J, Versteeg R, Thor T, Künkele A, Vandesompele J, Speleman F, Schorle H, Eggert A, Schramm A. MYCN and ALKF1174L are sufficient to drive neuroblastoma development from neural crest progenitor cells. Oncogene. 2012 Apr 9.

Chapter 5

Connexin36 is a Negative Regulator of Differentiation in Human Neuroblastoma

Mandeep Sidhu and Daniel J. Belliveau

Additional information is available at the end of the chapter

1. Introduction

Neuroblastoma is the most common extracranial solid tumor to present in children [1]. Neuroblastoma arises from bipotential sympathoadrenal progenitor cells of the trunk neural crest. During normal development, sympathoadrenal progenitors differentiate to form the sympathetic ganglia and adrenal medulla, however in neuroblastoma they form tumors at these sites instead [1, 2].

Retinoic acid is now employed in multi-modal therapy to treat high-risk neuroblastoma and eradicate minimal residual disease [3]. All-trans retinoic acid (ATRA) diminishes MYCN oncogene expression, arrests proliferation, and induces differentiation of neuroblastoma cells [4, 5].

Gap junctional intercellular communication (GJIC) and connexins (Cx) have been implicated in carcinogenesis and differentiation. GJIC is often perturbed and connexins are typically downregulated or aberrantly localized in cancer cells, including IMR-32 neuroblastoma cells [6, 7]. Many connexins have been identified as tumor suppressors when overexpressed in cancer cells [6]. For example, overexpression of Cx43 resulted in growth suppression of communication deficient Neuro-2A murine neuroblastoma cells [8]. In addition, connexins have been shown to enhance the differentiation of cancer cell lines [8, 9]. For example, overexpression of Cx32 and Cx43 resulted in enhanced nerve growth factor induced neurite outgrowth in PC12 cells [10].

Gap junctions are membrane channels that allow intercellular communication between adjacent cells [11]. GJIC involves the passage of ions, second messengers, and metabolites less than 1kDa in size between cells [11, 12]. Gap junctions and their constituent proteins, connexins, regulate cellular processes such as homeostasis, growth, and differentiation [6, 13]. Gap junctions are formed from the docking of two connexons or hemichannels contributed by adjacent cells. Each connexon in turn is comprised of a hexamer of connexin subunits [11]. There are 21 known members of the human connexin family, most with unique spatial and temporal expression patterns [14].

Cx36 is a recently identified connexin that is expressed in neurons and pancreatic beta cells [15-17]. Cx36 is highly expressed in the developing nervous system, however its expression is decreased or lost by the second post-natal week in many structures [18, 19]. In adults, Cx36 is the predominant connexin involved in electrical synapses [20].

The differentiating agent, retinoic acid, increases GJIC and Cx43 expression in multiple cell types [21-23]. Interestingly, the mouse *Cx36* gene contains a retinoid X receptor binding motif indicating that *Cx36* may be susceptible to transcriptional regulation by retinoic acid [24].

In this study, we explored the effect of the neuronal connexin, Cx36, on the differentiation of SH-SY5Y human neuroblastoma cells. SH-SY5Y cells are often utilized as a model system for studies of neural disease, as well as in studies of differentiation [25, 26]. The effect of ATRA on *Cx36* expression was first examined in SH-SY5Y cells. Furthermore, the effects of Cx36 on proliferation and features of differentiation including neuritogenesis and molecular differentiation marker expression were investigated by manipulating Cx36 expression.

2. Experimental procedures

2.1. Cell culture

The neuroblastoma cell line, SH-SY5Y was obtained from American Type Culture Collection. SH-SY5Y is a proliferative cell line with a documented doubling time of 48 hours. SH-SY5Y cells were maintained in Dulbecco's Modified Eagle Medium (DMEM, Invitrogen) with high glucose, and supplemented with 10% fetal bovine serum (FBS, HyClone), 100 U/ml penicillin and streptomycin (Invitrogen) and 2 mM L-glutamine (Invitrogen). For cell passage, cells were washed with Hank's Buffered Salt Solution (HBSS, Sigma), treated with 0.25% trypsin and incubated for 5 minutes at 37°C to disperse the cells. Five ml of growth medium was added to the cells, and they were resuspended in a 10 cm dish in fresh growth medium after pipetting several times.

2.2. Generation of stable cell lines

2.2.1. Overexpression

Cells were plated at a density of 1×10^6 cells per well in a 6-well dish. The following day, 4 µg of Cx36myc-DDK (Origene) or EGFP pcDNA3.1 were diluted in OPTI-MEM (Invitrogen) and mixed with 2.5 µl of lipofectamine 2000 (Invitrogen) in OPTI-MEM. The DNA and lipofectamine were mixed and the resulting complexes added to the cells after 20 minutes, which were also in OPTI-MEM. The cells and complexes were incubated for 6 hours and then returned to normal growth medium. The following day, transfected cells were passaged onto 10 cm dishes.

Kill curves were performed on wild-type cells to determine optimal antibiotic concentrations. For stable cell lines, 800 μg/ml G418 was added to the cells, and all viable cells were passaged to a 10 cm dish following two weeks of selection, and G418 was reduced to 200 μg/ml. However, cells were treated with 800 μg/ml G418 monthly to ensure purity of the culture.

2.2.2. Knockdown

shRNA knockdown: Cells were plated at a density of $5x10^5$ cells per well in a 6-well dish. The following day, 1 μg of one of four distinct shRNAs targeting Cx36 or non-effective (scrambled) control plasmids co-expressing GFP (Origene) were diluted in OPTI-MEM and mixed with 1.5 μl of lipofectamine 2000 in OPTI-MEM. The cells were then maintained as per the overexpression protocol. For stable cell lines, 800 ng/ml puromycin was added to the cells, and all viable cells were passaged to a 10 cm dish following two weeks of selection, and puromycin was further increased to 1.5 μg/ml. In addition, cells were treated with 2.5 μg/ml puromycin monthly to maintain purity of the culture due to the occasional appearance of non-fluorescent cells.

2.3. Differentiation assay

SHSY-5Y cells were plated on rat-tail collagen coated 6-well or 60 mm plates, at a density of 10 000 cells/cm² in growth medium. The following day, cells were treated with 10 μM of all trans-retinoic acid (Sigma) for 4 days, with medium and treatment refreshed every 2 days. Cells were then washed with HBSS and treated with 20 ng/ml of brain derived neurotrophic factor (BDNF) in serum-free DMEM for 6 days, with medium and BDNF replaced every 2 days (modified from [26]). Medium for transfected cells contained the appropriate antibiotic. RNA and protein were extracted at Days 0, 2, 4 and 10 of differentiation, and connexin and differentiation marker expression were analyzed. Images were taken at each timepoint with a Leica inverted epifluorescent microscope. The images were analyzed with the NeuronJ plugin for ImageJ [27, 28]. For each image, neurites within the 0.16 mm² field of view were traced. Neurites were classified as cell projections longer than one cell body length. For analysis of average neurite length, the mean length of all neurites in the field of view was computed. In order to calculate maximum neurite length, the length of the longest neurite in the field of view was analyzed. Finally, for neurite density, the number of neurites was divided by the number of cell bodies in the field of view.

2.4. Real-time PCR

RNA was extracted and purified using the Qiagen RNeasy mini kit, and 0.5 μg of RNA was reverse transcribed using the qScript cDNA synthesis kit (Quanta Biosciences). Connexin primers were designed using Primer-Blast yielding the following sense and anti-sense sequences: Cx36, 5'-AAG GCA TCT CCC GCT TCT ACA - 3' and 5'- GCC AAC CAG GAA CCC AAT TT- 3'; Cx45, 5'-CTG GAG GCT CTG CAG CGG GA- 3' and 5'-TCT CCC GGG GAC CAT GAG GG- 3'; Cx43, 5'-GGT TAC ACT TGC AAA AGA GAT C- 3', and 5'-GAG CAG CCA TTG AAA TAA GC- 3'. Differentiation markers: Neuropeptide Y (NPY), 5'- TCC AGC CCA GAG ACA CTG ATT-3' and 5'-AGG GTC TTC AAG CCG AGT TCT-3'; Growth associated protein 43 (Gap43), 5'-ACG ACC AAA AGA TTG AAC AAG ATG-3' and 5'-TCC ACG GAA GCT AGC CTG AA-3' (Origene). Adhesion molecule: Neural cell adhesion molecule (NCAM), 5'- CAT CAC CTG GAG GAC TTC TAC C-3' and 5'- CAG TGT ACT GGA TGC TCT TCA GG-3' (Origene). Inhibitor of DNA Binding 2 (ID2), 5'-TTGTCAGCCTGCATCACCAGAG-3' and 5'-AGCCACACAGTGCTTTGCTGTC-3' (Origene). Nestin, 5'-TCAAGATGTCCCT-CAGCCTGGA-3' and 5'-AAGCTGAGGGAAGTCTTGGAGC-3' (Origene). Values were normalized to those of the PPIA reference gene: cyclophillin A (PPIA), 5'-AGA CAA GGT CCC AAA GAC-3' and 5'ACC ACC CTG ACA CAT AAA-3'. All primer pairs were tested using standard curves with 10-fold serial dilutions, and selected only if the effiencies were within the 95-110% range over a minimum of 3 points. Three technical repeats were included for each biological replicate. The qPCR was performed in the CFX96 Real-Time PCR Detection System (Bio-Rad) using Perfecta Sybr Green Fastmix (Quanta Biosciences), and the data analyzed with CFX Manager software (Bio-Rad).

2.5. Western blot analysis

Protein was extracted using 18 mM Tris, 123mM NaCl, 10% glycerol, 1% NP40, and protease inhibitor cocktail (Calbiochem). Cell lysates were kept on ice for 5 minutes with frequent agitation, sonicated for 10 seconds, and lysates were cleared in a cold centrifuge at 10,000 rpm for 10 minutes. The supernatant was removed and used for western blotting. Protein concentration was measured using the BCA Protein Assay (Thermo Scientific). Thirty µg of protein were electrophoresed on 10% polyacrylamide gels and transferred to a nitrocellulose membrane. The membrane was blocked for one hour in 3% BSA in PBS with 0.05% Tween-20 (PBST), followed by incubation with primary antibodies: rabbit polyclonal Cx43 (Sigma) 1:2000 overnight at 4°C; mouse monoclonal Gap43 (Invitrogen) 1:500 overnight at 4°C; mouse monoclonal N-cadherin (BD) 1:2500 2 hours at room temperature; mouse monoclonal GAPDH (Millipore) 1:5000 for 2 hours at room temperature. Membranes were washed with PBST and incubated with secondary antibodies for one hour: horseradish peroxidase conjugated goat anti-mouse at a 1:5000 dilution (Thermo Scientific). Membranes were then washed with PBST and developed using enhanced chemiluminscence (Thermo Scientific). Zymed, Diatheva, Santa Cruz, and Sigma Cx36 antibodies were tested on blots with both positive and negative controls for Cx36. However, none of these antibodies were able to detect Cx36. Therefore, Cx36 expression was measured at the gene expression level. Protein expression was quantified with Quantity One software (Bio-Rad) by densitometric analysis. Protein levels were normalized to GAPDH.

2.6. MTT proliferation assay

Cells were plated at 20, 000 cells per well in a 48-well plate. At 0, 2, 4, and 6 days, 20 µl of MTT (Invitrogen) solution was added to each well and incubated for 4 hours. 200 µl of SDS-HCl was then added to each well and incubated for 14 hours. The absorbance was measured at 570 nm on a µQuant Biomolecular spectrophotometer (Bio-Tek). Increased absorbance indicates higher cell numbers. Four technical repeats were included in each biological replicate.

2.7. Statistical analysis

Student's t-test was conducted for aggregate and neuritogenesis analysis between EGFP and Cx36 overexpressing cells. One-way analysis of variance (ANOVA) was conducted for the following experiments: gene expression analysis between wild-type cells, and neuritogenesis analysis between non-effective shRNA and Cx36 shRNAs. Tukey's multiple comparison post-hoc test was used to assess differences in means between groups.

Two-way ANOVA was conducted for the following experiments: All gene and protein expression analysis and proliferation assays between transfected cells (overexpression and knockdown). Bonferroni's post-hoc test was conducted to assess differences in means between groups. $p < 0.05$ was considered significant for all tests. All statistical analysis was performed with GraphPad Prism 4.0 software.

3. Results

3.1. Retinoic acid induces differentiation and upregulates Cx36 expression of SH-SY5Y neuroblastoma cells

SH-SY5Y human neuroblastoma cells were induced to differentiate with all-trans retinoic acid to determine whether neuronal connexins are regulated by retinoic acid. Neuritogenesis, and Gap43 and NPY expression were assessed in order to evaluate the differentiation status of cells. Neuritogenesis is the process of morphological differentiation of neuronal cells whereby the cytoskeleton reorganizes and forms neurites, which are extensions of the cell body that serve as precursors of axons and dendrites [29]. Gap43 is found at high concentrations in the growth cone during neuritogenesis [30] and consequently it is often used as marker of neuronal differentiation [25, 31]. NPY is a sympathetic peptide neurotransmitter and is also often used as a marker for differentiated neurons [31, 32].

SH-SY5Y cells were exposed to retinoic acid and BDNF treatment to induce cell differentiation. Neurite outgrowth was observed in treated cells beginning at day 2 (Figure 1A). Neuritogenesis continued through day 4, and within 10 days extensive neurite networking was observed (Figure 1A). Untreated cells began to cluster and form aggregates by day 2, and continued to form large aggregates by day 10 (Figure 1A). Thus, retinoic acid and BDNF treatment induces the morphological differentiation of SH-SY5Y cells.

In order to determine whether retinoic acid regulates the expression of neuronal connexins, the effect of the differentiation treatment on Cx36 and Cx45 transcript expression was examined. Gap43 transcript expression was also assessed to confirm differentiation at the molecular level. RNA was isolated from untreated and treated cells at each timepoint, and real-time PCR was used to quantify gene expression. Messenger RNA for the growth cone marker, Gap43, was upregulated at days 4 and 10 of treatment compared to untreated cells (Figure 1B). Cx36 mRNA was increased in treated cells at 2, 4, and 10 days compared to untreated cells (Figure 1C). Cx45 mRNA, however, did not increase in treated cells (Figure 1D). These results indicate that transcription of the gene encoding *Cx36* is upregulated by retinoic acid signaling, while *Cx45* mRNA expression is unaffected.

3.2. Cx36 suppresses neuritogenesis

Cx36 mRNA was either stably overexpressed or knocked down in SH-SY5Y cells to determine the effect of Cx36 on differentiation. SH-SY5Y cells were transfected and selected to stably overexpress *Cx36* mRNA. Three weeks post-transfection, Cx36 overexpressing cells expressed 150 fold (141 +/- 27) more *Cx36* mRNA than EGFP transfected cells (Figure 2A). Cx36 shRNA expressing cells exhibited an 88-99% reduction in *Cx36* mRNA levels in comparison to non-effective shRNA control prior to our differentiation studies (Figure 2B). Since all shRNA constructs coexpressed GFP, fluorescence was visualized to ensure continued expression of the construct during differentiation. The majority of differentiating cells (>85%) continued to express all constructs during the ten day experiments (Figure 2C). Therefore, all constructs were successfully transfected and expressed by SH-SY5Y cells. In addition, Cx43 expression was analyzed following Cx36 overexpression and knockdown to ensure that Cx43 did not compensate for changes in Cx36 expression. Since Cx43 expression was not altered by changes in Cx36 expression, Cx43 does not appear to compensate for Cx36 in SH-SY5Y cells.

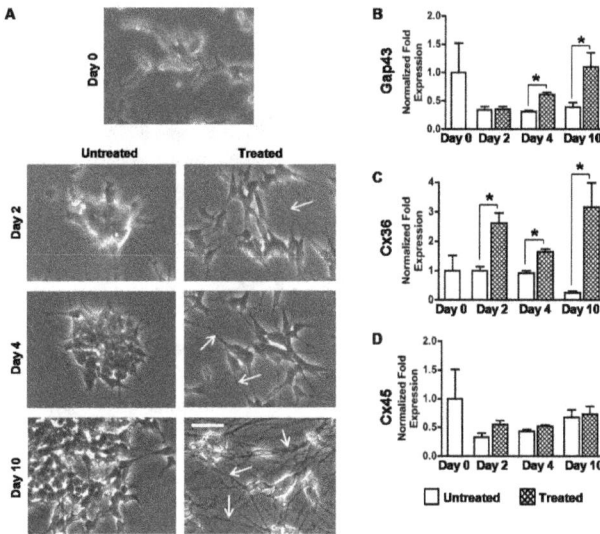

Figure 1. Retinoic acid induces differentiation of SH-SY5Y cells and upregulates *Gap43* and *Cx36* expression. Cells were seeded on rat-tail collagen coated dishes and treated with 10 µM of retinoic acid the following day. During days 5-10, cells were treated with 20 ng/ml of BDNF in serum-free medium. **(A)** Untreated cells formed increasingly larger aggregates over time. Neurite outgrowth (arrows) was observed beginning at days 2 and 4 of treatment, and dense neurite networks were formed following 10 days of treatment. Scale bar = 50 µm. **(B-D)** RNA was isolated from SH-SY5Y cells at days 0, 2, 4, and 10 of treatment. Real-time PCR was used to quantify mRNA expression. **(B)** *Gap43* expression increased following 4 and 10 days of treatment. **(C)** *Cx36* expression increased following 2, 4 and 10 days

of treatment, as compared to untreated cells. **(D)** *Cx45* expression did not increase in either treated or untreated cells. mRNA levels were normalized to *PPIA*. N=3 (Day10, N=5). * p<0.05. Bars show mean +/- S.E.

Cx36 overexpressing cells were induced to differentiate in order to determine the effect of Cx36 on neuritogenesis. EGFP and Cx36 overexpressing cells were seeded for differentiation, and imaged at 0, 2, 4, and 10 days following differentiation treatment. EGFP expressing cells showed intense neurite networking by day 10 of differentiation treatment, while Cx36 overexpression diminished neuritogenesis (Figure 3A). There was no significant difference between EGFP and Cx36 overexpressing cells in average neurite length (Figure 3B). However, Cx36 overexpressing cells had significantly reduced neurite density compared to EGFP expressing cells (Figure 3C). Thus, our findings indicate that Cx36 downregulates retinoic acid induced neuritogenesis.

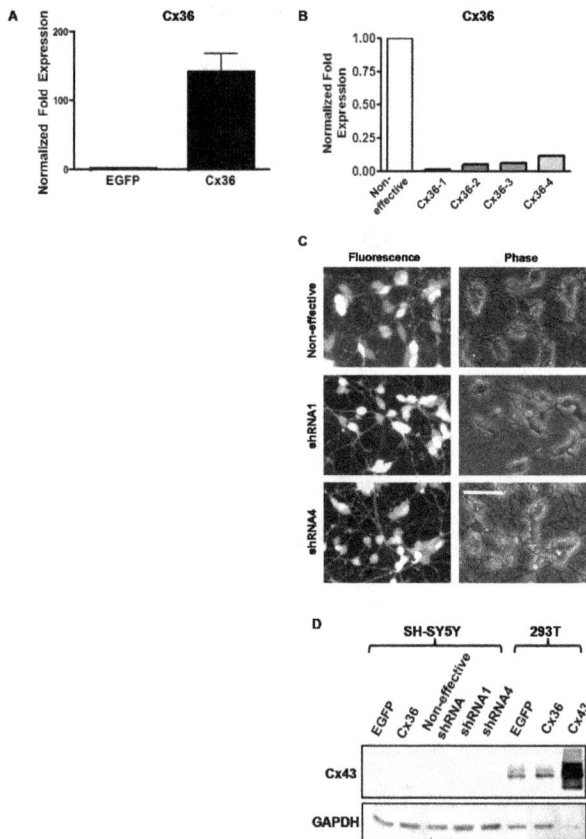

Figure 2. Cx36 overexpression and knockdown are maintained throughout differentiation. (A) SH-SY5Y cells were transfected and selected to stably overexpress Cx36 or EGFP as a transfection control. RNA was isolated from transfected cells over the 10 day differentiation treatment, and Cx36 overexpressing cells showed at least 150 fold

greater Cx36 expression levels than the EGFP control. **(B, C)** In addition, cells were transfected and selected to express four distinct Cx36 shRNA's and a non-effective shRNA transfection control, all of which coexpressed GFP. **(B)** RNA was isolated to determine expression levels prior to seeding cells for experiments. Cx36 shRNA expressing cells had decreased *Cx36* transcript levels compared to non-effective control. RNA expression levels were normalized to *PPIA* mRNA. N=3 (B, N=1). *p<0.05. Bars show mean +/-S.E. **(C)** Most of the cell population expressed GFP, and thus the shRNA construct through ten days of differentiation treatment. Scale bar = 50 μm. **(D)** Cx43 expression was not detected and did not change following Cx36 overexpression or knockdown in SH-SY5Y cells.

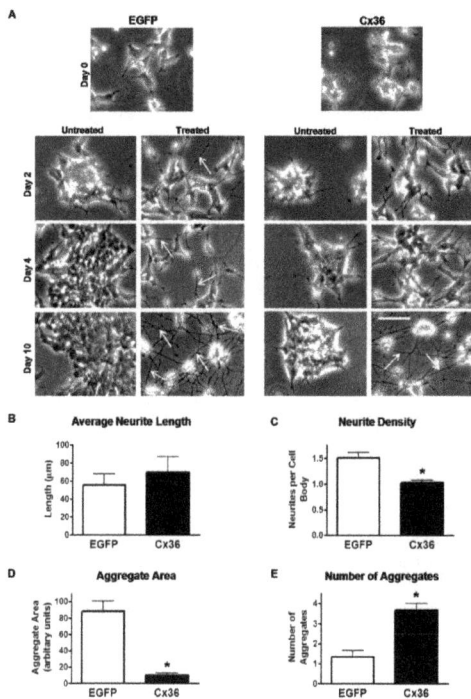

Figure 3. Cx36 overexpression diminishes neurite density and increases cell clumping in SH-SY5Y cells. Stably transfected EGFP and Cx36 overexpressing SH-SY5Y cells were treated with retinoic acid and BDNF. **(A)** EGFP expressing cells formed denser neurite networks (arrows) than Cx36 overexpressing cells following treatment. Untreated Cx36 overexpressing cells formed numerous small cell clumps whereas EGFP expressing cells formed larger aggregates. Scale Bar = 50 μm. **(B,C)** Treated cells were imaged at day 10 and neurite length and density were measured using Neuron J. **(B)** There was no significant difference in average neurite length between EGFP control and Cx36 overexpressing cells. **(C)** However, neurite density was diminished in Cx36 overexpressing cells. **(D,E)** Aggregate area and number were measured for untreated cells at day 10 using Image J. **(D)** Cx36 overexpressing cells formed aggregates with significantly smaller area, **(E)** however developed more numerous aggregates per field of view than EGFP expressing cells. * p<0.05. Bars show mean +/- S.E

To further demonstrate that Cx36 negatively regulates neuritogenesis, the effect of Cx36 knockdown on neuritogenesis was determined. An identical experimental design as the overexpression study was conducted between non-effective shRNA and Cx36 shRNA expressing cells. In these experiments, Cx36 shRNA expressing cells showed enhanced neuritogenesis (Figure 4A). There was no significant difference in average neurite length between Cx36 shRNA expressing and non-effective shRNA expressing cells (Figure 4B). However, neurite density was significantly increased in Cx36 shRNA expressing cells compared to non-effective shRNA expressing cells (Figure 4C). Therefore, knockdown of Cx36 enhanced retinoic acid induced neuritogenesis. These findings confirm that Cx36 diminishes retinoic acid induced neuritogenesis of SH-SY5Y cells.

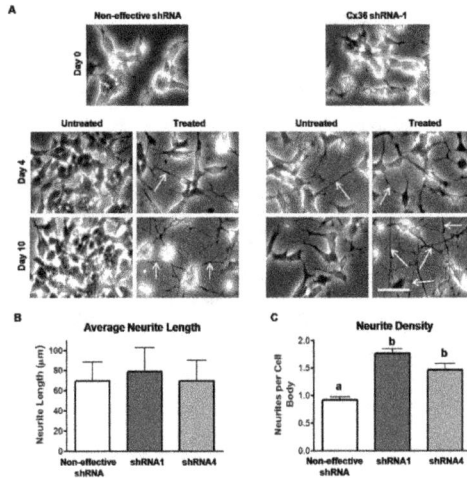

Figure 4. Knockdown of Cx36 increases neurite density and suppresses aggregate formation in SH-SY5Y cells. Cx36 shRNA expressing cells were plated and subjected to differentiation treatment over 10 days. (A) Treated Cx36 shRNA expressing cells exhibit enhanced neuritogenesis compared to non-effective control. Untreated non-effective shRNA expressing cells aggregate on collagen, while Cx36 shRNA expressing cells remain dispersed. Scale bar = 50 μm. (B,C) Differentiating cells were imaged at day 10 and neurite length and density were measured using Neuron J software. (B) There was no significant difference in average neurite length between non-effective shRNA expressing control and Cx36 shRNA expressing cells. (C) However, neurite density was higher in Cx36 shRNA expressing cells than in control. N=3. Different letters indicate statistical significance. p<0.05. Bars show mean +/- S.E.

3.3. Cx36 suppresses differentiation marker expression

In order to determine whether Cx36 also negatively regulates other indicators of differentiation, the effect of Cx36 on the expression of molecular differentiation markers, Gap43 and NPY, was assessed. Transcript expression of the *Gap43* differentiation marker was significantly reduced in Cx36 overexpressing cells at days 2 and 4 of treatment in comparison with EGFP expressing cells (Figure 5A). *NPY* mRNA levels were also significantly decreased in Cx36 overexpressing cells at days 2 and 10 of treatment compared to EGFP expressing cells (Figure 5B). Gap43 protein expression significantly increased upon differentiation treatment in EGFP expressing cells, however Cx36 overexpressing cells failed to significantly increase Gap43 expression following treatment (Figure 5 C & D). Thus, Cx36 overexpression diminished the retinoic acid induced expression of molecular differentiation markers.

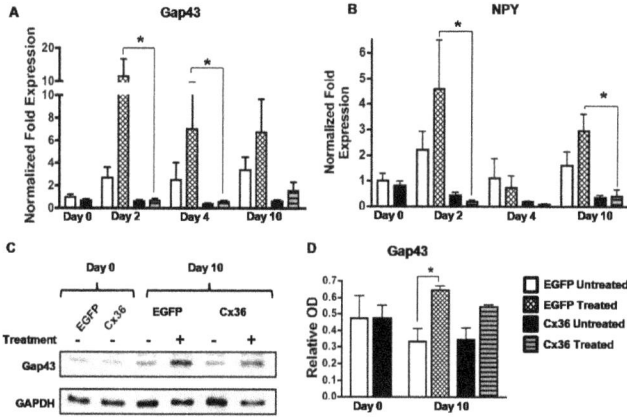

Figure 5. Cx36 overexpression diminishes retinoic acid induced Gap43 and NPY expression. (A,B) RNA was isolated from cells at day 0, 2, 4, and 10 of differentiation treatment, and real-time PCR was used to quantify changes in mRNA expression. **(C,D)** Protein was extracted from cells at 0 and 10 days of treatment and western blot analysis was used to quantify protein expression. **(A)** *Gap43* expression was diminished in Cx36 overexpressing cells at days 2 and 4 of treatment. **(B)** *NPY* expression is diminished at days 2 and 10 of treatment in Cx36 overexpressing cells. **(C,D)** Gap43 protein expression did not significantly differ between Cx36 overexpressing and EGFP expressing cells. Gap43 expression significantly increased upon treatment in EGFP cells, however it failed to significantly increase in treated Cx36 overexpressing cells. mRNA levels were normalized to *PPIA* and protein levels to GAPDH. N=3. *p<0.05. Bars show mean +/- S.E.

The impact of Cx36 knockdown on expression of differentiation markers was assessed to confirm the effect of Cx36 on differentiation. Non-effective shRNA and Cx36 shRNA expressing cells were subjected to the 10 day differentiation treatment, and RNA was isolated at days 0, 4, and 10. Cx36 shRNA expressing cells exhibited significantly increased levels of *Gap43* mRNA expression at day 10 of treatment compared with non-effective shRNA expressing cells (Figure 6A). In addition, Cx36 shRNA expressing cells had significantly higher *NPY* mRNA expression at day 0 and day 10 of differentiation treatment compared to non-effective shRNA expressing cells (Figure 6B). Untreated and treated Cx36 knockdown cells also expressed higher levels of Gap43 protein (Figure 6 C & D). Furthermore, untreated Cx36 shRNA expressing cells expressed as much Gap43 protein as treated non-effective control, while treated Cx36 shRNA expressing cells expressed the highest levels of Gap43. Our findings show that Cx36 knockdown enhances retinoic acid induced differentiation marker expression.

3.4. Cx36 promotes cell clumping

An unexpected finding of our study was that Cx36 overexpression affected the adhesion and aggregation properties of cells on collagen coated dishes. Untreated EGFP and Cx36 overexpressing cells were plated on collagen coated plates for ten days. EGFP expressing cells behaved like wild-type cells, where they formed large cell aggregates over time, while Cx36 overexpressing cells formed cell clumps that were susceptible to lifting off the plate (Figure 3A). Cx36 overexpressing cells formed significantly smaller aggregates than EGFP expressing

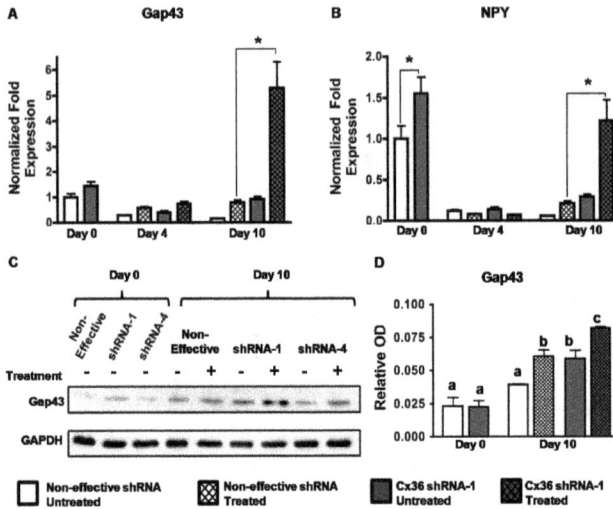

Figure 6. Cx36 knockdown enhances retinoic acid induced Gap43 expression and upregulates *NPY* expression. RNA and protein were isolated from cells at days 0, 4, and 10 of differentiation treatment. Real-time PCR and western blotting were used to quantify mRNA and protein expression respectively. (A) Gap43 expression is increased at day 10, (B) while NPY expression is increased at 0 and 10 days of treatment in Cx36 shRNA expressing cells compared to non-effective control. (C,D) Gap43 protein expression is enhanced in untreated and untreated Cx36 shRNA expressing cells compared to non-effective control at day 10 of treatment. mRNA levels were normalized to *PPIA* and protein normalized to GAPDH. N=3. Asterisks and different letters denote a statistically significant difference. $p<0.05$. Bars show mean +/- S.E.

cells (Figure 3D) in addition to significantly higher numbers of cell clumps than EGFP expressing cells (Figure 3E). Expression levels of two distinct cell adhesion molecules, *NCAM* and N-cadherin, were examined to determine whether altered expression of these proteins mediated the cell clumping in Cx36 overexpressing cells. However, neither *NCAM* mRNA nor N-cadherin protein levels showed any significant changes in Cx36 overexpressing cells during differentiation or in their untreated state (Figure 7). Therefore, Cx36 overexpression resulted in increased formation of small cell clumps, although the adhesion molecules involved in this process have not yet been identified.

In order to further explore the effect of Cx36 on cell clumping, the effect of Cx36 knockdown on aggregate formation was assessed in a comparable study between non-effective shRNA and Cx36 shRNA expressing SH-SY5Y cells. The untreated non-effective shRNA expressing cells formed large aggregates over ten days, similar to wild-type cells (Figure 4A). However, Cx36 shRNA expressing cells did not form aggregates, and maintained a dispersed phenotype (Figure 4A). *NCAM* expression was significantly higher in treated non-effective shRNA expressing cells than all other conditions (Figure 8A). N-cadherin expression did not meaningfully change between constructs (Figure 8 B & C). Therefore, Cx36 knockdown prevents aggregate and cell clump formation in SH-SY5Y cells. However, the molecules through which Cx36 exerts its effect on cell aggregation have not yet been determined.

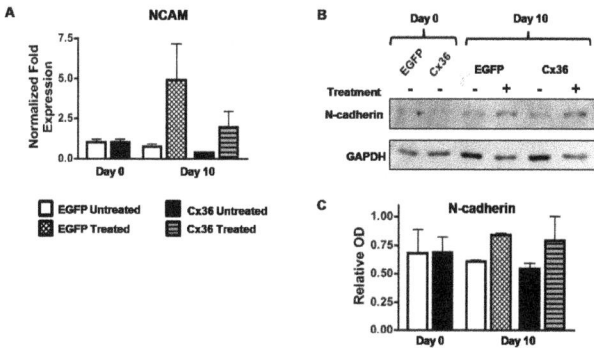

Figure 7. NCAM and N-cadherin expression were not altered in differentiating Cx36 overexpressing cells. RNA and protein were isolated from cells at day 0 and 10 of treatment, and real-time PCR was used to quantify mRNA expression and western blotting to quantify protein expression. **(A)** *NCAM* mRNA expression levels were not significantly different between any condition. **(B,C)** N-cadherin protein expression levels did not change between differentiation treatment or overexpression conditions (B & C). mRNA levels were normalized to *PPIA* mRNA and protein levels to GAPDH. N=3. Bars show mean +/- S.E.

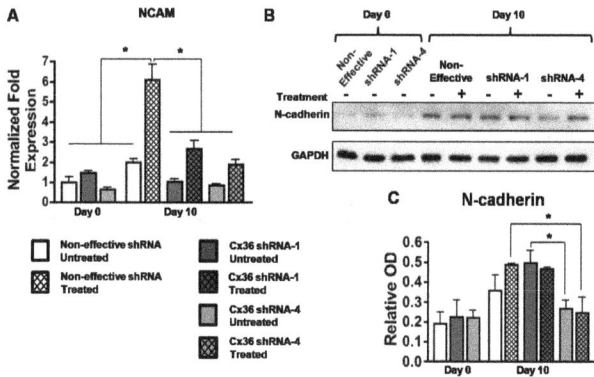

Figure 8. NCAM expression was reduced in Cx36 shRNA expressing cells and N-cadherin expression was only decreased in shRNA-4 expressing cells. RNA and protein were isolated from cells at day 0 and 10 of differentiation treatment, and real-time PCR was used to quantify mRNA expression and western blots to quantify protein expression. (A) *NCAM* mRNA expression was higher in treated non-effective control cells than all other conditions. (B,C) N-cadherin protein expression levels were decreased in shRNA-4 but not shRNA-1 expressing cells in comparison to non-effective control. mRNA levels were normalized to *PPIA* mRNA and protein levels to GAPDH. *p< 0.05. N=3. Bars show mean +/- S.E.

3.5. Cx36 increases SH-SY5Y cell proliferation

Neurons typically exit the cell cycle in order to terminally differentiate. Thus, cell proliferation was assessed in Cx36 overexpressing and knockdown cells to determine if changes in proliferation rate are a consequence of Cx36 manipulation of differentiation. The proliferation rates of EGFP and Cx36 overexpressing cells were assessed using the MTT proliferation assay. Absorbance was measured at 0, 2, 4, and 6 days in culture. At day 6, Cx36 overexpressing cells had significantly higher absorbance than EGFP expressing cells implying enhanced cell proliferation in these cells (Figure 9A).

The identical assay was performed for non-effective shRNA and Cx36 shRNA expressing cells to confirm that Cx36 stimulates cell proliferation. At day 6, Cx36 shRNA expressing cells had significantly reduced absorbance in comparison to non-effective shRNA expressing cells (Figure 9B). Therefore, our findings indicate that Cx36 promotes proliferation of SH-SY5Y neuroblastoma cells.

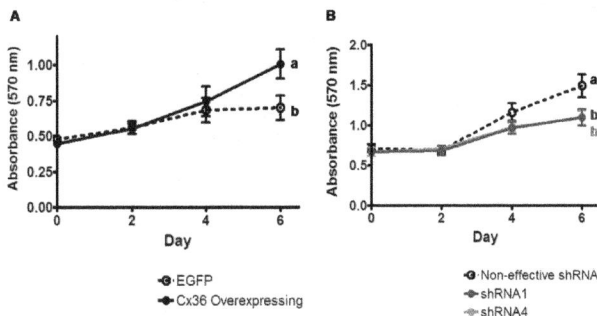

Figure 9. Cx36 overexpression increases SH-SY5Y cell proliferation while knockdown of Cx36 suppresses cell proliferation. Cells were seeded at 20,000 cells per well in 48-well plates and the MTT proliferation assay was conducted according to manufacturer's guidelines. (A) Following 6 days in culture, Cx36 overexpressing cells had a significantly higher proliferation rate than EGFP control cells. In contrast, Cx36 shRNA expressing cells had a significantly lower rate of proliferation than non-effective control. Different letters indicate significant difference. p< 0.05. N=3. Points show mean +/-S.E.

Since high proliferation and lack of differentiation are traits of stem cells, the effect of Cx36 overexpression and knockdown on stem cell marker expression was assessed. ID2 and Nestin mRNA expression were upregulated following Cx36 overexpression (Figure 10 A & B), but did not change upon Cx36 knockdown (Figure 10 C & D). These findings suggest that Cx36 overexpression may cause SH-SY5Y cells to adopt a stem-cell like phenotype.

4. Discussion

4.1. Retinoic acid induces upregulation of Cx36

Retinoic acid is often used as a therapeutic agent in the treatment of neuroblastoma to induce differentiation. In current neuroblastoma therapy, patients are given 13-cis retinoic acid during remission following treatment with chemotherapeutics to eradicate minimal residual disease [3, 33]. Retinoic acid has been shown to upregulate Cx43 expression [21, 22], however there have been no reports of its effect on the neuronal connexins, Cx36 and Cx45. The SH-SY5Y human neuroblastoma cell line is known to undergo extensive differentiation in response to retinoic acid treatment [4, 25]. Therefore, the effect of retinoic acid on these neuronal connexins was investigated in the SH-SY5Y neuroblastoma cell line. We also investigated the IMR32 neuroblastoma cell line and while it expressed Cx36 and was responsive to retinoic acid, it had limited differentiation potential, consistent with previous findings by others [34]. Our study indicates that *Cx36* may be a target of retinoic acid signaling, since it is upregulated upon retinoic acid induced differentiation and *Cx36* contains a retinoid X receptor binding motif similar to that of the *Cx43* gene [24]. Conversely, *Cx45* does not appear to be regulated by retinoic acid. In fact, the influence of retinoic acid in either of its configurations, *cis*-retinoic acid or all-trans retinoic acid appears to have similar effects on connexins in a particular cellular context, however that effect can be very different depending on cellular environment, with examples of enhanced expression on Cx32 protein in LNCaP prostate cancer cells [35] versus suppression of Cx26 or 43 mediated coupling in squamous cell carcinoma cells [36]. Thus, we have identified *Cx36* as a novel potential transcriptional target in retinoic acid signaling. In addition, since *Cx36* expression increased upon retinoic acid induced differentiation, *Cx36* gene expression was manipulated to ascertain its effects on the differentiation and proliferation of SH-SY5Y cells.

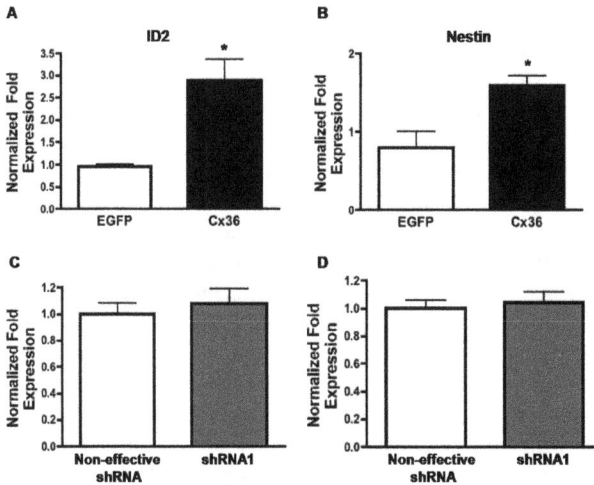

Figure 10. Cx36 overexpression results in increased stem cell marker expression, while Cx36 knockdown has no effect. RNA was isolated from cells and real-time PCR was used to quantify mRNA expression. (A,B) ID2 and Nestin expression increased following Cx36 overexpression. (C,D) However, ID2 and Nestin were unaffected by knockdown of Cx36. mRNA levels were normalized to *PPIA*. N=3. Asterisks denote a statistically significant difference. p<0.05. Bars show mean +/- S.E.

4.2. Cx36 negatively regulates SH-SY5Y cell differentiation

Cx36 appears to negatively regulate differentiation of SH-SY5Y human neuroblastoma cells. Accordingly, overexpression of Cx36 dimishes differentiation while knockdown of Cx36 enhances differentiation. This appears to be in contradiction with the upregulation of Cx36 upon retinoic acid induced differentiation. However, since we were unable to measure protein expression, it is possible that although Cx36 mRNA is upregulated in response to retinoic acid, Cx36 protein expression is unaffected. Conversely, this discrepancy may also be due to the requirement of an optimal level of Cx36 for proper differentiation. Accordingly, the small increase in Cx36 expression induced by retinoic acid in wild-type cells does not appear to interfere with differentiation. However, since Cx36 overexpressing cells exhibit diminished differentiation and Cx36 knockdown enhances differentiation, it is apparent that substantial changes in Cx36 expression alter the process of differentiation.

The effect of Cx36 on SH-SY5Y differentiation is in contrast with what Hartfield et al (2011) have recently shown on Cx36 and neuronal progenitor cells [37]. Progenitors isolated from the rat hippocampus and striatum and grown in neurospheres showed increased differentiation with Cx36 overexpression, and diminished differentiation with Cx36 knockdown [37]. Although neuroblastoma arises from progenitor cells, these cancer cells likely respond differently to Cx36 levels than healthy progenitors. It is also possible that neuronal cells of the peripheral nervous system react differently to Cx36 than those of the central nervous system. The effect of Cx36 on differentiation is also in contrast with other connexins, which are known to enhance differentiation [8, 9]. For example, overexpression of Cx43 and Cx32 enhanced nerve growth factor induced differentiation of PC12 cells [10]. Although connexin overexpression usually enhances differentiation, Todorova et al (2008) have shown that GJIC and Cx43 are required to maintain pluripotency of embryonic stem cells. Inhibition of GJIC or Cx43 knockdown resulted in reduced proliferation and stem cell marker expression, with a concomitant increase in differentiation marker expression [38]. Thus, in certain environments, as with our Cx36 overexpression study, connexin expression may be required to maintain the stem cell or cancer phenotype. This is further demonstrated in human breast cancer where gap junctions and GJIC are usually associated with tumor suppression however in aggressive breast cancers they may facilitate disease progression [39]. Our finding of Cx36 knockdown enhancing differentiation in fact parallels the natural expression patterns of Cx36, where it is highly expressed in many neural structures of the developing fetus but is subsequently downregulated during postnatal differentiation and maturation of the nervous system [18, 19]. This downregulation may be due in part to replacement of electrical synapses with chemical synapses [40], or it may indicate that Cx36 is actually detrimental in the process of terminal differentiation of certain tissues or cell types, as was shown in this study.

4.2.1. Cx36 promotes clumping of SH-SY5Y cells

A surprising finding was that altering Cx36 expression dramatically changed the adhesion and aggregation properties of SH-SY5Y cells. Cx36 overexpression led to the formation of small cell clumps susceptible to lifting off the dish and growing in suspension. This type of growth is similar to that of neurospheres, which are suspended clusters of neural stem cells [41]. In fact, it is characteristic of the neuroblast subpopulations of SH-SY5Y cells to aggregate, lift off, and grow in suspension [42]. This neuroblastic phenotype appears to be stimulated by overexpression of Cx36, which is in accordance with our findings of Cx36 induced downregulation of differentiation. Interestingly, knockdown of Cx36 resulted in a dispersed cell phenotype.

NCAM and N-cadherin expression were assessed as potential mediators of the differential aggregate formation in Cx36 overexpressing and knockdown cells. Cx43 is known to colocalize with N-cadherin and regulate its localization at the cell surface [43]. Although there have been no documented reports of Cx36 and N-cadherin interaction, we investigated whether manipulation of Cx36 expression resulted in changes to N-cadherin expression. In addition, we explored the effect of Cx36 expression on NCAM mRNA expression, as NCAM is upregulated in poorly differentiated and aggressive neuroblastomas [44]. Based on our studies, N-cadherin and NCAM are unlikely to be the primary adhesion molecule involved in this process. Therefore, while Cx36 expression has a dramatic effect on cell aggregation, the adhesion molecules mediating this process are yet to be identified.

4.2.2. Cx36 increases cell proliferation

There is a substantial linkage between connexin expression and cell growth and proliferation [6]. Our findings of increased cell proliferation with Cx36 overexpression, and diminished cell proliferation following knockdown of Cx36 are in contrast to other connexins, which typically act as tumor suppressors [6, 8]. However, in certain environments, connexins and gap junctional intercellular communication are required to maintain the proliferative ability of cells. For example, extravillous trophoblasts lost the ability to proliferate when GJIC was inhibited by a gap junction blocker or Cx40 antisense cDNA [45].

Additionally, Cx36 has been implicated in retinal cell survival following injury [46]. In light of the role of Cx36 in cell survival and its high expression during development when neural precursors are proliferating, it is not surprising to find that Cx36 serves to increase proliferation. It is also important to consider that Cx36 is regulated in a different manner from other connexins. For example, Cx36 channels show differential pH gating and experience very low sensitivity to voltage gating [47, 48]. This pH gating may be important under pathological conditions such as ischemia, where Cx36 expression has been shown to be upregulated and involved in cell survival [49]. Therefore, the differential regulation mechanisms of Cx36 channels may suggest a different role for Cx36 in key cellular processes from that of other connexins.

In relation to differentiation, as neurons do not retain a capacity to divide, cells must exit the cell cycle and stop proliferating in order to terminally differentiate into neurons. Retinoic acid also exerts part of its differentiation inducing effects by inhibiting cell proliferation [50]. Therefore, the enhanced differentiation observed in Cx36 shRNA expressing cells may be partially due to their decreased proliferative ability.

SH-SY5Y cells overexpressing Cx36 adopt several characteristics of stem cells, including aggregation, high proliferation, and lack of differentiation. To determine whether these cells were also more stem cell like at the molecular level, the expression levels of ID2 and Nestin were assessed. ID2 is expressed in neural crest cells and is also known to increase proliferation and inhibit differentiation of neuroblastoma cells [51]. Nestin is often used as a neural stem cell marker as it is highly expressed in progenitor cells during development, but is downregulated in adults [52]. The upregulation of both ID2 and Nestin upon Cx36 overexpression suggests that increased levels of Cx36 push SH-SY5Y cells towards a stem cell phenotype.

This study is the first to determine the effects of Cx36 in a cancer cell context. We have identified *Cx36* as a novel potential transcriptional target of retinoic acid signaling. However, further research is required to determine whether *Cx36* is a direct target of retinoic acid signaling. In addition, Cx36 negatively regulates SH-SY5Y differentiation, which is in contrast to the effects of other connexins on differentiation. Furthermore, it appears that Cx36 promotes a neural stem cell like phenotype based on the diminished differentiation, enhanced clumping and increased proliferation in overexpressing cells, and the reversal of this phenotype in cells where Cx36 is knocked down.

However, it is unknown whether Cx36 mediates these changes in a gap junctional intercellular communication dependent manner or through interaction of Cx36 with binding partners, and thus downstream signaling pathways. Therefore, further research is required to elucidate the mechanisms underlying Cx36 mediated regulation of differentiation.

Acknowledgements

Supported by the National Sciences and Engineering Research Council of Canada to DJB.

Author details

Mandeep Sidhu and Daniel J. Belliveau*

*Address all correspondence to: dbellive@uwo.ca

Department of Anatomy and Cell Biology, Schulich of Medicine & Dentistry and School of Health Studies, Faculty of Health Sciences, Western University, London, Ontario, Canada

References

[1] Brodeur, G. M. Neuroblastoma: biological insights into a clinical enigma. Nature reviewsCancer. (2003). Mar;PubMed PMID: PMID: 12612655; nrc1014 [pii]., 3(3), 203-16.

[2] Huber, K. The sympathoadrenal cell lineage: specification, diversification, and new perspectives. Developmental biology. (2006). Oct 15;PubMed PMID: PMID: 16928368; S0012-1606(06)00992-4 [pii]., 298(2), 335-43.

[3] Wagner, L. M, & Danks, M. K. New therapeutic targets for the treatment of high-risk neuroblastoma. Journal of cellular biochemistry. (2009). May 1;PubMed PMID: PMID: 19277986., 107(1), 46-57.

[4] Thiele, C. J, Reynolds, C. P, & Israel, M. A. Decreased expression of N-myc precedes retinoic acid-induced morphological differentiation of human neuroblastoma. Nature. (1985). Jan 31-Feb 6;PubMed PMID: PMID: 3855502., 313(6001), 404-6.

[5] Sidell, N, Altman, A, Haussler, M. R, & Seeger, R. C. Effects of retinoic acid (RA) on the growth and phenotypic expression of several human neuroblastoma cell lines. Experimental Cell Research. (1983). Oct;PubMed PMID: 6313408. Epub 1983/10/01. eng., 148(1), 21-30.

[6] Naus, C. C, & Laird, D. W. Implications and challenges of connexin connections to cancer. Nature Reviews Cancer. (2010). Jun;PubMed PMID: 20495577. Epub 2010/05/25. eng., 10(6), 435-41.

[7] Arnold, J. M, Phipps, M. W, Chen, J, & Phipps, J. Cellular sublocalization of Cx43 and the establishment of functional coupling in IMR-32 neuroblastoma cells. Molecular carcinogenesis. (2005). Mar;PubMed PMID: PMID: 15605363., 42(3), 159-69.

[8] Mao, A. J, Bechberger, J, Lidington, D, Galipeau, J, Laird, D. W, & Naus, C. C. Neuronal differentiation and growth control of neuro-2a cells after retroviral gene delivery of connexin43. The Journal of biological chemistry. (2000). Nov 3;PubMed PMID: PMID: 10924505; M003917200 [pii]., 275(44), 34407-14.

[9] Banks, E. A, Yu, X. S, Shi, Q, & Jiang, J. X. Promotion of lens epithelial-fiber differentiation by the C-terminus of connexin 45.6 a role independent of gap junction communication. Journal of cell science. (2007). Oct 15;PubMed PMID: PMID: 17895360; jcs.000935 [pii]., 120(20), 3602-12.

[10] Belliveau, D. J, Bani-yaghoub, M, Mcgirr, B, Naus, C. C, & Rushlow, W. J. Enhanced neurite outgrowth in PC12 cells mediated by connexin hemichannels and ATP. The Journal of biological chemistry. (2006). Jul 28;PubMed PMID: PMID: 16731531; M600026200 [pii]., 281(30), 20920-31.

[11] Laird, D. W. The life cycle of a connexin: gap junction formation, removal, and degradation. Journal of Bioenergetics and Biomembranes. (1996). Aug;PubMed PMID: 8844328. Epub 1996/08/01. eng., 28(4), 311-8.

[12] Saez, J. C, Connor, J. A, Spray, D. C, & Bennett, M. V. Hepatocyte gap junctions are permeable to the second messenger, inositol 1,4,5-trisphosphate, and to calcium ions. Proceedings of the National Academy of Sciences of the United States of America. (1989). Apr;PubMed PMID: 2784857. Epub 1989/04/01. eng., 86(8), 2708-12.

[13] Vinken, M, Vanhaecke, T, Papeleu, P, Snykers, S, Henkens, T, & Rogiers, V. Connexins and their channels in cell growth and cell death. Cell Signal. (2006). May;PubMed PMID: 16183253. Epub 2005/09/27. eng., 18(5), 592-600.

[14] Laird, D. W. Life cycle of connexins in health and disease. The Biochemical journal. (2006). Mar 15;PubMed PMID: PMID: 16492141; BJ20051922 [pii]., 394(3), 527-43.

[15] Sohl, G, Degen, J, Teubner, B, & Willecke, K. The murine gap junction gene connexin36 is highly expressed in mouse retina and regulated during brain development. FEBS Letters. (1998). May 22;428(1-2):27-31. PubMed PMID: 9645468. Epub 1998/06/30. eng.

[16] Condorelli, D. F, Parenti, R, & Spinella, F. Trovato Salinaro A, Belluardo N, Cardile V, et al. Cloning of a new gap junction gene (Cx36) highly expressed in mammalian brain neurons. European Journal of Neuroscience. (1998). Mar;PubMed PMID: 9753189. Epub 1998/09/30. eng., 10(3), 1202-8.

[17] Serre-beinier, V, Bosco, D, Zulianello, L, Charollais, A, Caille, D, Charpantier, E, et al. Cx36 makes channels coupling human pancreatic beta-cells, and correlates with insulin expression. Human molecular genetics. (2009). Feb 1;PubMed PMID: 19000992. Epub 2008/11/13. eng., 18(3), 428-39.

[18] Belluardo, N, Mudo, G, & Trovato-salinaro, A. Le Gurun S, Charollais A, Serre-Beinier V, et al. Expression of connexin36 in the adult and developing rat brain. Brain Research. (2000). May 19;PubMed PMID: 10814742. Epub 2000/05/18. eng., 865(1), 121-38.

[19] Gulisano, M, Parenti, R, Spinella, F, & Cicirata, F. Cx36 is dynamically expressed during early development of mouse brain and nervous system. Neuroreport. (2000). Nov 27;PubMed PMID: 11117498. Epub 2000/12/16. eng., 11(17), 3823-8.

[20] Connors, B. W, & Long, M. A. Electrical synapses in the mammalian brain. Annual Review of Neuroscience. (2004). PubMed PMID: PMID: 15217338., 27, 393-418.

[21] Bertram, J. S, & Vine, A. L. Cancer prevention by retinoids and carotenoids: independent action on a common target. Biochimica et biophysica acta. (2005). May 30;PubMed PMID: PMID: 15949684; S0925-4439(05)00003-7 [pii]., 1740(2), 170-8.

[22] Stahl, W, & Sies, H. The role of carotenoids and retinoids in gap junctional communication. International journal for vitamin and nutrition research. (1998). PubMed PMID: 9857261. Epub 1998/12/19. eng., 68(6), 354-9.

[23] Vine, A. L, & Bertram, J. S. Upregulation of connexin 43 by retinoids but not by non-provitamin A carotenoids requires RARs. Nutrition and cancer. (2005). PubMed PMID: PMID: 16091010., 52(1), 105-13.

[24] Cicirata, F, Parenti, R, Spinella, F, Giglio, S, Tuorto, F, Zuffardi, O, et al. Genomic organization and chromosomal localization of the mouse Connexin36 (mCx36) gene. Gene. (2000). Jun 27;PubMed PMID: 10876089. Epub 2000/07/06. eng., 251(2), 123-30.

[25] Encinas, M, Iglesias, M, Liu, Y, Wang, H, Muhaisen, A, Cena, V, et al. Sequential treatment of SH-SY5Y cells with retinoic acid and brain-derived neurotrophic factor gives rise to fully differentiated, neurotrophic factor-dependent, human neuron-like

cells. Journal of Neurochemistry. (2000). Sep;PubMed PMID: 10936180. Epub 2000/08/11. eng., 75(3), 991-1003.

[26] Agholme, L, Lindstrom, T, Kagedal, K, Marcusson, J, & Hallbeck, M. An in vitro model for neuroscience: differentiation of SH-SY5Y cells into cells with morphological and biochemical characteristics of mature neurons. J Alzheimers Dis. (2010). PubMed PMID: 20413890. Epub 2010/04/24. eng., 20(4), 1069-82.

[27] Abramoff, M. D, Magelhaes, P. J, & Ram, S. J. Image Processing with ImageJ. Biophotonics International. (2004). , 11(7), 36-42.

[28] Meijering, E, Jacob, M, Sarria, J. C, Steiner, P, Hirling, H, & Unser, M. Design and validation of a tool for neurite tracing and analysis in fluorescence microscopy images. Cytometry A. (2004). Apr;PubMed PMID: 15057970. Epub 2004/04/02. eng., 58(2), 167-76.

[29] Clagett-dame, M, Mcneill, E. M, & Muley, P. D. Role of all-trans retinoic acid in neurite outgrowth and axonal elongation. Journal of neurobiology. (2006). Jun;PubMed PMID: PMID: 16688769., 66(7), 739-56.

[30] Larsson, C. Protein kinase C and the regulation of the actin cytoskeleton. Cell Signal. (2006). Mar;PubMed PMID: 16109477. Epub 2005/08/20. eng., 18(3), 276-84.

[31] Edsjo, A, Lavenius, E, Nilsson, H, Hoehner, J. C, Simonsson, P, Culp, L. A, et al. Expression of trkB in human neuroblastoma in relation to MYCN expression and retinoic acid treatment. Laboratory investigation; a journal of technical methods and pathology. (2003). Jun;PubMed PMID: PMID: 12808116., 83(6), 813-23.

[32] Hokfelt, T, Stanic, D, Sanford, S. D, Gatlin, J. C, Nilsson, I, Paratcha, G, et al. NPY and its involvement in axon guidance, neurogenesis, and feeding. Nutrition. (2008). Sep;PubMed PMID: PMID: 18725084; S0899-9007(08)00276-1 [pii]., 24(9), 860-8.

[33] Reynolds, C. P, Matthay, K. K, Villablanca, J. G, & Maurer, B. J. Retinoid therapy of high-risk neuroblastoma. Cancer letters. (2003). Jul 18;197(1-2):185-92. PubMed PMID: PMID: 12880980; S0304383503001083 [pii].

[34] Haussler, M, Sidell, N, Kelly, M, Donaldson, C, Altman, A, & Mangelsdorf, D. Specific high-affinity binding and biologic action of retinoic acid in human neuroblastoma cell lines. Proceedings of the National Academy of Sciences of the United States of America. (1983). Sep;PubMed PMID: 6310582. Pubmed Central PMCID: PMC384290. Epub 1983/09/01. eng., 80(18), 5525-9.

[35] Kelsey, L, Katoch, P, Johnson, K. E, Batra, S. K, & Mehta, P. P. Retinoids regulate the formation and degradation of gap junctions in androgen-responsive human prostate cancer cells. PloS one. (2012). e32846. PubMed PMID: 22514600. Pubmed Central PMCID: PMC3326013. Epub 2012/04/20. eng.

[36] Rudkin, G. H, Carlsen, B. T, Chung, C. Y, Huang, W, Ishida, K, Anvar, B, et al. Retinoids inhibit squamous cell carcinoma growth and intercellular communication. The

Journal of surgical research. (2002). Apr;PubMed PMID: 11922733. Epub 2002/04/02. eng., 103(2), 183-9.

[37] Hartfield, E. M, Rinaldi, F, Glover, C. P, Wong, L. F, Caldwell, M. A, & Uney, J. B. Connexin 36 expression regulates neuronal differentiation from neural progenitor cells. PloS one. (2011). e14746. PubMed PMID: 21408068. Epub 2011/03/17. eng.

[38] Todorova, M. G, Soria, B, & Quesada, I. Gap junctional intercellular communication is required to maintain embryonic stem cells in a non-differentiated and proliferative state. Journal of cellular physiology. (2008). Feb;PubMed PMID: PMID: 17654515., 214(2), 354-62.

[39] Mclachlan, E, Shao, Q, & Laird, D. W. Connexins and gap junctions in mammary gland development and breast cancer progression. The Journal of membrane biology. (2007). Aug;218(1-3):107-21. PubMed PMID: 17661126. Epub 2007/07/31. eng.

[40] Lee, S. C, Cruikshank, S. J, & Connors, B. W. Electrical and chemical synapses between relay neurons in developing thalamus. Journal of Physiology. (2010). Jul 1;588(Pt 13):2403-15. PubMed PMID: 20457735. Epub 2010/05/12. eng.

[41] Bez, A, Corsini, E, Curti, D, Biggiogera, M, Colombo, A, Nicosia, R. F, et al. Neurosphere and neurosphere-forming cells: morphological and ultrastructural characterization. Brain Research. (2003). Dec 12;993(1-2):18-29. PubMed PMID: 14642827. Epub 2003/12/04. eng.

[42] Ross, R. A, Spengler, B. A, & Biedler, J. L. Coordinate morphological and biochemical interconversion of human neuroblastoma cells. Journal of the National Cancer Institute. (1983). Oct;PubMed PMID: 6137586. Epub 1983/10/01. eng., 71(4), 741-7.

[43] Wei, C. J, Francis, R, Xu, X, & Lo, C. W. Connexin43 associated with an N-cadherin-containing multiprotein complex is required for gap junction formation in NIH3T3 cells. Journal of Biological Chemistry. (2005). May 20;PubMed PMID: 15741167. Epub 2005/03/03. eng., 280(20), 19925-36.

[44] Jensen, M, & Berthold, F. Targeting the neural cell adhesion molecule in cancer. Cancer Letters. (2007). Dec 8;PubMed PMID: 17949897. Epub 2007/10/24. eng., 258(1), 9-21.

[45] Nishimura, T, Dunk, C, Lu, Y, Feng, X, Gellhaus, A, Winterhager, E, et al. Gap junctions are required for trophoblast proliferation in early human placental development. Placenta. (2004). Aug;PubMed PMID: 15193866. Epub 2004/06/15. eng., 25(7), 595-607.

[46] Striedinger, K, Petrasch-parwez, E, Zoidl, G, Napirei, M, Meier, C, Eysel, U. T, et al. Loss of connexin36 increases retinal cell vulnerability to secondary cell loss. European Journal of Neuroscience. (2005). Aug;PubMed PMID: 16101742. Epub 2005/08/17. eng., 22(3), 605-16.

[47] Gonzalez-nieto, D, Gomez-hernandez, J. M, Larrosa, B, Gutierrez, C, Munoz, M. D, Fasciani, I, et al. Regulation of neuronal connexin-36 channels by pH. Proceedings of

the National Academy of Sciences of the United States of America. (2008). Nov 4;PubMed PMID: PMID: 18957549; 0804189105 [pii]., 105(44), 17169-74.

[48] Srinivas, M, Rozental, R, Kojima, T, Dermietzel, R, Mehler, M, Condorelli, D. F, et al. Functional properties of channels formed by the neuronal gap junction protein connexin36. Journal of Neuroscience. (1999). Nov 15;PubMed PMID: 10559394. Epub 1999/11/13. eng., 19(22), 9848-55.

[49] Oguro, K, Jover, T, Tanaka, H, Lin, Y, Kojima, T, Oguro, N, et al. Global ischemia-induced increases in the gap junctional proteins connexin 32 (Cx32) and Cx36 in hippocampus and enhanced vulnerability of Cx32 knock-out mice. Journal of Neuroscience. (2001). Oct 1;PubMed PMID: 11567043. Epub 2001/09/22. eng., 21(19), 7534-42.

[50] Voigt, A, & Zintl, F. Effects of retinoic acid on proliferation, apoptosis, cytotoxicity, migration, and invasion of neuroblastoma cells. Medical and pediatric oncology. (2003). Apr;PubMed PMID: 12555246. Epub 2003/01/30. eng., 40(4), 205-13.

[51] Lofstedt, T, Jogi, A, Sigvardsson, M, Gradin, K, Poellinger, L, Pahlman, S, et al. Induction of ID2 expression by hypoxia-inducible factor-1: a role in dedifferentiation of hypoxic neuroblastoma cells. Journal of Biological Chemistry. (2004). Sep 17;PubMed PMID: 15252039. Epub 2004/07/15. eng., 279(38), 39223-31.

[52] Wiese, C, Rolletschek, A, Kania, G, Blyszczuk, P, Tarasov, K. V, Tarasova, Y, et al. Nestin expression--a property of multi-lineage progenitor cells? Cellular and molecular life sciences. (2004). Oct;61(19-20):2510-22. PubMed PMID: 15526158. Epub 2004/11/05. eng.

Chapter 6

Pathways of Intrinsic Apoptosis in Neuroblastoma: Targets for Therapeutics and New Drug Development

Fieke Lamers and Aru Narendran

Additional information is available at the end of the chapter

1. Introduction

Neuroblastoma (NB) is one of the most difficult to treat malignancies of early childhood that originates from the sympathetic nervous system and ranks high among the diseases with unacceptable fatality rates in paediatrics. Currently, children with high risk NB are treated with intensive multi-modal therapeutic regimens, but often endure disease recurrence that is refractory to further treatment. Hence, research strategies are urgently needed to discover novel therapeutic targets to advance the timely development of innovative treatment approaches for these children.

In general, growth and survival of tumors are thought to be defined largely by deregulated genetic processes such as cell cycle checkpoints, DNA damage repair mechanisms, oncogenes and tumor suppressor genes, resulting in enhanced and unregulated malignant cellular proliferation. These findings have contributed significantly to the development of various chemotherapeutic agents and current treatment protocols. In addition, recent studies have provided evidence for enhanced tumor survival as a consequence of the breakdown of the cell death mechanisms that otherwise safeguard the integrity of normal tissue homeostasis while evading over-proliferation.

Reports from several laboratories have shown that NB cells carry defective or silenced proapoptotic factors, such as caspases (cysteinyl aspartate-specific proteases; CASP) and have enhanced expression and activity of a range of pro-survival factors [1]. These observations led to the reasoning that better understanding of the apoptotic mechanisms that sustain the survival of NB cells could aid in the development of novel therapeutic approaches. The potential to target and modulate the life or death signals in cancer cells carries immense therapeutic potential and therefore research continues to focus on the understanding of the apoptosis process that intersects the growth and survival pathways of NB. It is hoped that this information will facilitate effective therapeutic drug discoveries.

2. Apoptosis

Under normal circumstances, cell death processes are characterized by distinct morphological changes and are classified as necrotic, apoptotic, autophagic or those coupled with mitotic catastrophe. Among these, apoptosis relates to programmed cell death that occurs in response to distinct signals such as hypoxia, excessive oncogene activation or chemotherapeutic agents. The mechanistic basis for this process involves the concerted activity of caspases, which inactivate or activate target substrates in a cascade of enzymatic activities. This sequence of activities is broadly grouped as the "extrinsic" and the "intrinsic" apoptotic pathway. The extrinsic pathway involves the engagement of cell surface "death receptors", activated by extra-cellular signals, which induce apoptosis by directly activating the caspase cascade. The "intrinsic" pathway, also known as the mitochondrial apoptotic pathway, is activated from within the cell in response to signals of cellular stress. This may occur as a result of deprivation of cell survival factors, DNA damage and increased levels of abnormally folded cellular proteins and reactive oxygen species [2], Figure 1. This process, in conjunction with the pro-apoptotic BCL2 family mediated pore formation, leads to the release of mitochondrial mediators such as DIABLO (SMAC) and CYCS (cytochrome c) [2]. Once released, CYCS complexes with APAF1 to mediate dATP/ATP dependent activation of APAF1 and pro-CASP9, leading to subsequent caspase activation, cell death and more release of DIABLO. However, this process also lends to the liberation of inhibitor-of-apoptosis protein (IAP) mediated inhibition of the pro-caspases [3-5]. Currently, however, it appears that in some cell types, alternate pathways can contribute to the cellular apoptotic activity.

3. BCL2 family of apoptosis regulators

By virtue of their ability to localize to mitochondrial membranes, the BCL2 family of proteins play a pivotal role in the regulation of mitochondrial apoptotic pathways [6]. They share at least one of four homologous regions known as BCL homology (BH) domains (BH1-BH4), which enable the formation of homo- and heterotypic dimers among these molecules. All anti-apoptotic effectors and members and some pro-apoptotic members, such as BAX and BAK1, share sequence homology of three or more of such domains, whereas the BH3-only proteins show sequence homology only within the BH3 domain [6, 7]. Such interactions are thought to form the mechanistic basis for the activity of BCL2 proteins. These proteins can be divided into anti-apoptotic members, including BCL2, BCL2L1 (BCL-XL), MCL1 and BCL2L2 (BCL-W), and pro-apoptotic members. The pro-apoptotic members can be divided into three groups: 1. proteins with multi-domain members: BAX and BAK1, which form pores in the mitochondrial membrane through which CYCS and DIABLO can be released, 2. the group of BH3-only members including proteins that inhibit anti-apoptotic members by binding directly, such as

PMAIP1 (NOXA), BAD and BIK and 3. the collection of pro-apoptotic BH3-only proteins that can either inhibit the anti-apoptotic members or induce BAX/BAK pore formation directly. This last group consists of BID, BCL2L11 (BIM) and BBC3 (PUMA) [6-8].

In cancer cells, the BCL2 family of proteins contribute to enhanced cell survival and expansion by blocking physiologically relevant cell death processes. Up-regulated BCL2 proteins also play a key role in the generation of resistance to chemotherapeutic drugs and radiotherapy by interfering with tumor cell death induced by cytotoxic agents [9]. In addition, they also offer protection against cell death pathways that are activated during conditions such as cytokine withdrawal. An altered expression of BCL2 proteins has been found in many cancers, including NB [10, 11]. Furthermore, transfection mediated over-expression of BCL2 or BCL2L1 in NB cells has been shown to generate a phenotype with acquired resistance to therapeutic agents [12]. Overall, current experimental evidence suggest that BCL2 expression critically regulates apoptosis and plays an important role in the tumorigenesis and survival of NB [13].

B-cell lymphoma-extra-large (BCL2L1, BCL-XL) is a mitochondrial membrane protein and a member of the BCL2 family. BCL2L1 has been shown to exhibit its anti-apoptotic properties by regulating mitochondrial homeostasis. Over-expression of BCL2L1 confers a multidrug resistance phenotype and protects tumor cells from chemotherapy induced differentiation and apoptosis. A recent study has shown that, in NB cells, repression of BCL2L1 by the proteasome inhibitor bortezomib resulted in the activation of pro-apoptotic PMAIP1, thereby triggering cell death [14]. Additional studies have shown that targeted inhibition of BCL2L1 in combi-nation with 4-HPR (a synthetic retinoid) can work synergistically to significantly increase differentiation and apoptosis in BCL2L1 bountiful NB cells [15, 16]. These data provide rationale for targeting regulatory pathways of BCL2 proteins in therapeutic approaches for NB patients.

4. Inhibitor of Apoptosis Proteins (IAPs)

The inhibitor of apoptosis proteins are a group of conserved molecules that are frequently over-expressed in tumors that confer survival properties and chemotherapy resistance [17, 18]. Structurally, these proteins are characterized by one to three baculoviral IAP repeats (BIR) domains, which carry characteristic caspase inhibitory activity. The known members of the human IAP family include, NAIP (BIRC1), c-IAP1 (BIRC2), c-IAP2 (BIRC3), XIAP (BIRC4), survivin (BIRC5), Apollon/Bruce (BIRC6) ML-IAP (BIRC7 or livin) and ILP-2 (BIRC8) [19]. IAPs appear to control both extrinsic and intrinsic apoptotic pathways. By virtue of their ubiquitin ligase activity, BIRC2 and BIRC3 regulate the extrinsic apoptotic pathway [20]. As for the effects on the intrinsic pathway, XIAP inhibits CASP3, CASP7 and CASP9 by direct binding. However, this activity can be diminished by DIABLO binding to XIAP through its N-terminal IAP-binding motif (IBM) [21]. Furthermore, the activity of DIABLO can be blocked by BIRC5 which can also bind and stabilize XIAP [22, 23].

BIRC5 (MW 16.5-kDa) is an IAP member protein found in dividing cells that carries at least one BIR domain and normally exists as a homodimer [24]. The expression of BIRC5 has been demonstrated in many diverse tumor types, including neuroblastoma and appears to correlate with poor prognosis [25]. Many potential mechanisms have been postulated for the regulation of cellular expression of BIRC5 in cancer cells, including its transcriptional repression by wild-type p53, gene amplification, hypomethylation, increased promoter activity, and loss of p53 function [26, 27]. BIRC5 appears to have multiple functions in the growth and survival of tumor cells [28]. Although not shown in all experimental systems, some studies have indicated a role for BIRC5 in the regulation of cellular caspase activity. For example, a report by Tamm and colleagues showed that BIRC5 can be co-immunoprecipitated with CASP3, CASP7, and CASP9 and it suppresses apoptosis following over-expression of these caspases [29]. In staurosporine (STS)–induced apoptosis in NB model, BIRC5 has been shown to exert its phase specific anti-apoptotic effect by inhibiting CASP9 activity [30]. Recently, using affymetrix mRNA expression analysis, a strong up-regulation of BIRC5 in NB cells compared to normal and fetal adrenal tissues and adult tumor specimens has been demonstrated [31]. Increased BIRC5 levels were also found to be associated with poorer prognosis, independent of chromosome 17q gain. Furthermore, antisense mediated silencing of BIRC5 in ten NB cell lines showed significantly increased apoptotic cell death defined by PARP cleavage and loss of cell viability.

In addition to its influence on programmed cell death, BIRC5 has also been shown to be a component of the chromosome passage protein complex (CPC), which is needed for chromosome alignment and segregation during mitosis and cytokinesis. The remaining constituents of CPC include AURKB (Aurora-B kinase), CDCA8 (Borealin), and INCENP [32]. Based on localization findings, *it has been postulated that* nuclear BIRC5 is involved in the control cell division, whereas cytoplasmic/mitochondrial BIRC5 is cytoprotective [33]. Constitutive expression of BIRC5 has also been demonstrated in a number of neuroblastoma cell lines [27]. BIRC5 knockdown in SK-N-BE2 and SH-SY-5Y NB cells caused an increase in expression of pro-apoptotic BAX and a decrease in anti-apoptotic BCL2 expression. A recent study by Miller and colleagues examined the relationship between CASP8 and BIRC5 levels and outcomes in neuroblastoma patients [34]. In this investigation, increased BIRC5 was found to be associated with poor overall survival and an increased BIRC5 to CASP8 ratio was associated with unfavorable histology and high risk stratification, indicating a combined influence of these two apoptosis associated factors in the clinical consequences of NB. Moreover, additional studies have shown that CASP8 is often hypermethylated in neuroblastoma tumors resulting in an inactive extrinsic apoptotic pathway [35-37].

BIRC7 is a member of the IAP family that has been found to play a notable role in apoptosis [38]. The expression of BIRC7 has been demonstrated in NB tumor specimens and cell lines [39]. Although the expression of BIRC7 by itself does not appear to be a prognostic marker, patients with increased BIRC7 expression and MYCN amplification had significantly poorer survival compared to those lacking both or either one of these markers. This suggests that NB patients with increased BIRC7 and MYCN may constitute a worse prognosis subset within the *MYCN* amplified group. Subsequently it has been shown that in cells that have increased MYCN and BIRC7, the suppression of MYCN leads to loss of BIRC7 [40]. An opposite effect was also seen when NB cells with low MYCN were induced to up-regulate MYCN, which led to increased BIRC7 levels. Furthermore, these studies also detected a consensus MYCN binding domain within the 5' proximal sequence of the putative BIRC7 promoter, indicating that MYCN is involved in the expression of BIRC7 and that BIRC7 may offset the effects of MYCN. Normally, NB cells with *MYCN* amplification show increased proliferation and paradoxically, increased sensitivity to apoptosis by chemotherapeutic agents [41]. Data provided by Dasgupta and colleagues suggest that MYCN may act as a transcriptional activator of BIRC7 expression and in cells co-expressing these genes, the anti-apoptotic effect of BIRC7 may counteract the apoptotic effects of *MYCN* amplification, thus enabling tolerance to cytotoxic agents and enhancing tumor growth and survival properties [42].

BIRC6 (also known as BIR-containing protein 6, Bruce or Apollon) is a giant 528 kDa highly conserved protein that has been implicated as a modulator of the intrinsic apoptotic pathway promoting cell survival. The apoptosis inhibitory functions of BIRC6 is mediated by its ability to bind to caspases through its BIR domain. In humans, BIRC6 has been shown to be involved in the generation of chemotherapy resistance in cancer cells [43]. *In vitro* studies have shown its ability to ubiquitylate DIABLO and consequently cause hindrance to apoptosis caused by DIABLO [44]. In addition, BIRC6 also binds to pro-CASP9 and inhibits its cleavage and activation [45]. The expression of BIRC6 in cancer has been investigated in a number of recent studies. For example, an up-regulation of BIRC6 has been found in gliomas that are resistant to treatment [43] and in pediatric ALL [46], where its over-expression appears to be associated with poor overall and disease free survivals. Gene copy number gains and increased expression of BIRC6 in primary NB specimens have been shown the silencing of BIRC6 leads to cell death in the NB cell line SKNSH [47]. Importantly, these studies have demonstrated that in neuroblastoma cells, BIRC6 binds to DIABLO and that DIABLO levels increase upon silencing of BIRC6, indicating a mechanism for the degradation of cytoplasmic DIABLO by BIRC6.

5. Targeted drug development

Experimental evidence regarding the role of the BCL2 family of proteins in the intrinsic apoptotic pathway of NB led to the evaluation of agents that are BH3 mimetics. These drugs compete with BH3 domains for interaction with the apoptosis inhibitors and prevent the inhibitors from sequestering the pro-apoptotic members [Reviewed in 48]. Prominent among these are ABT-737 and it's orally bioavailable analog, ABT-263. These small molecule inhibitors bind to BCL2, BCL2L1 and BCL2L2 with high affinity and induce apoptosis as single agents or in combination with chemotherapeutic agents based on the priming status of the inhibitors [49]. Studies by Klymenko et al showed that ABT-737 sensitizes NB cells to clinically relevant cytotoxic agents under normoxic conditions and maintains its activity under hypoxia, when tumor cells show resistance to these agents [49]. Using a BH3 profiling approach with mito-chondria isolated from NB cells, Goldsmith and colleagues have demonstrated that such profiles can accurately predict whole cell sensitivity to small molecule BCL2 family antagonists and may be useful in predicting response to agents, thereby targeting chemoresistance in NB [50]. Several studies have evaluated the mechanisms of potential emergence of resistance to ABT-737. MCL1 has been shown to confer resistance to ABT-737 because of the reduced affinity of ABT-737 for MCL1. Studies by Lestini, and co-workers have shown that in NB cells, resistance to ABT-737 can be overcome by MCL1 knockdown [51]. Currently, available data suggest the utility of effective target identification on tumor specimens to stratify responders and the formulation of drug combination regimens with MCL1 antagonists to enhance the clinical effectiveness of agents such as ABT-737 in future clinical trials [51, 52]. Compared to many NB cell lines, NB tumor specimens expressed high BCL2 [53]. The anti-tumor activity of ABT263 against cell lines with high BCL2 cell lines suggested the potential of targeting BCL2 for effective therapeutics [53].

Agents that target IAPs have also been evaluated in preclinical models of NB. Generally, two distinct approaches are being taken in the development and identification of effective inhibitors of IAP: antisense oligonucleotides and small molecular weight inhibitors [54]. Antisense oligonucleotides against XIAP and BIRC5 are already been evaluated in preclinical and early phase clinical trials for adult malignancies. YM155 (1-(2-Methoxyethyl)-2-methyl-4,9-dioxo-3-(pyrazin-2-ylmethyl)-4,9-dihydro-1H-naphtho[2,3-d]imidazolium bromide) has been shown to inhibit BIRC5 expression in a dose and time dependent manner leading to the activation of caspases in a variety of tumor models. Currently, YM155 has been evaluated in early phase clinical trials for adult tumors [55]. The effect of YM155 against a panel of NB cell lines have been examined, which showed that YM155 induced effective cytotoxicity in 14 of the 23 neuroblastoma cell lines, with an IC_{50} in the low nM range, although a direct correlation between the IC_{50} values in individual cell lines and extent of BIRC5 expression was not noted in this study [56]. However, mRNA array studies identified the expression of ABCB1 (MDR1) as the most predictive gene for the generation of resistance to YM155 and it was possible to sensitize resistant cells by ABCB1 knockdown.

Recently, a number of innovative screening approaches have been attempted to identify agents and drug combinations that target apoptotic pathways in NB. Tsang and colleagues have used a synthetic lethal screen approach to discover targets for effective therapeutic combinations with topotecan [57]. Their studies have found a number of genes whose suppression synergized with toptecan to enhance cell death. Notable among these were the NF-κB target genes. Furthermore, in drug combinations, known NF-κB inhibitors such as bortezomib were also found to induce caspase-3 activity in NB cell lines and delay tumor formation in xenograft mouse models. Specific molecular aberrations in NB and associated anti-apoptotic changes have also been used in drug screening studies. Recently, Zirath et al. have screened a library of 80 cytotoxic compounds to identify those that preferentially targeted the cells with MYC over-expression [58]. These studies have shown that MYC also increases sensitivity to targeted inhibition of certain cellular mechanisms including the activity of topoisomerases and the mitotic control machinery. In addition to cell lines, methods to screen for agents that selectively target patient-derived stem-like or tumor-initiating cells (TICs) have also been described [59]. The dequalinium analogue, C-14 linker (DECA-14), and rapamycin showed selective inhibition of NB TICs *in vitro* and a reduction in xenograft tumor growth and tumor initiating capacity.

6. Discussion

In comparison to the progress made in the treatment outcomes of a number of common pediatric malignancies, the survival rates of children diagnosed with NB with unfavorable biological features still remains unacceptably low. Hence, in the recent past a significant amount of research effort has been focused on the development of effective novel therapeutic approaches for the treatment of these children. With the application of cutting edge molecular technologies, recent years have seen a significant advancement in new knowledge regarding the complex molecular components and pathways involved in the diversity, growth, survival, differentiation, metastasis and treatment resistance of this disease. It is becoming evident that the over-expression of oncogenic survival factors and effective interference with normal cell death pathways appear to be key strategic characteristics of aggressive NB. As details of the components, role and regulators of the intrinsic apoptotic pathway in cancer emerge, it is expected that newer agents and novel therapeutic approaches, especially those with mecha-nistically validated drug combination regimens, will be developed for the treatment of refractory NB. In addition, the advent of molecular screening techniques such as Whole Genome Sequencing and Comparative Genomic Hybridization arrays may facilitate the screening of NB specimens from individual patients in high-throughput approach for target validation to advance future individualized therapeutic regimens.

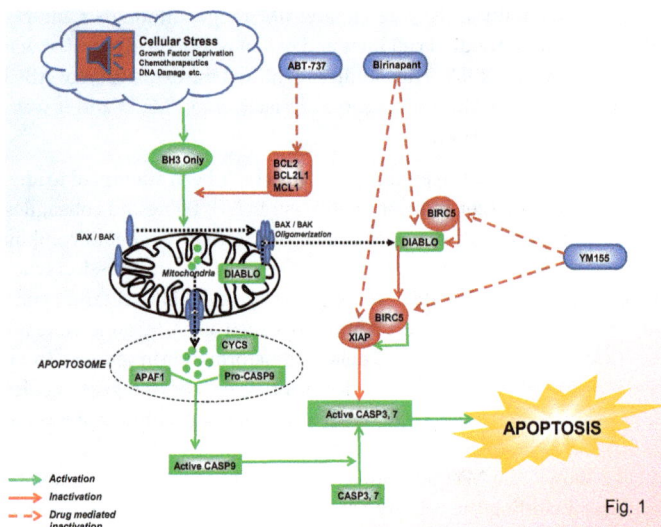

Figure 1. Schematic representation of key events of intrinsic apoptotic pathways.

The intrinsic pathway is triggered by stimuli from cytotoxic stress which leads to the up-regulation of BH3 only proteins and consequently the mitochondrial translocation and oligomerization of BAX/ BAK. This results in the release of cytochrome c which then binds to the pro-apoptotic factor Apaf-1 to form apoptosomes. Aptoptosomes then activate caspase-9, which in turn leads to the activation of caspases-3, 7 and subsequently to apoptosis. This process can be regulated by XIAP. In addition, the mitochondrial activation also leads to the release of SMAC /DIABLO which promotes apoptosis by directly interacting with IAPs and disrupting their ability to inactivate the caspases but itself can be modulated by BIRC5. In addition to IAPs, mitochondrial apoptosis can also be inhibited by the anti-apoptotic BCL2 family members such as BCL2, MCL1 and BCL-X$_L$. The points at which different targeted agents may interfere with their activities are also indicated.

Acknowledgements

We thank Prof. H.N. Caron, Prof. R. Versteegand and Dr. Molenaar for providing the research training that was invaluable in writing this review (FL). We acknowledge the technical assistance of Gaya Narendran in the preparation of Fig. 1.

This study was supported in part by a grant for AN from the Alberta Children's Hospital Foundation, Calgary, Alberta, Canada.

Author details

Fieke Lamers[1] and Aru Narendran[2]

1 Department of Oncogenomics, Academic Medical Center, University of Amsterdam, AZ Amsterdam, The Netherlands

2 Laboratory for Preclinical and Drug Discovery Studies, Pediatric Oncology Experimental Therapeutics Investigators' Consortium (POETIC). Division of Pediatric Oncology, Alberta Children's Hospital, University of Calgary, Calgary, Alberta, Canada

References

[1] Goldsmith, K. C. Hogarty MD Targeting programmed cell death pathways with ex-perimental therapeutics: opportunities in high risk neuroblastoma. Cancer Lett. (2005). Oct 18;228(1-2):133-41.

[2] Ouyang, L, Shi, Z, Zhao, S, Wang, F. T, Zhou, T. T, Liu, B, & Bao, J. K. Programmed cell death pathways in cancer: a review of apoptosis, autophagy and programmed necrosis. Cell Prolif. (2012). Dec;, 45(6), 487-98.

[3] García-sáez, A. J. The secrets of the Bcl-2 family. Cell Death Differ. (2012). Nov;, 19(11), 1733-40.

[4] Li, P, Nijhawan, D, Budihardjo, I, Srinivasula, S. M, Ahmad, M, Alnemri, E. S, & Wang, X. Cytochrome c and dATP-dependent formation of Apaf-1/caspase-9 com-plex initiates an apoptotic protease cascade. Cell. (1997). Nov 14;, 91(4), 479-89.

[5] Adams, J. M, & Cory, S. Apoptosomes: engines for caspase activation. Curr Opin Cell Biol. (2002). Dec;, 14(6), 715-20.

[6] Huang, Z. Bcl-2 family proteins as targets for anticancer drug design. Oncogene. (2000). Dec 27;, 19(56), 6627-31.

[7] Danial, N. N. BCL-2 family proteins: critical checkpoints of apoptotic cell death. Clin Cancer Res. (2007). Dec 15;, 13(24), 7254-63.

[8] Wang, K, Yin, X. M, Chao, D. T, Milliman, C. L, & Korsmeyer, S. J. BID: a novel BH3 domain-only death agonist. Genes Dev. (1996). Nov 15;, 10(22), 2859-69.

[9] Chao, D. T, & Korsmeyer, S. J. BCL-2 family: regulators of cell death. Annu Rev Immunol. (1998). , 16, 395-419.

[10] Reed, J. C. Dysregulation of apoptosis in cancer. J Clin Oncol. (1999). Sep;, 17(9), 2941-53.

[11] Coultas, L. Strasser A The role of the Bcl-2 protein family in cancer. Semin Cancer Biol. (2003). Apr;, 13(2), 115-23.

[12] Fulda, S, & Debatin, K. M. Caspase activation in cancer therapy, in: M. Los, H. Walczak (Eds.), Caspases-Their Role in Cell Death and Cell Survival, Kluwer Academic Press, (2002).

[13] Ikeda, H, Hirato, J, Akami, M, Matsuyama, S, Suzuki, N, Takahashi, A, & Kuroiwa, M. Bcl-2 oncoprotein expression and apoptosis in neuroblastoma. J Pediatr Surg. (1995). Jun;, 30(6), 805-8.

[14] Hagenbuchner, J, Ausserlechner, M. J, Porto, V, David, R, Meister, B, Bodner, M, Villunger, A, Geiger, K, & Obexer, P. The anti-apoptotic protein BCL2L1/Bcl-xL is neutralized by pro-apoptotic PMAIP1/Noxa in neuroblastoma, thereby determining bortezomib sensitivity independent of prosurvival MCL1 expression. J Biol Chem. (2010). Mar 5;, 285(10), 6904-12.

[15] Mohan, N, Banik, N. L, & Ray, S. K. Synergistic efficacy of a novel combination therapy controls growth of Bcl-x(L) bountiful neuroblastoma cells by increasing differentiation and apoptosis. Cancer Biol Ther. (2011). Nov 1;, 12(9), 846-54.

[16] Mohan, N, Banik, N. L, & Ray, S. K. Synergistic efficacy of a novel combination therapy controls growth of Bcl-x(L) bountiful neuroblastoma cells by increasing differentiation and apoptosis. Cancer Biol Ther. (2011). Nov 1;, 12(9), 846-54.

[17] Tamm, I, Kornblau, S. M, Segall, H, Krajewski, S, Welsh, K, Kitada, S, Scudiero, D. A, Tudor, G, Qui, Y. H, Monks, A, Andreeff, M, & Reed, J. C. Expression and prognostic significance of IAP-family genes in human cancers and myeloid leukemias. Clin Cancer Res. (2000). May;, 6(5), 1796-803.

[18] Cossu, F, Milani, M, Vachette, P, Malvezzi, F, Grassi, S, Lecis, D, Delia, D, Drago, C, Seneci, P, Bolognesi, M, & Mastrangelo, E. Structural insight into inhibitor of apopto-

sis proteins recognition by a potent divalent smac-mimetic. PLoS One. (2012). e49527. doi:journal.pone.0049527.

[19] De Almagro, M. C, & Vucic, D. The inhibitor of apoptosis (IAP) proteins are critical regulators of signaling pathways and targets for anti-cancer therapy. Exp Oncol. (2012). Oct;, 34(3), 200-11.

[20] Vucic, D, Dixit, V. M, & Wertz, I. E. Ubiquitylation in apoptosis: a post-translational modification at the edge of life and death. Nat Rev Mol Cell Biol. (2011). Jun 23;, 12(7), 439-52.

[21] Vaux, D. L, & Silke, J. Mammalian mitochondrial IAP binding proteins. Biochem Biophys Res Commun. (2003). May 9;, 304(3), 499-504.

[22] Song, Z, Yao, X, & Wu, M. Direct interaction between survivin and Smac/DIABLO is essential for the anti-apoptotic activity of survivin during taxol-induced apoptosis. J Biol Chem. (2003). Jun 20;, 278(25), 23130-40.

[23] Dohi, T, Okada, K, Xia, F, Wilford, C. E, Samuel, T, Welsh, K, Marusawa, H, Zou, H, Armstrong, R, Matsuzawa, S, Salvesen, G. S, Reed, J. C, & Altieri, D. C. An IAP-IAP complex inhibits apoptosis. J Biol Chem. (2004). Aug 13;, 279(33), 34087-90.

[24] Kelly, R. J, Lopez-chavez, A, Citrin, D, Janik, J. E, & Morris, J. C. Impacting tumor cell-fate by targeting the inhibitor of apoptosis protein survivin. Mol Cancer. (2011). Apr 6;10:35.

[25] Islam, A, Kageyama, H, Takada, N, Kawamoto, T, Takayasu, H, Isogai, E, Ohira, M, Hashizume, K, Kobayashi, H, Kaneko, Y, & Nakagawara, A. High expression of Survivin, mapped to 17q25, is significantly associated with poor prognostic factors and promotes cell survival in human neuroblastoma. Oncogene. (2000). Feb 3;, 19(5), 617-23.

[26] Hoffman, W. H, Biade, S, Zilfou, J. T, Chen, J, & Murphy, M. Transcriptional repression of the anti-apoptotic survivin gene by wild type J Biol Chem. (2002). Feb 1;277(5):3247-57., 53.

[27] Hossain, M. M, Banik, N. L, & Ray, S. K. Survivin knockdown increased anti-cancer effects of (-)-epigallocatechin-3-gallate in human malignant neuroblastoma SK-N-BE2 and SH-SY5Y cells. Exp Cell Res. (2012). Aug 1;, 318(13), 1597-610.

[28] Zangemeister-wittke, U, & Simon, H. U. An IAP in action: the multiple roles of survivin in differentiation, immunity and malignancy. Cell Cycle. (2004). Sep;, 3(9), 1121-3.

[29] Tamm, I, Wang, Y, Sausville, E, Scudiero, D. A, Vigna, N, Oltersdorf, T, & Reed, J. C. IAP-family protein survivin inhibits caspase activity and apoptosis induced by Fas (CD95), Bax, caspases, and anticancer drugs. Cancer Res. (1998). Dec 1;, 58(23), 5315-20.

[30] Chandele, A, Prasad, V, Jagtap, J. C, Shukla, R, & Shastry, P. R. Upregulation of sur-
      vivin in G2/M cells and inhibition of caspase 9 activity enhances resistance in stauro-
      sporine-induced apoptosis. Neoplasia. (2004). Jan-Feb;, 6(1), 29-40.

[31] Lamers, F, Van Der Ploeg, I, Schild, L, Ebus, M. E, Koster, J, Hansen, B. R, Koch, T,
      Versteeg, R, Caron, H. N, & Molenaar, J. J. Knockdown of survivin (BIRC5) causes
      apoptosis in neuroblastoma via mitotic catastrophe. Endocr Relat Cancer. (2011). Oct
      27;, 18(6), 657-68.

[32] Lens, S. M, Vader, G, & Medema, R. H. The case for Survivin as mitotic regulator.
      Curr Opin Cell Biol. (2006). Dec;, 18(6), 616-22.

[33] Li, F, Yang, J, Ramnath, N, Javle, M. M, & Tan, D. Nuclear or cytoplasmic expression
      of survivin: what is the significance? Int J Cancer. (2005). Apr 20;, 114(4), 509-12.

[34] Miller, M. A, Ohashi, K, Zhu, X, Mcgrady, P, London, W. B, Hogarty, M, & Sandler,
      A. D. Survivin mRNA levels are associated with biology of disease and patient sur-
      vival in neuroblastoma: a report from the children's oncology group. J Pediatr Hema-
      tol Oncol. (2006). Jul;, 28(7), 412-7.

[35] Teitz, T, Lahti, J. M, & Kidd, V. J. Aggressive childhood neuroblastomas do not ex-
      press caspase-8: an important component of programmed cell death. J Mol Med
      (Berl). (2001). Aug;, 79(8), 428-36.

[36] Eggert, A, Grotzer, M. A, Zuzak, T. J, Wiewrodt, B. R, Ho, R, Ikegaki, N, & Brodeur,
      G. M. Resistance to tumor necrosis factor-related apoptosis-inducing ligand (TRAIL)-
      induced apoptosis in neuroblastoma cells correlates with a loss of caspase-8 expres-
      sion. Cancer Res. (2001). Feb 15;, 61(4), 1314-9.

[37] Van Noesel, M. M, Van Bezouw, S, Voûte, P. A, Herman, J. G, Pieters, R, & Versteeg,
      R. Clustering of hypermethylated genes in neuroblastoma. Genes Chromosomes
      Cancer. (2003). Nov;, 38(3), 226-33.

[38] Kasof, G. M, & Gomes, B. C. Livin, a novel inhibitor of apoptosis protein family
      member. J Biol Chem. (2001). Feb 2;, 276(5), 3238-46.

[39] Kim, D. K, Alvarado, C. S, Abramowsky, C. R, Gu, L, Zhou, M, Soe, M. M, Sullivan,
      K, George, B, Schemankewitz, E, & Findley, H. W. Expression of inhibitor-of-apopto-
      sis protein (IAP) livin by neuroblastoma cells: correlation with prognostic factors and
      outcome. Pediatr Dev Pathol. (2005). Nov-Dec;, 8(6), 621-9.

[40] Dasgupta, A, Peirce, S. K, & Findley, H. W. MycN is a transcriptional regulator of li-
      vin in neuroblastoma. Oncol Rep. (2009). Oct;, 22(4), 831-5.

[41] Fulda, S, Lutz, W, Schwab, M, & Debatin, K. M. MycN sensitizes neuroblastoma cells
      for drug-induced apoptosis. Oncogene. (1999). Feb 18;, 18(7), 1479-86.

[42] Dasgupta, A, Alvarado, C. S, Xu, Z, & Findley, H. W. Expression and functional role of inhibitor-of-apoptosis protein livin (BIRC7) in neuroblastoma. Biochem Biophys Res Commun. (2010). Sep 10;, 400(1), 53-9.

[43] Chen, Z, Naito, M, Hori, S, Mashima, T, Yamori, T, & Tsuruo, T. A human IAP-family gene, apollon, expressed in human brain cancer cells. Biochem Biophys Res Commun. (1999). Nov 2;, 264(3), 847-54.

[44] Hao, Y, Sekine, K, Kawabata, A, Nakamura, H, Ishioka, T, Ohata, H, Katayama, R, Hashimoto, C, Zhang, X, Noda, T, Tsuruo, T, & Naito, M. Apollon ubiquitinates SMAC and caspase-9, and has an essential cytoprotection function. Nat Cell Biol. (2004). Sep;, 6(9), 849-60.

[45] Qiu, X. B, & Goldberg, A. L. The membrane-associated inhibitor of apoptosis protein, BRUCE/Apollon, antagonizes both the precursor and mature forms of Smac and caspase-9. J Biol Chem. (2005). Jan 7;, 280(1), 174-82.

[46] Ismail, E. A, Mahmoud, H. M, Tawfik, L. M, Habashy, D. M, Adly, A. A, Sherif, N. H, & Abdelwahab, M. A. BIRC6/Apollon gene expression in childhood acute leukemia: impact on therapeutic response and prognosis. Eur J Haematol. (2012). Feb;, 88(2), 118-27.

[47] Lamers, F, Schild, L, Koster, J, Speleman, F, Ora, I, Westerhout, E. M, Van Sluis, P, Versteeg, R, Caron, H. N, & Molenaar, J. J. Identification of BIRC6 as a novel intervention target for neuroblastoma therapy. BMC Cancer. (2012). Jul 12;12:285.

[48] Stamelos, V. A, Redman, C. W, & Richardson, A. Understanding sensitivity to BH3 mimetics: ABT-737 as a case study to foresee the complexities of personalized medicine. J Mol Signal. (2012). Aug 16;7(1):12. doi:

[49] Klymenko, T, Brandenburg, M, Morrow, C, Dive, C, & Makin, G. The novel Bcl-2 inhibitor ABT-737 is more effective in hypoxia and is able to reverse hypoxia-induced drug resistance in neuroblastoma cells. Mol Cancer Ther. (2011). Dec;, 10(12), 2373-83.

[50] Goldsmith, K. C, Lestini, B. J, Gross, M, Ip, L, Bhumbla, A, Zhang, X, Zhao, H, Liu, X, & Hogarty, M. D. BH3 response profiles from neuroblastoma mitochondria predict activity of small molecule Bcl-2 family antagonists. Cell Death Differ. (2010). May;, 17(5), 872-82.

[51] Lestini, B. J, Goldsmith, K. C, Fluchel, M. N, Liu, X, Chen, N. L, Goyal, B, Pawel, B. R, & Hogarty, M. D. Mcl1 downregulation sensitizes neuroblastoma to cytotoxic chemotherapy and small molecule Bcl2-family antagonists. Cancer Biol Ther. (2009). Aug;, 8(16), 1587-95.

[52] Goldsmith, K. C, Gross, M, Peirce, S, Luyindula, D, Liu, X, Vu, A, Sliozberg, M, Guo, R, Zhao, H, Reynolds, C. P, & Hogarty, M. D. Mitochondrial Bcl-2 family dynamics

define therapy response and resistance in neuroblastoma. Cancer Res. (2012). May 15;, 72(10), 2565-77.

[53] Lamers, F, Schild, L, Koster, J, Versteeg, R, Caron, H. N, & Molenaar, J. J. Targeted BIRC5 silencing using YM155 causes cell death in neuroblastoma cells with low ABCB1 expression. Eur J Cancer. (2012). Mar;, 48(5), 763-71.

[54] Schimmer, A. D, & Dalili, S. Targeting the IAP family of caspase inhibitors as an emerging therapeutic strategy. Hematology Am Soc Hematol Educ Program. (2005). , 2005, 215-9.

[55] Tolcher, A. W, Mita, A, Lewis, L. D, Garrett, C. R, Till, E, Daud, A. I, Patnaik, A, Papadopoulos, K, Takimoto, C, Bartels, P, Keating, A, & Antonia, S. Phase I and pharmacokinetic study of YM155, a small-molecule inhibitor of survivin. J Clin Oncol. (2008). Nov 10;, 26(32), 5198-203.

[56] Lamers, F, Schild, L, Koster, J, Versteeg, R, Caron, H. N, & Molenaar, J. J. Targeted BIRC5 silencing using YM155 causes cell death in neuroblastoma cells with low ABCB1 expression. Eur J Cancer. (2012). Mar;, 48(5), 763-71.

[57] Tsang, P. S, Cheuk, A. T, Chen, Q. R, Song, Y. K, Badgett, T. C, Wei, J. S, & Khan, J. Synthetic lethal screen identifies NF-κB as a target for combination therapy with topotecan for patients with neuroblastoma. BMC Cancer. (2012). Mar 21;12:101

[58] Frenzel, A, Zirath, H, Vita, M, Albihn, A, & Henriksson, M. A. Identification of cytotoxic drugs that selectively target tumor cells with MYC overexpression. PLoS One. (2011). e27988. doi:journal.pone.0027988. Epub 2011 Nov 23.

[59] Smith, K. M, Datti, A, Fujitani, M, Grinshtein, N, Zhang, L, Morozova, O, Blakely, K. M, Rotenberg, S. A, Hansford, L. M, Miller, F. D, Yeger, H, Irwin, M. S, Moffat, J, Marra, M. A, Baruchel, S, Wrana, J. L, & Kaplan, D. R. Selective targeting of neuroblastoma tumour-initiating cells by compounds identified in stem cell-based small molecule screens. EMBO Mol Med. (2010). Sep;, 2(9), 371-84.

Chapter 7

Analysis of Apoptotic and Autophagic Pathways in Neuroblastoma by Treatment with Copper Compounds

Enrique Hernández-Lemus,
Anllely Grizett Gutiérrez, Adriana Vázquez-Aguirre,
M. Lourdes Palma-Tirado, Lena Ruiz-Azuara and
Carmen Mejía

Additional information is available at the end of the chapter

1. Introduction

Neuroblastoma (NB) is the most common extra-cranial tumor of childhood with more than 600 new cases per year in the United States. The clinical presentation is heterogeneous and dependent on age at diagnosis, staging, histology, and alterations such as *MYCN* amplification and chromosome 1p loss or 17q gain. High-risk patients with evidence of metastases have an overall survival rate of less than 40% despite intensive multimodality treatment. This highlights the urgent need for new therapeutic intervention strategies. However due to NB characteristic molecular features, in about 10% of patients with metastases, tumors disappear by apoptosis [1].

In the search of new anticancer agents with increased chemotherapeutic spectrum, and lower toxicity, new substances based on metals have shown initial promising results. Casiopeínas® (Cas) are a family of compounds with a central Cu^{2+} core atom and an amino acid acidates or α, β-diketonates to seem give them tumor specificity [2]. To date, their action mechanisms are still not completely understood. A possible mechanism may be envisaged however, since it has been described that metals such as Copper and some complexes of them, participate in redox reactions that may generate reactive oxygen species (ROS) including Hydrogen peroxide (H_2O_2), hydroxyl radical (HO●) and superoxide (O_2^-●) [3] that are probably the main factors, leading to apoptosis in cells exposed to these anti-tumor compounds [4-6]

Programmed cell death is an important process for the regulation of different pathways such as cellular homeostasis, embryonic development or regulation of the immune system [7-9].

Apoptosis, a form of programmed cell death, is a highly cotrolled process which includes several well-characterized morphological changes, like membrane blebbing and cell shrinkage, chromatic condensation and nuclear fragmentation [10].The induction of apoptosis may involve either extracellular triggering signals as tumor necrosis factor or endogenous signals such as a cytochrome c (cyt C) release [11], followed by caspase-and endonuclease-activation [12], resulting in the disassembly of nuclear chromatin and degradation of oligonucleosomal DNA.

Several studies have identified other cell death programs clearly distinct from apoptosis [13], and even if we know they are genetically regulated and often have morphological features resembling necrosis, their underlying molecular mechanisms remain unclear. Autophagy is a process that regulates the amount of cell death that occurs in response to specific stimuli like blocking apoptosis after growth factor depletion [14-15] or external insults as DNA damaging agents [16] protecting against caspase-independent death [17] and also by the action of a large variety of anticancer drugs [18].

2. Casiopeínas, a new compound against cancer

Copper is an essential transition metal involved in diverse biological functions, quite especially in redox balance processes [19]. Due to its properties, Copper and its complexes have the ability to catalyze the generation of ROS by means of the Fenton reaction [20]. This process might cause oxidative modification of cellular components like lipids, DNA and proteins, thus disturbing the redox balance and interfering with the redox-related cellular signaling pathways [21].

Casiopeínas is a family of new antineoplastic agents that have been synthesized, characterized and patented in base of chelated Copper (II) complexes. Their general formula is [Cu(N–N)(a-L-aminoacidate)]NO$_3$ and [Cu(N–N)(O-O)]NO$_3$, where the N–N donor is an aromatic substituted diimine (1,10-phenanthroline or 2,20-bipyridine) and the O-O donor is acac or salal (Figure 1). The underlying hypothesis is that nature, number and position of the substituents on the diimine ligands, and modification of a-L-amino acidate or O–O donor will have an effect either on the selectivity or on the degree of biological activity shown by the mixed ternary Copper (II) complexes. Chemical data for Casiopeínas are: Cas IIgly [elemental analysis data: calculated (%) for CuC16H16O5N4 2H20 (443.90 g/mol)]: C, 43.29; N, 12.62; H, 4.54. Found (%): C, 43.59; N, 12.61; H, 4.52); Cas IIIia [(elemental analysis data: calculated (%) for CuC17H19O5N3 2H20 (444.93 g/mol): C, 45.89; N, 9.44; H, 5.21. Found (%): C, 46.59; N, 9.80; H 4.93)] and Cas IIIEa [(elemental analysis data: calculated (%) for CuC19-H19O5N3 H20 (450.94 g/mol): C, 50.61; N, 9.32; H, 4.69. Found (%): C, 51.37; N, 9.40; H 4.46)] [22].

Cas have been tested, both *in vitro* and *in vivo*, and have shown cytotoxic, genotoxic [23] and antitumor activity [5, 24]. Cas have been shown good therapeutic indexes in human ovarian carcinoma (CH1), murine leukemia (L1210), AS-30D rat hepatoma, cervix-uterine (HeLa), breast, colon (HCT40) carcinomas, murine glioma C6, and human medulloblastoma (Daoy)

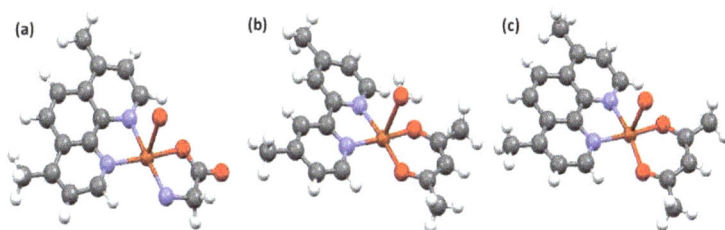

Figure 1. Structures of Casiopeínas.(a) Cas IIgly [Cu (4,7-dimethyl-1,10-phenantroline) (glycinato) (H$_2$O)] NO$_3$; **(b)** Cas IIIia [4,4'-dimethyl-2,2'-bipiridina) (acetylacetonato) (NO$_3$)]. **(c)** Cas IIIEa [Cu (4,7-dimetyl-1,10-phenantroline) (acetylacetonato) (H$_2$O)] NO$_3$

and neuroblastoma (CHP-212 and SK-N-SH) cells [25-29]. As well as in animal tumor models such isolated rat hearts [30], dogs [31-32], and nude mice models [5].

The precise mechanism of action for each Cas is still not completely understood and a detailed description of the events that lead to cell death remains unexplained. However, there is evidence that supports that these compounds are able to inhibit cell proliferation and produce cell death by apoptosis by means of mechanisms dependent of caspases activation and independent of caspases throughout ROS generation [24, 26, 29]. It has been shown that Cas are able to block oxidative phosphorylation and to bind DNA by adenine and thymine interactions [33-35], and computational modeling has been done in order to explain such an interaction [36-37]. This suggests that there is more of than one biochemical action mechanism for Cas.

3. Apoptosis by means of Casiopeínas in neuroblastoma

According to previous research results of our group, neuroblastoma cell lines CHP-212 and SK-N-SH have showed that Cas IIgly, IIIia and IIIEa, were active even at very low concentrations (8 μg/ml) when compared to cisplatin, their more efficient competing treatment [29]. These NB cells also showed a differential sensitivity for every Cas treatment and cell lineage at 24 h. This last finding may be due a selectivity given for the specific ligands in the Copper core. For instance, Cas IIgly and Cas IIIEa contain the same imine (4,7-dimethyl,1,10-phenanthroline) with a different charged ligand (glycine *vs* acetylacethonate). Then Cas IIIEa turned out to be more active for CHP-212, whereas Cas IIgly is more active for SK-N-SH cell line. Cellular origin of NB cell lines or even the lack of caspase-8 cleaved expression [38], are features that may define the behavior of NB towards Cas.

Since caspase-8 is commonly silenced in NB, mitochondrial apoptosis is the preferential route to apoptotic cell death, which may involve endogenous process such as cyt C release from mitochondria, resulting in disruption of the mitochondrial transmembrane potential (Δψm) [39]. This event generates a reduction in ATP levels with an influx of ions that leads to decreased mitochondrial activity, and opening of the mitochondrial permeability transition pores [40]. This is an essential component for caspase-3 activation [41].

Under stress conditions such as those produced by Cas, the cell could promote several survival *Stimuli*, one of them is expression of the Bcl-2 family of proteins. Even when Bcl-2 protein is found in the cytoplasmic fraction of treated cells, its expression does not result enough to stop the apoptotic process. In contrast, the expression of the well-known apoptosis promoter Bax is decreased in neuroblastoma cells treated with Cas. Casiopeínas then possess several mitochondrial targets in NB. The main effects of these is production of ROS that in turn provoke $\Delta\psi m$ loss, with an augmented Bcl-2 and cyt C release and a massive entrance of Bax protein. By considering, all this body of evidence together we may support the position that the apoptotic pathway favored by Casiopeínas in NB is the intrinsic route [29].

4. Autophagy and Copper compounds in neuroblastoma

Autophagy is a dynamic process that involves the arrest of cytoplasmic portions and intra-cellular organelles in large double-membrane vesicles (autophagosomes). When these vesicles are fused with lysosomes they generate autophagolysosomes and mature lysosomes, where the arrested material is degraded, inducing cell death [42-43].

Constitutive autophagy enables the physiologic turnover of intracellular components, thus playing an important function in cell homeostasis. However, autophagy can be rapidly induced as a defensive stress response [44-45]. Although apoptosis and autophagic cell death present distinct morphological features among themselves, the two pathways overlap at the level of various signaling steps and may converge and be integrated at the level of the same organelles (i.e. the lysosome and the mitochondrion) [48].

Another molecule involved in the autophagic process is the cytoplasmic form of LC3-I, which during the formation of autophagosomes is cleaved and liquefied to give rise to the membra-nous form LC3-II. The expression levels of LC3-II can be used to estimate the abundance of autophagosomes before they are degraded by lysosomal hydrolases and the subcellular localization of LC3 redistributes from a cytosolic diffuse pattern to punctuate staining in vacuolar membranes when autophagy is induced. Increased autophagic activity is then reflected by the enhanced conversion of LC3-I to LC3-II.

In a model of rat glioma C6 treated with Cas IIIia were found augmented levels of LC3, particularly of LC3-II, leading to an increased ratio of LC3-II/LC3-I. These results indicate that Cas IIIia induced autophagy promoters such as LC3-II and Beclin-1 [47]. When autophagy was subsequently prevented with 3-methyladenine (3-MA), localization of LC3 at the autophago-somal membrane was inhibited and tumor cells were rescued from cell death [48]. Meanwhile, when neuroblastoma cells (CHP-212) were treated with Cas IIgly, Cas IIIia, Cas IIIEa and cisplatin, LC3-II increases protein at 2 h and 10 h were observed. However at 24 h this molecule was absent, indicating that there was another event different to cellular death [50].

Beclin-1 is a clue regulator of autophagy that directly interacts with Bcl-2, because when they are bound, Beclin-1 is incapable of activating autophagy. However, autophagy is induced by the release of Beclin-1 from Bcl-2 by pro-apoptotic BH3 proteins, Beclin-1 phosphorylation by

DAP kinase (DAPK), or Bcl-2 phosphorylation by JNK [50-51]. Conversely, over-expression of Bcl-2 or Bcl-X_L can inhibit autophagy [52-54]. Another Beclin-1-dependent mechanism by which apoptosis can inhibit autophagy is through caspase-3 cleavage of Beclin-1 to produce a truncated protein that is unable to promote autophagy, thus leading to the overall inhibition of autophagy [55].

Depending of the *status* of caspase-3, neuroblastoma cells may switch between autophagic and apoptotic cell death. It was found that a targeted toxin kills glioma cells *via* a caspase-independent mechanism, and when autophagy is inhibited, this increases (modestly) the amount of death, but changes dramatically the mode of death by allowing the toxin to activate caspases. These data show that autophagy can alter the way cells die, not just whether they die or not [56].

Autophagy in cells treated with Casiopeínas may be result of a diminished effect of this compound that on low doses may not be efficient enough to produce apoptosis. Thus, caspase-3 activity was found in neuroblastoma cells, yet at very early times (2 and 4 h); whilst at 24 h this protein was totally absent [29]. This event is probably seemed to point out that low doses of Cas treatments enable the physiologic turnover of the tumoral cells. In a model of C6 rat glioma cells treated with low doses (5-10 µg/ml) of Casiopeína IIIa, effects at 24 h were also compatible with autophagic features [32].

5. The role of ROS in apoptosis and autophagy in NB

Among several effector mechanisms are involved in the control and regulation of cell death pathways, including autophagy and apoptosis, it seems that the starting point is related with changes in the cellular redox *status*. In the cell, this stage is determined by the balance between rates of production and breakdown of ROS, including free radicals such as superoxide, hydroxyl radical and non-radicals capable of to generate free radicals (i.e., H_2O_2) [57].

A deeper understanding of the mechanisms linking the oxide-radicals-induced autophagy response to cell death pathways, may suggest new therapeutic strategies for the treatment of oxidative stress-associated diseases and phenotypic conditions. For instance, apoptosis observed with Cas treatments, might be the result of one or several events which lead to this final effect: these signals could be mediated by generation of ROS [23-24, 29], by mitochondrial toxicity [58], or both, and might play –either alone or cooperatively- an important role in the regulation of cell death induced by this type of complexes. Several studies have shown that inhibition of cell proliferation and DNA degradation [59-60]) in the presence of reducing agents is simultaneous to ROS generation, suggesting that DNA oxidation observed on cells might also be triggering cell death.

Exposure of C6 glioma cells to Cas IIIa resulted in cell death, with structural and biochemical features consistent with autophagy and apoptosis. Furthermore, the involvement of ROS generation and JNK activation, were showed to be the main features of the autophagic and apoptotic pathways [47]. Hydrogen peroxide reacts with the superoxide radical to constitute itself into a non-radical reactive species. Even toughH_2O_2 is less reactive than radical oxygen it can produce higher levels of cellular damage. Since it hydrolyzes metals -specially iron Fe(II) and Copper Cu(I)- giving rise to Fenton reactions, a phenomenon already documented in Cas-therapy [6, 58].

On the other hand, it has been reported that low H_2O_2 concentrations (as low as 100µM), are able to induce several events including morphological cell changes, DNA fragmentation and caspase-activation in leukemia cell lines [61]. For this reason H_2O_2 increase by Cas treatment might be implied, either in apoptosis induction or participating as a substrate in Fenton's reaction, producing hydroxyl radical which is a highly reactive and affecting different biomolecules, which not only may cause an apoptotic process but also secondary necrosis. ROS increase could then promote p53-mediated increase of both Bax messenger and protein, implicating cyt C release and consequently promoting caspase-3 activation [62]. In neuroblastoma cells, Cas treatments can induce ROS expression that in turn is related with mitochondrial apoptosis [29].

Superoxide radical is produced when molecular oxygen accepts an electron which remains unpaired. Within the cell this process takes place mainly in the mitochondria, since as a consequence of metabolism, oxygen receive transported electrons [63]. Superoxide synthesis is increased by the influence of factors as radiation or chemicals like pharmaceutical drugs and narcotics. Treatment by Cas increase the concentrations of superoxide thus promoting an unusually high oxidizing environment. This highly oxidant environment cannot be regulated by means of the usual antioxidant defense mechanisms of the cell [6, 23]. For this reason oxidative stress appears, thus damages biomolecules, in particular mitochondrial DNA [58]. As a consequence, cells die *via* the intrinsic route to apoptosis [29, 49]

Previous findings suggest that Copper–phenanthroline complexes react in a redox-cycle with thiols and H_2O_2, resulting in ROS production [64]. On the other hand, glutathione (GSH) indexes haves been related directly to apoptosis due to the ROS expression. In order to maintain the basal concentrations of GSH in the cell, glutathione reductase (Grd) reduces GSS to GSH [65]. Intracellular GSH decrement is thus related to ROS production, because the sulphydril group of Cas is charged in order to trap reactive species that forms a coordinated covalent link with the metal, thus reducing GSH to GSS, by means of a nucleophilic substitution reaction. Platinum is, in the other hand, a soft metal which has affinity to soft donors like those in glutathione's cysteine group. This link may be the mechanism by which the cells eliminate cisplatin. Such processes are implied in producing the low levels of GSH detected in both cell lines after cisplatin treatment, since elimination of cisplatin related to GSS avoids Grd regeneration of the basal levels of GSH. This effect has been reported in several neoplasic lines after the treatment with cisplatin [6, 58].

In fact, Copper has been reported as reacting with GSH to form a stable complex [58]. Nevertheless, it is not clear if this is the elimination mechanism for Cas, or if this complex interferes with the process of GSH regeneration. Decrease in intracellular levels of GSH has been reported in murine melanoma and pulmonary cancer cells treated with Cas IIgly, since Cas catalyzes Fenton's reaction and GSH acts catching the produced ROS [6, 29, 58]. These results allow us to explain the decreased intracellular levels of GSH resulting after treatment with Cas. This comes as a result of a pro-oxidant atmosphere, which could be produced since Fenton's reaction is catalyzed through the active Copper core in Casiopeínas. Our results support the hypothesis that, under certain conditions, GSH can be a substrate for pro-oxidant reactions in the cell. CasII gly has been previously shown to interfere directly with the mitochondrial respiratory chain, another effect that could account for an increase in ROS [66]. However, both, delayed ROS burst and mitochondrial depolarization observed by flow cytometry, support Cas IIgly-mediated indirect effects, i.e. GSH depletion and disruption of the mitochondrial respiratory chain due to mitochondrial DNA damage. Given the fast drop in GSH levels, such delay may be due to the ability of the cells to initially control ROS levels, including O_2-● and HO●; however, after some time this ability results exhausted.

The activation of either the pro-survival or the pro-death pathways by oxidative stress depends on the type of ROS and the site of its generation [65, 67], the dose and length of exposure, as well as on the genetic and metabolic background of the target cell [68-73]. Understanding the mechanisms linking the oxide-radicals-induced autophagy response to cell death pathways could suggest new therapeutic strategies for the treatment of neuroblastoma.

6. Pathways and biological processes

As we have seen the action mechanisms of Cas-based chemotherapeutics involves system-level interactions of a number of biochemical processes in the cell, including apoptosis, autophagy, and response to oxidative stress as main motifs; but also involving (to some extent) signaling pathways such as NGF, SCF-KIT, interleukins, and FGFR. Immune response processes involving interferon (alpha/beta), PI3K/AKT; as well as B-cell activation and phosphorylation cascades. With so many complex processes interacting one may wonder what the driving forces (and what the 'side-effects') are.

In order to acquire a closer understanding of these processes, we performed computational and data-mining analyses in both protein-protein interactions and biochemical pathway enrichment. Particular emphasis has been paid to molecular interactions related with the turnover between apoptosis and autophagy since these are the main mechanisms of cell death observed in NB cells after Cas treatment.

6.1. Protein interaction networks

Computational mining in protein-protein interaction databases (String) was performed in a curated list of molecules associated with apoptosis. The results may be seen in Figure 2. Panel A presents the associated protein-protein (physical) interaction network. Panel B renders a visualization of the same network color- and size-coded according with their connectivity degree: big red circles represent protein that are highly connected within such network (i.e. proteins that may interact in a large number of macromolecular assemblies and other functional roles) while small green nodes are less connected proteins.

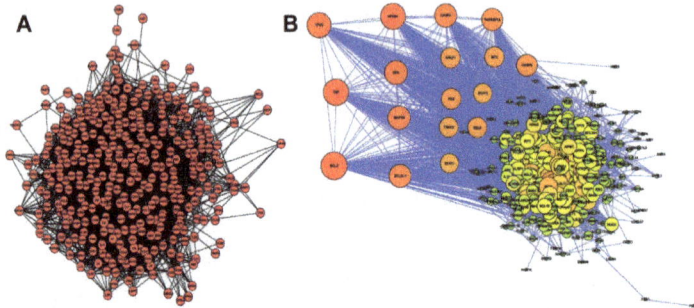

Figure 2. Protein interaction network of apoptotic molecules Panel A displays the protein-protein (physical) interaction network for molecules playing a role in apoptotic processes. Panel B renders a visualization of the same network color- and size-coded according with their number of known interactions. Big, red circles are thus highly interacting apoptotic molecules.

One may hypothesize that highly connected proteins (or hubs) perform central roles in their corresponding biochemical pathways [73]. In fact, by considering the hubs in Figure 2 B we may see this. Molecules such as TP53, TNF, BCL2, NFKB1, BAX, MAPK8, BCL2L1, CASP3, APAF1, FAS, TRAF2, STAT1, TNFRSF1A, MYC, STAT3, RELA, and CASP8 seem to be the main players in the pro-apoptotic/anti-apoptotic molecular switching. These general trends may vary from one tissue/phenotype to another (for instance CASP8 is usually absent or mildly expressed in NB cells) yet their compact interaction structure allows for biological robustness, as displayed for instance in the complementary roles of intrinsic and extrinsic apoptosis.

A similar analysis was performed for molecules associated with autophagy; in Figure 3 we can see the protein interaction network for these molecules. Again panel A shows the protein-protein network. Panel B also displays the network color- and size-coded according with the individual connectivity degree. The key players in this process seem to be MTOR, TP53, UBA52, BCL2, BECN1, AKT1, FAM48 A, and to a lesser extent PTEN, ULK1, PIK3C3, ATG5, HSP90AA1 and JUN. Interestingly enough this network is not so densely connected as the one corresponding to apoptosis (Figure 2) a fact that may result in important outcomes: the network is less robust to removal of one of its key players hence the regulatory mechanisms should be more strict. This may be a reason for apoptosis (and not autophagy) as the main mechanism of cell death.

Given the fact that treatment by Casiopeínas in NB may involve a turn-over between apoptotic and autophagic cell death, it results appealing to analyze the protein interaction network of molecules common to both processes since these molecules may serve as switches between both regimes. In Figure 4 we can see the depiction of a (much simpler) protein interaction network involving molecules related both to apoptosis and autophagy: main players in both processes are BCL2, TP53, and AKT1 with TNFSF10, TRAF6, BNIP3 and BECN1 also associated. Again, response to oxidative stress, DNA damage and cell signaling are represented in

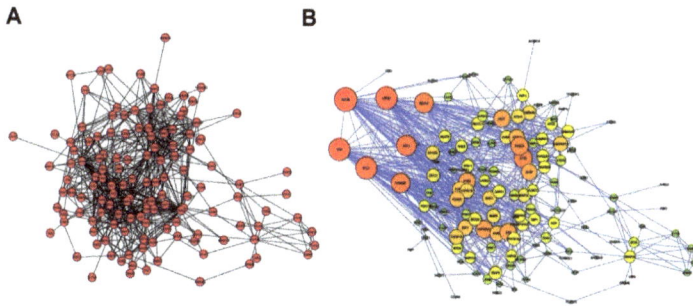

Figure 3. Protein interaction network of autophagic molecules Panel A displays the protein-protein (physical) interaction network for molecules playing a role in authphagy. Panel B renders a visualization of the same network color- and size-coded according with their number of known interactions. Big, red circles are highly interacting autophagic molecules.

this set. Especially intriguing results the role of AKT1 since it is known that some survival factors, induce transcription-independent anti-apoptotic behavior by activation of the oncogene-homolog RAC. AKT1 in turn, phosphorylates inactivating components of the apoptotic machinery.

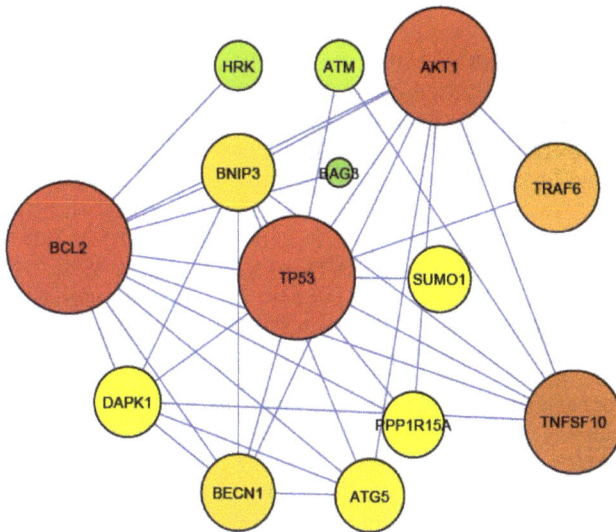

Figure 4. Protein interaction network of molecules involved both in apoptotic and autophagic pathways Molecules are again size and color-coded according with the number of interactions. The role of BCL2, TP53 and AKT1 as strongly interacting molecules centrally-involved both in apoptosis and autophagy may point to these molecules as concertators for the transition between these processes.

6.2. Coupled biochemical pathways

After considering physical interactions between proteins related both to apoptosis and autophagy, we may wonder which are the most common cellular processes involving such molecules. Resorting to data-mining and enrichment analyses in the REACTOME database we found the following pathways (see Fig.4).

7. Conclusions

In the search for new keys to undermine neuroblastoma, our knowledge of the pathways limiting tumor growth, as well as a deeper understanding of the molecules involved in these processes result essential. Based on years of research, our experience is that chemotherapeutic interventions based in Copper compounds as an essential metal, have opened new possibilities to understand not only the pharmacology but indeed some of the biology behind neuroblastoma's behavior. In this sense, we consider of extreme importance to understand, for instance, how Casiopeínas affect neuroblastoma cells in such a way that they finally undergo cellular death by apoptosis, or either -in what resembles a failed attempt of cellular rescue- resort to autophagy. By identifying key molecules for these processes by means of functional genomics and similar analyses we may be able to determine if there are other routes involved in neuroblastoma's final-fate decision processes.

With regards to apoptosis associated molecules, these also take part in biological functions such as: NGF-signaling (TRIB3, MAPK7, RAF1, PRKAR1A, MDM2, BCL2L11, DUSP6, NFKBIA, NGFR, RIPK2, BRAF, NGFRAP1, MYD88, **MAPK8**, NFKB1, **AKT1**, PIK3R1, CASP9, CHUK, GSK3B, SRC, CASP2, MLLT7, AKT3, FOXO1A, **STAT3**, FOXO3A, MAGED1, TRAF6, MAPK1, BAD, CDKN1A, RELA, **CASP3**, HRAS, NTRK1, AATF, YWHAE, NGFB, GRB2), Interleukin-signaling (IL6ST, IL18, STAT5A, RAF1, IL3, CARD15, CSF2RB, HRAS, RIPK2, MYD88, STAT5B, NFKB1, **STAT1**, PIK3R1, CARD4, CHUK, IL1A, JAK1, IL2RG, IL6, STAT3, CASP1, TRAF6, IL1R1, MAPK1, GRB2, IL7), SCF-KIT signaling (BAD, TRIB3, CDKN1A, STAT5A, RAF1, MDM2, HRAS, STAT5B, **AKT1**, **STAT1**, PIK3R1, CASP9, CHUK, GSK3B, SRC, MLLT7, FOXO1A, AKT3, STAT3, FOXO3A, MAPK1, GRB2) and activation of BAD and translocation to the mitochondria (BAD, **AKT1**, **BCL2**, BID); amongst others (full enrichment analysis –more than 500 statistically significant (p<0.05) processes- available upon request).

In the case of autophagic molecules, they also participate in the following biological processes: PI3K/AKT activation (PTEN, PDK1, Lst8, FoxO3, PKB, FoxO1, **MTOR**), adaptive immune system (TAK1, **ATG5**, LRSAM1, **BCL2**, ATG7, ATG12, PKR, Rab7, PDK1, FoxO1, CD46, HMGB1, **PTEN**, RAGE, JNK1, FoxO3, Lst8, Vps34, PKB, TRAF6, **MTOR**), as well as in the regulation of apoptosis (JNK1, **BCL2**, ZIPK, PKB, TRAIL, HMGB1, DAPK) by activation of BAD and translocation to mitochondria (**BCL2**, PKB) also among many others [full enrichment analysis of more than 200 statistically significant (p<0.05) pathways available upon request].

One interesting case for study in the analysis of apoptotic and autophagic pathways as an effect of Cas therapy, is the biochemical processes (other than apoptosis and autophagy) involving apoptotic/autophagic molecules, these involve autodegradation of the E3 ubiquitin ligase COP1 (**ATM, TP53**) related to DNA damage repair, NOD-like receptor signaling (**BCL2, TRAF6**) closely associated with inflammatory processes, and immune system preparation (**AKT1, BCL2, SUMO1, TRAF6, ATG5**). In all the biological response of NB to treatment with Cas seem to involve oxidative stress causing immune response, cytokine inflammation and DNA damage leading to cell death initiation either by apoptosis or autophagy depending on the specific kinase signaling present.

Acknowledgements

This work was supported by grants from ICYTDF (PICSA10-61 and PIUTE 10-92) and PAPIIT-UNAM 204511.

Author details

Enrique Hernández-Lemus[1,2], Anllely Grizett Gutiérrez[3], Adriana Vázquez-Aguirre[3], M. Lourdes Palma-Tirado[4], Lena Ruiz-Azuara[5] and Carmen Mejía[3]

*Address all correspondence to: maria.c.mejia@uv.es

1 Computational Genomics Department, National Institute of Genomic Medicine, México, D.F, México

2 Center for Complexity Sciences, National Autonomous University of México, México, D.F, México

3 Genomic Medicine and Environmental Toxicology Department, Institute of Biomedical Research, National Autonomous University of México, México, D.F, México

4 Microscopy Unit, Neurobiology Institute, Campus Juriquilla, National Autonomous University of México, Querétaro, México

5 Inorganic and Nuclear Chemistry Department, School of Chemistry, National Autonomous University of México, México, D.F, México

References

[1] Uccini S, Colarossi C, Sccarpino S, Boldrini R, Natali PG, Nicotra MR, *et al.* Morpho logical and molecular assessment of apoptotic mechanisms in peripheral neuroblastic tumours. British J Cancer 2006; 95,49-55.

[2] Ruiz-Azuara L, Bravo-Gómez ME. Copper compounds in cancer chemotherapy. Current Med Chem 2010; 17(31):3606-3615.

[3] Ferrer-Sueta G, Ruiz-Ramírez L, Radi R. Ternary Copper complexes and manganese (III) tetrakis (4-benzoic acid) porphyrin catalyze peroxynitrite-dependent nitration of aromatics. *Chem Res Toxicol* 1997; 10,1338–1344.

[4] De Vizcaya-Ruiz A, Rivero-Müller A, Ruiz-Ramirez L, Howarth JÁ, Dobrota M. Hematotoxicity response in rats by the novel Copper-based anticancer agent: casio peina II. Toxicology 2003; 194, 103–113.

[5] Carvallo-Chaigneau F, Trejo-Solís C, Gómez-Ruiz C, Rodríguez-Aguilera E, Macías-Rosales L, Cortés-Barberena E, Cedillo-Pelaez C, Gracia-Mora I, Ruiz-Azuara L, Madrid-Marina V, Constantino-Casas F. Casiopeina III-ia induces apoptosis in HCT-15 cells in vitro through caspase-dependent mechanisms and has antitumor effect in vivo. Biometals 2008; 21(1),17-28.

[6] Alemón-Medina R, Bravo-Gómez ME, Gracia-Mora MI, Ruiz-Azuara L. Comparison between the antiproliferative effect and intracellular glutathione depletion induced by Casiopeína IIgly and cisplatin in murine melanoma B16 cells. Toxicol in Vitro *2011;* 25,868–873

[7] Degterev A, Boyce M, Yuan J. A decade of caspases. Oncogene 2003; 22, 53,8543–8567.

[8] Jacobson MD, Weil M, Raff MC. Programmed cell death in animal development. Cell 1997; 88 (3),347–354.

[9] Nicholson DW, Thornberry NA. Apoptosis. Life and death decisions. Science 2003; 299(5604),214–215.

[10] Susin SA, Daugas E, Ravagnan L, Samejima K, Zamzami N, Loeffle N, Constantini P, Ferri KF, Irinopoulou T, Prevost MC, Brothers G, Mak TW, Penninger J, Earnshaw WC, Kroemer G. Two distinct pathways leading to nuclear apoptosis. J Exp Med 2000; 192(4),571-580.

[11] Bossy-Wetzel E, Newmeyer DD, Green DR. Mitochondria cytochrome *c* release in apoptosis occurs upstream of DEVD-specific caspase activation and independently of mitochondrial transmembrane depolarization. EMBO J 1998; 17(1), 37-49.

[12] Sakahira H, Enari M, Nagata S. Cleavage of CAD inhibitor in CAD activation and degradation during apoptosis. Nature 1998; 391(6662),96-99

[13] Leist M, Jäättelä M. Four deaths and a funeral: from caspases to alternative mechanisms. Nat Rev Mol Cell Biol 2001; 8,589–598.

[14] Boya P, Gonzalez-Polo RA, Casares N, Perfettini JL, Dessen P, Larochette N, Métivier D, Meley D, Souquere S, Yoshimori T, Pierron G, Codogno P, Kroemer G. Inhibition of macroautophagy triggers apoptosis. *Mol Cell Biol* 2005; 25, 1025–1040.

[15] Lum JJ, Bauer, DE, Kong M, Harris MH, Li C, Lindsten T, Thompson CB. Growth factor regulation of autophagy and cell survival in the absence of apoptosis. Cell 2005; 120(2),237-248.

[16] Shimizu S, Kanaseki T, Mizushima N, Mizuta T, Arakawa-Kobayashi S, Thompson CB, Tsujimoto Y. Role of Bcl-2 family proteins in a non-apoptotic programmed cell death dependent on autophagy genes. Nat Cell Biol 2004; 6(12),1221-1228.

[17] Colell A, Ricci JE, Tait S, Milasta S, Maurer U, Bouchier-Hayes L, Fitzgerald P, Guio-Carrion A, Waterhouse NJ, Li CW, Mari B, Barbry P, Newmeyer DD, Beere HM, Green DR. GAPDH and autophagy preserve survival after apoptotic Cytochrome c release in the absence of caspase activation. Cell 2007; 129(5),983-997.

[18] Kondo Y, Kanzawa T, Sawaya R, Kondo S. The role of autophagy in cancer development and response to therapy. Nat Rev Cancer 2005; 5,726-734.

[19] Fraústo da Silva JJJR, Williams RJP. The Biological Chemistry of theElements – The Inorganic Chemistry of Life. Oxford UniversityPress, Oxford, 1991.

[20] Valko M, Morris H, Cronin MT. Metals, toxicity and oxidative stress. Curr Med Chem 2005; 12,1161-1208.

[21] Huang R, Wallqvist A, Covell DG. Anticancer metal compounds in NCI's tumor-screening database: putative mode of action. Biochem Pharmacol 2005; 69(7), 1009-1039.

[22] Ruiz Azuara, L. Patente, Enero 26, (1994) no. 172967; SECOFI 18802. P. I. (1990). Patente Dic.9 (1993) no. 172248; US Patent Ap 21 (1992) Number 5, 107, 005. Re35, 458, Feb. 18 (1997); U. S. Patent Pat.No. 5,576,326. Nov. 19 (1996) [®Trade Mark: Casiopeína. Reg. 407543 SECOFI (1992), renewal (2002), (2012)]

[23] Alemón-Medina R, Muñoz-Sánchez JL, Ruiz-Azuara L, Gracia-Mora I. Casiopeína IIgly induced cytotoxicity to HeLa cells depletes the levels of reduced glutathione and is prevented by dimethyl sulfoxide. Toxicol in Vitro 2008; 22,710-715.

[24] Trejo-Solis C, Palencia G, Zuniga S, Rodriguez-Ropon A, Osorio-Rico L, Luvia ST, Gracia-Mora I, Marquez-Rosado L, Sanchez A, Moreno-Garcia ME, Cruz A, Bravo-Gomez ME, Ruiz-Ramirez L, Rodriguez-Enriquez S, Sotelo J. CasIIgly induces apoptosis in glioma C6 cells in vitro and in vivo through caspase dependent and – independent mechanisms. Neoplasia 2005; 7(6),563-574.

[25] Ruiz-Ramírez L, De La Rosa ME, Gracia-Mora I, Mendoza A, Pérez G, Ferrer-Sueta G, Tovar A, Breña M, Gutierrez P, Cruces-Martinez MP. Casiopeinas, metal-based drugs a new class of antineoplastic and genotoxic compounds. J Inorganic Biochem 1995; 207,2-3.

[26] De Vizcaya-Ruiz A, Rivero-Muller A, Ruiz-Ramirez L, Kass GE, Kelland LR, Orr RM, Dobrota M. Induction of apoptosis by a novel copper-based anticancer compound,

casiopeina II, in L1210 murine leukaemia and CH1 human ovarian carcinoma cells. Toxicol in Vitro 2000; 14, 1,1-5.

[27] Gracia-Mora I, Ruiz-Ramírez L, Gómez-Ruiz C, Tinoco-Méndez M, Márquez-Quiñones A, Romero de Lira L, Marín-Hernández A, Macías-Rosales L, Bravo-Gómez ME. Knight's move in the periodic table, from copper to platinum, novel antitumor mixed chelate copper compounds, casiopeinas, evaluated by an in vitro human and murine cancer cell line panel. Metal Based Drug 2001; 8, 1,19-29.

[28] Mejia C, Ruiz-Azuara L. Casiopeinas IIgly and IIIia Induce Apoptosis in Medulloblas- toma Cells. Pathol Oncol Res 2008; 14,467–472.

[29] Gutiérrez AG. Apoptosis mediante especies reactivas de oxígeno en el neuroblastoma, por efecto de Casiopeinas®. M.D. thesis. Universidad Nacional Autónoma de México; 2012.

[30] Hernández-Esquivel L, Marín-Hernández A, Pavón N, Carvajal K, Moreno-Sánchez R. Cardiotoxicity of copper-based antineoplastic drugs casiopeinas is related to inhibition of energy metabolism. Toxicol Appl Pharmacol 2006; 212(1),79-88.

[31] Cañas-Alonso RC, Fuentes-Noriega I, Ruiz-Azuara L. Pharmacokinetics of Casiopeína IIgly in Beagle Dog: A Copper Based Compound with Antineoplastic Activity. J Bioanal Biomed 2010; 2,028-034.

[32] Leal-García M, García-Ortuño L, Ruiz-Azuara L, Gracia-Mora I, Luna-Delvillar J, Sumano H. Assessment of acute respiratory and cardiovascular toxicity of casiopeinas in anaesthetized dogs. Basic Clin Pharmacol Toxicol 2007; 101(3), 151-158.

[33] Rivero-Müller A, De Vizcaya-Ruiz A, Plant N, Ruiz L, Dobrota M. Mixed chelate Copper complex, CasiopeinaIIgly®, binds and degrades nucleic acids: A mechanism of cytotoxicity. Chemico-Biol Inter 2007; 165(3),189–199.

[34] Rodríguez-Enríquez S, Gallardo-Pérez JC, Avilés-Salas A, Marín-Hernández A, Carreño-Fuentes L, Maldonado-Lagunas V, Moreno-Sánchez R. Energy metabolism transition in Multi-Cellular Human Tumor Spheroids. J Cell Physiol 2008; 216,189–197.

[35] Marín-Hernández A, Gallardo-Pérez JC, López-Ramírez SY, García-García JD, Rodríguez-Zavala JS, Ruiz-Ramírez L, Gracia-Mora I, Zentella-Dehesa A, Sosa-Garrocho M, Macías-Silva M, Moreno-Sánchez R, Rodríguez-Enríquez S. Casiopeina II-gly and bromo-pyruvate inhibition of tumor hexokinase, glycolysis, and oxidative phosphorylation. Arch Toxicol 2012; 86(5),753-766.

[36] García-Ramos JC, Tovar-Tovar A, Hernández-Lima J, Cortés-Guzmán F, Moreno-Esparza R, Ruiz-Azuara L. A new kind of intermolecular stacking interaction between Copper (II) mixed chelate complex (Casiopeína III-ia) and adenine. Polyhedron 2011; 2697-2703.

[37] Galindo-Murillo R, Hernández-Lima J, González-Rendón M, Cortés-Guzmán F, Ruiz-Azuara L, Moreno-Esparza R. Stacking between Casiopeinas ® and DNA bases. *Phys Chem Chem Phys* 2011; 13,14510-14515.

[38] Li LC, Sheng JR, Mulherkar N, Prabhakar BS, Meriggioli MN. Regulation of apop- tosis and caspase-8 expression in neuroblastoma cells by isoforms of the IG20 gene. Cancer Res 2008; 68,7352-7361.

[39] Rincheval V, Bergeaud M, Mathieu L, Leroy J, Guillaume A, Mignotte B, Le Floch N, Vayssière JL. Differential effects of Bcl-2 and caspases on mitochondrial permeabilization during endogenous or exogenous reactive oxygen species-induced cell death: A comparative study of H(2)O (2), paraquat, t-BHP, -induced cell death. Cell Biol Toxicoletoposide and TNF- 2012; 4,239-253.

[40] Garcia-Saez AJ, Chiantia S, Salgado J, Schwille P. Pore formation by a Bax-derived peptide: effect on the line tension of the membrane probed by AFM. Biophys J 2007; 93,103-112.

[41] Budd SL, Tenneti L, Lishnak T, Lipton SA. Mitochondrial and extramitochondrial apoptotic signaling pathways in cerebrocortical neurons. Proc Natl Acad Sci U S A 2000; 97(11):6161-6166.

[42] Baehrecke EH. Autophagy dual roles in life and death?. Nat Rev Mol Cell Biol 2005; 6(6),505-510.

[43] Eskelinen EL, Saftig P. Autophagy: a lysosomal degradation pathway with a central role in health and disease. Biochim Biophys Acta 2009; 1793(4):664-673.

[44] Kim EH, Sohn S, Kwon HJ, Kim SU, Kim MJ, Lee SJ, Choi KS. Sodium selenite induces ces superoxide-mediated mitochondrial damage and subsequent autophagic cell death in malignant glioma cells. Cancer Res 2007; 67(13):6314-6324.

[45] Williams A, Jahreiss L, Sarkar S, Saiki S, Menzies FM, Ravikumar B, Rubinsztein DC. Aggregate-prone proteins are cleared from the cytosol by autophagy: therapeutic implications. Curr Top Dev Biol 2006; 76:89-101.

[46] Kurz T, Eaton JW, Brunk UT. Redox activity within the lysosomal compartment: implications for aging and apoptosis. Antioxid Redox Signal 2010; 13(4):511-523.

[47] Trejo-Solís C, Jimenez-Farfan D, Rodriguez-Enriquez S, Fernandez-Valverde F, Cruz-Salgado A, Ruiz-Azuara A, Sotelo J. Copper compound induces autophagy and apoptosis of glioma cells by reactive oxygen species and jnk activation. BMC Cancer 2012; 12,156.

[48] Kanzawa T, Germano IM, Komata T, Ito H, Kondo Y, Kondo S. Role of autophagy in temozolomide-induced cytotoxicity for malignant glioma cells. Cell Death Differ 2004; 11(4),448–457.

[49] Vázquez-Aguirre A, Gutiérrez A, Bravo-Gómez ME, Ruiz-Azaura L, Mejía C. Advan-
      ces in Neuroblastoma Research 2012: Determination of apoptosis and autophagy in
      neuroblastoma by Casiopeínas®, June 17-22, 2012, Toronto, Canada; 2012.

[50] Wei Y, Pattingre S, Sinha S, Bassik M, Levine B. JNK1-mediated phosphorylation of
      Bcl-2 regulates starvation-induced autophagy. Mol Cell 2008; 30(6):678-688.

[51] Pattingre S, Tassa A, Qu X, Garuti R, Liang XH, Mizushima N, Packer M, Schneider
      MD, Levine B. Bcl-2 antiapoptotic proteins inhibit Beclin 1-dependent autophagy.
      Cell 2005; 122(6):927-939

[52] Chipuk JE, Moldoveanu T, Llambi F, Parsons MJ, Green DR. The BCL-2 family reun-
      ion. Mol Cell 2010; 37(3):299-310.

[53] Erlich S, Mizrachy L, Segev O, Lindenboim L, Zmira O, Adi-Harel S, Hirsch JA, Stein
      R, Pinkas-Kramarski R. Differential interactions between Beclin 1 and Bcl-2 family
      members. Autophagy 2007; 3(6):561-568

[54] Levine B, Sinha S, Kroemer G. Bcl-2 family members: dual regulators of apoptosis
      and autophagy. Autophagy. 2008;4(5):600-606.

[55] Luo S, Rubinsztein DC. Apoptosis blocks Beclin 1-dependent autophagosome syn
      thesis: an effect rescued by Bcl-xL. Cell Death Differ 2010; 17(2):268-277.

[56] Thorburn J, Horita H, Redzic J, Hansen K, Frankel AE, Thorburn A. A. Autophagy
      regu23 lates selective HMGB1 release in tumor cells that are destined to die. Cell
      Death Dif- fer 2009; 16(1):175–183.

[57] Kamata H, Honda S, Maeda S, Chang L, Hirata H, Karin M. Reactive oxygen species
      promote TNF alpha-induced death and sustained JNK activation by inhibiting MAP
      kinase phosphatases. Cell 2005; 120(5),649–661.

[58] Kachadourian R, Brechbuhl HM, Ruiz-Azuara L, Gracia-Mora I, Day BJ. Casiopeína
      IIgly-induced oxidative stress and mitochondrial dysfunction in human lung cancer
      A549 and H157 cells. *Toxicol* 2010; 268,176–183.

[59] Becco L, Rodríguez A, Bravo ME, Prieto MJ, Ruiz-Azuara L, Garat B, Moreno V,
      Gambino D. New achievements on biological aspects of copper complexes Casiopeí
      nas®: interaction with DNA and proteins and anti-Trypanosoma cruzi activity. J In
      org Biochem 2012; 109:49-56.

[60] Serment-Guerrero J, Cano-Sanchez P, Reyes-Perez E, Velazquez-Garcia F, Bravo-Go-
      mez ME, Ruiz-Azuara L. Genotoxicity of the copper antineoplastic coordination
      com- plexes casiopeinas. Toxicol In Vitro. 2011 Oct; 25(7):1376-1384.

[61] Gruss-Fischer T, Fabian I. Protection by ascorbic acid from denaturation and release
      of cytochrome c, alteration of mitochondrial membrane potential and activation of
      multiple caspases induced by H(2)O(2), in human leukemia cells. Biochem Pharma-
      col 2002; 63(7):1325-1335.

[62] Chantara W, Watcharasit P, Thiantanawat A, Satayavivad J. Acrylonitrile-induced extracellular signal-regulated kinase (ERK) activation via protein kinase C (PKC) in SK-N-SH neuroblastoma cells. J Appl Toxicol 2006; 26,517-523.

[63] Michel H. Cytochrome c oxidase: catalytic cycle and mechanisms of proton pumping-a discussion. Biochem 1999; 16,15129-15140.

[64] Antholine WE, Kalyanaraman B, Petering DH. ESR of copper and iron complexes with antitumor and cytotoxic properties. Environ Health Perspect 1985; 64:19-35.

[65] Circu ML, Aw TY. Reactive oxygen species, cellular redox systems, and apoptosis. Free Rad Biol Med 2010; 48,749-762.

[66] Marin-Hernandez A, Gracia-Mora I, Ruiz-Ramírez L, Moreno-Sánchez R. Toxic effects of Copper-based antineoplastic drugs (Casiopeinas) on mitochondrial functions. Biochem Pharmacol 2003; 65,1979-1989.

[67] Groeger G, Quiney C, Cotter TG. Hydrogen peroxide as a cell-survival signaling molecule. Antioxid Redox Signal 2009; 11(11):2655-2671.

[68] Castino R, Isidoro C, Murphy D. Autophagy-dependent cell survival and cell death in an autosomal dominant familial neurohypophyseal diabetes insipidus in vitro model. FASEB J 2005; 19(8):1024-1026.

[69] Brieger K, Schiavone S, Miller J, Krause K. Reactive oxygen species: from health to disease. Swiss Med Wkly 2012; 142:0. doi: 10.4414/smw.2012.13659.

[70] Choi K, Kim J, Kim GW, Choi C. Oxidative stress-induced necrotic cell death via mitochondira-dependent burst of reactive oxygen species. Curr Neurovasc Res 2009; 6(4):213-222.

[71] Chen J, Gusdon AM, Thayer TC, Mathews CE. Role of increased ROS dissipation in prevention of T1D. Ann N Y Acad Sci 2008; 1150:157-166.

[72] Huang Q, Shen HM. To die or to live: the dual role of poly(ADP-ribose) polymerase-1 in autophagy and necrosis under oxidative stress and DNA damage. Autophagy 2009; 5(2):273-276.

[73] Barabási AL, Oltvai ZN. Network biology: understanding the cell's functional organization. Nat Rev Genet 2004; 5(2):101-113.

Neuroblastoma, Biology - 2

Chapter 8

Neuroblastoma Integrins

Shanique A. Young, Ryon Graf and
Dwayne G. Stupack

Additional information is available at the end of the chapter

1. Introduction

In the body, cells are surrounded and supported by an intricate network of glycoproteins and proteoglycans that make up a complex extracellular matrix, or ECM. Many constituents, such as collagen, laminin, and fibronectin, are locally produced within the tissues, where they act as physical scaffolds, growth factor depots, and points of anchorage [1]. The local rigidity and composition of the matrix also provide environmental cues that govern cell behavior.

The ECM surrounding cells can be considered in two broad classes. On one hand, there exists a 'physiologic' ECM, present in all tissues, that aids in structuring and maintaining homeostasis. Typical ECM components include several collagens and laminins, as well as proteoglycans. On the other hand, there is a provisional ECM that is deposited during wounding, hemostasis and tissue remodeling. This ECM is typically deposited, digested and replaced in a very dynamic manner, and contains proteins such as fibronectin, fibrin, vitronectin and even residual fragments of collagen and laminin. This type of ECM promotes tissue remodeling as well as cellular survival, proliferation and invasion. In both types of ECM, however, the diversity in the type and quantity of each individual ECM component present determines the physical properties of these tissues. In so doing, this modulates the mechanical forces sensed by cells that bind to the ECM, and provides yet another layer of information relayed to cells. This 'mechanosensation' requires integrins, receptors that can transmit extracellular forces to the actin cytoskeleton.

Although many classes of receptors can interact with components of the ECM, the integrins are regarded as the principle receptors mediating anchorage and attachment to the ECM [2]. The name integrin was derived from initial observations that these receptors permitted a realignment of the actin cytoskeleton to match that of an underlying ECM. Integrins are transmembrane glycoprotein receptors that are composed of a heterodimer of α and β subunits

[3]. There are 18 different α subunits and 8 β subunits, but there are a limited number of possible combinations that can form from these subunits. To date, at least 24 unique integrin complexes have been identified, each with its own binding specificity for different subsets of ligands (Figure 1). Cells will generally express only a limited number of integrins, perhaps 10 of these combinations. The particular repertoire of integrins expressed by a given cell varies, but is typically closely tied to a cell's particular extracellular microenvironment. Differences in integrin binding to a ligand can be subtle. For example, approximately one third of human integrins bind to an arginine-glycine-aspartic acid (RGD) sequence of amino acid residues, but this can be profoundly conformation specific, and thus not all 'RGD-binding' integrins are capable of binding all RGD sequences with appreciable affinity.

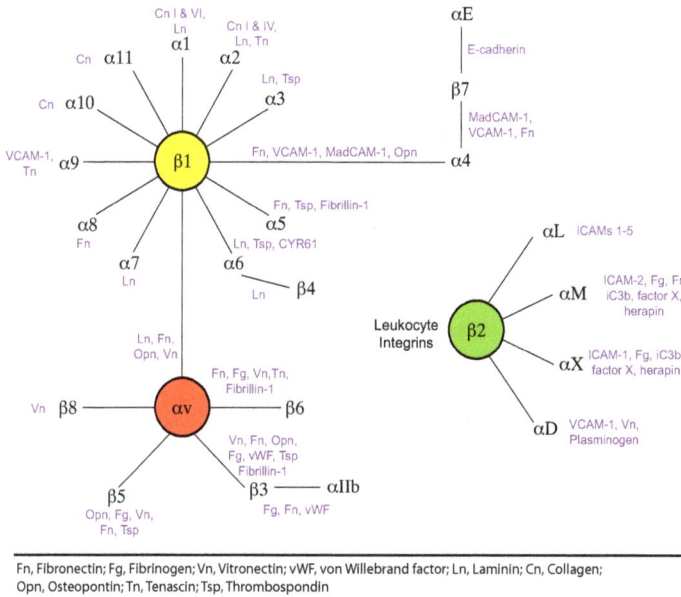

Fn, Fibronectin; Fg, Fibrinogen; Vn, Vitronectin; vWF, von Willebrand factor; Ln, Laminin; Cn, Collagen; Opn, Osteopontin; Tn, Tenascin; Tsp, Thrombospondin

Figure 1. Integrin heterodimers and their ligands This diagram shows the 24 known heterodimers and their ligands. Integrin heterodimers are represented by an α and a β subunit connected by a black line. For example, the β1 subunit dimerizes with 12 different α subunits. The ligands for each heterodimer are written in purple.

1.1. Integrin structure

Each integrin is composed of a large extracellular region of 600-1000 amino acids, as well as a single transmembrane domain. The extracellular regions can be broadly thought of in terms of a head and stalk (leg/thigh) region; the head is the critical site for ligand binding and divalent cation binding, as well as heterodimerization between the α and β subunits. Most integrins also have a small (~30-50 amino acid) cytosolic domain, with the singular exception being integrin β4, which has a large cytosolic domain that interacts with intermediate filaments [4]. Integrins are cysteine–rich proteins, and have extensive crosslinking within domains that stabilize domain structure. Thus, integrins appear at different sizes when analyzed on reducing and non-reducing gels, and detection of integrins by some antibodies may require either condition, depending upon the linearity or conformation dependence of an epitope.

The integrin extracellular domains are required for and sufficient to bind to ECM or to 'receptor-ligands' present on the surface of adjacent cells. However, the binding of integrins to their ligands is controlled by their conformation, which is influenced by the stalk and cytosolic regions of the molecule. Inactive integrins adapt a 'folded back' conformation at a region halfway up the stalk (at the 'genou,' or knee, between the thigh and leg). Active integrins are extended molecules with stalks separated, and intermediates between these states tend to have intermediate affinities for ligands. Integrin-ligand binding requires the presence of divalent cations, with a typical preference for manganese, magnesium and calcium, although the relative preference for optimal affinity varies among the different heterodimers. These divalent cations, and Mn^{+2} in particular, directly influence integrin conformation, stabilizing them in the extended and high affinity conformation (Figure 2).

With the exception of circulating hematopoietic cells, which tend to maintain their integrins in an inactive conformation, most cells that have been examined express both active and inactive integrins. Active integrins tend to form higher order clusters on the cell surface, which promotes their localization to sites of ligation. There, the integrins are further stabilized by interaction with ligand. The accumulation of integrins in these sites creates a 'Velcro-like' effect, with groups of integrins (rather than individual molecules) collaborating to strengthen anchorage and to induce downstream signaling points of extracellular matrix contact. This clustering effect is called integrin 'avidity' regulation, which is distinct from affinity. This permits the stable interaction with the ECM required for sustained cellular anchorage and signaling via the assembly of a 'focal adhesion complex' that accumulates proximal to the membrane.

The focal adhesion complex that forms is multifunctional, and is capable of signaling directly, scaffolding additional or alternative signals, and engaging the actin/myosin system. Thus, despite the absence of intrinsic kinase or proteolytic activity, integrins transform mechanical and chemical cues from the extracellular environment into intracellular signals that profoundly impact cell behavior and function.

The focal adhesion complex contains a complicated array of non-receptor kinases and adaptor proteins that mediate downstream signaling events. As will be discussed in more detail below, integrin effectors in the focal adhesion include diverse signaling elements such as: focal adhesion kinase (FAK), src kinase, cytoskeletal elements including talin, paxillin and vinculin, phosphoinositide 3 kinase, and small GTPases of the Ras and Rho families and their effectors [5, 6]. Importantly, as part of the clustering process, integrins tend to undergo lateral associations with other cell surface receptors such as the receptor tyrosine kinases, EGFR and VEGFR, which are important for other global cellular signaling events. This type of signaling, in which the integrin ectodomain is ligated and transforms information from the extracellular environment into cues for cytosolic signaling events has been termed "outside-in signaling."

However, in some cases, signals from inside the cell result in changes in integrin conformation. These are typically associated with cytosolic proteins binding to the cytosolic domains of the integrins. This type of regulation of integrin conformation is called "inside-out signaling." Both types of signaling are important for understanding the role of integrins in normal tissues and in disease pathology.

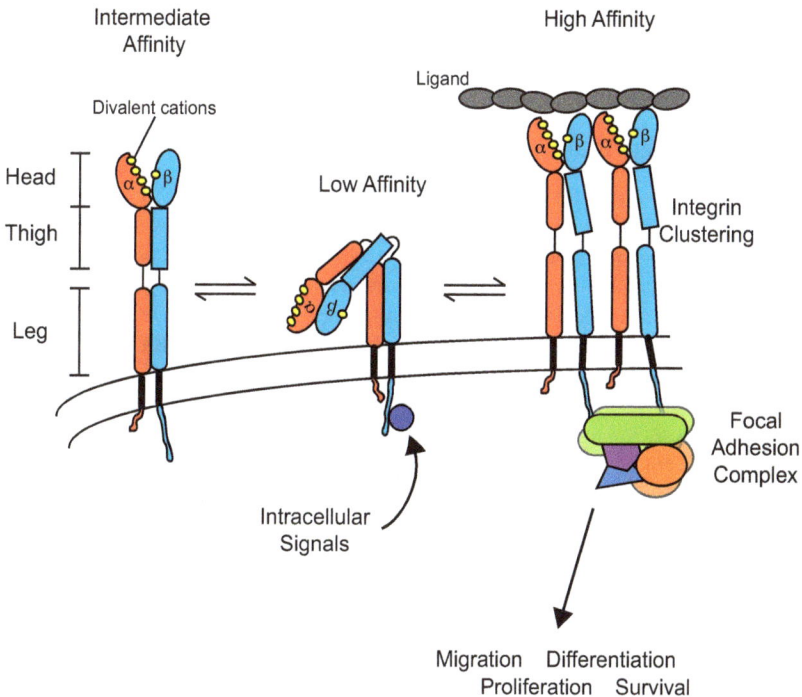

Figure 2. Integrin structure and activation Integrins are composed of a large extracellular domain and short intra-cellular tails (with the exception of the β4 tail). The extracellular domain comprises a head region and a stalk region, which includes the "thigh" and "leg" areas of the integrin. Ligand binding occurs at the head region and requires the presence of divalent cations such as manganese, magnesium, and calcium. Integrins on the cell surface can exist in a range of conformations that affect their affinity for ligand. In the low affinity conformation, the extracellular domain is folded back at the knee (between the thigh and leg areas) and the intracellular tails are clasped together. In the high affinity conformation the extracellular stalk is straight, the subunits are slightly separated and the tails shift apart as well. Conformations between these low and high affinity states confer intermediate affinity for ligand. Changes in conformation can be regulated by intracellular signaling events such as the binding of cytosolic proteins to integrin tails leading to integrin clustering, focal adhesion formation and further interaction of cytoskeletal proteins.

2. Integrins and development

2.1. Integrins in early development

The ability of cells to interact with their extracellular environment is crucial for most developmental processes. Consequently, it is perhaps not surprising that integrins, as mediators of the interplay between cells, the ECM and the microenvironment, have critical roles in early development. The early physiological relevance is evident in defects observed in murine genetic models lacking proper integrin function or expression. Overall, the loss of the β1, α5, and α4 subunits leads to an embryonic lethal phenotype. The loss of the αv or α3 subunits permits initial and subsequent development, but results in perinatal lethality. Other integrin subunits do not appear to be essential during development.

Nonetheless, loss, misregulation, or improper function of integrins can lead to other abnormalities [7]. (Table 1)

2.2. Integrins in nervous system development

The development of the nervous system is dependent on integrin function, in part, because it involves extensive migration of neuronal precursors which is mediated by integrins. During the process of neurulation, the neural crest forms in the region of the neural plate border. Upon formation of the neural tube, neural crest cells undergo an 'epithelial-to-mesenchymal-like transition' which permits them to move along migratory tracks. These tracks lead cells to a variety of destinations where they differentiate and help to form several different tissue types. During development, collagens, laminins, fibronectin and vitronectin are expressed along these migratory pathways [28]. Disruption of integrin-ligand binding inhibits neural crest cell migration and results in impaired function in the peripheral nervous system. Following the initial gross exodus of neurons from the neural crest, integrins also play other key roles in the development of the peripheral nervous system, including the establishment of Schwann cell polarity [29], neurite outgrowth [30, 31] and myelination [32].

In addition to the requirement for integrins to support migration, integrins are also important for arresting migration at the proper time and place. In the central nervous system, for example, the presence of the α6 and β1 subunits appears to serves as stop signals for neuronal cells when they reach a laminin rich region. This is critical for cortical plate formation. In the absence of these integrins, neuronal precursors migrating outward to the outermost layer of the cortical plate overshoot their destination and disrupt the cortical plate structure [33, 34].

2.3. Integrin expression in the dorsal root ganglion and in neuroblasts

Neuroblastoma is a tumor that is considered to arise from ganglion or pre-ganglion cells. To begin to understand the pathological roles of integrins in this disease, it is helpful to be familiar with the normal expression patterns of these receptors in neural crest cells and how that expression changes over time. Neural crest cells express subsets of integrins that allow them to adhere to the fibrillar proteins that line their migratory pathways. Truncal neural crest cells, which give rise to dorsal root ganglia, sympathetic ganglia, and the adrenal medulla express

Integrin subunit	Genetic Defect (KO)	Expressed on NB tumors	Notes
α1	Viable	Yes	Normal; [8]
α2	Viable	Yes	Abnormal mammary branching morphogenesis; [9]
α3	Perinatal lethality	Yes	Abnormal kidneys; [10]
α4	Lethal, by E14.5	Yes	Abnormal placenta and heart formation; [11]
α5	Lethal, E11	Yes	Abnormal mesoderm morphogenesis; [12]
α6	Perinatal lethality	Yes	Skin blistering; [13]
α7	Viable	Yes	Muscular dystrophy; [14]
α8	Perinatal lethality	No*	Abnormal kidneys and lungs; [15, 16]
α9	Perinatal lethality	No	Bilateral chylothorax; [17]
α10	Viable	No	Improper function of growth plate chondrocytes; [18]
α11	Viable	No	Dwarfism; [18]
αv	Perinatal lethality	Yes	Brain and bladder, hemorrhages; [19]
αL	Viable	No	Impaired leukocyte recruitment; [18]
αM	Viable	No	Impaired phagocytosis; obesity; [18]
αE	Viable	No	Inflammatory skin lesions; [18]
αIIb	Viable	No	Impaired platelet aggregation; [18]
β1	Lethal, E5.5	Yes	Abnormal mesoderm morphogenesis; [20]
β2	Viable	No	Impaired leukocyte recruitment; [21]
β3	Viable	Yes	Glanzmann's thrombasthenia; osteosclerotic; [22]
β4	Perinatal lethality	No	Skin blistering; [23]
β5	Viable	Yes	No apparent phenotype; [24]
β6	Viable	No	Macrophage infiltration in skin and lungs; [25]
β7	Viable	No	No gut-associated lymphoid tissue; [26]
β8	Lethal, E12 - birth	No*	Abnormal placenta; defects in neurovascular homeostasis; [27]

*Subunit found on neural crest cells but not yet reported on NB tumor cells

Table 1. Effects of Integrin Deletion in Murine Models

receptors for vitronectin ($\alpha v\beta 1$, $\alpha v\beta 3$, and $\alpha v\beta 5$: [35]), laminin ($\alpha 1\beta 1$, $\alpha 3\beta 1$,: [36] [37]), and fibronectin and associated molecules ($\alpha 4\beta 1$, $\alpha 5\beta 1$, $\alpha 8\beta 1$, $\alpha v\beta 1$ and $\beta 8$ integrin: [37], [38]). Antibody blockade of any one type of these integrins is unable to completely abolish cell migration, consistent with a multi-receptor and complex ligand system. However, in studies on avian truncal neural crest cells, the $\alpha 3\beta 1$, $\alpha 4\beta 1$, and αv integrins appear to be the most crucial to maintain migration [38]. In particular, inhibition of the interaction between $\alpha 4\beta 1$ and its ligands via blocking antibodies or ligand-mimicking peptides, leads to a marked reduction in neural crest cell migration [37].

As neural crest cells reach their target tissues and differentiate, their integrin expression changes. For example, neural crest cells do not express detectable levels of α6β1 until they differentiate into a peripheral nervous system cell type such as a Schwann cell precursor [39]. Conversely, neural crest cells express α1β1 but Schwann cell precursors do not [40, 41]. This induction of expression of one class of integrins while another is eliminated is not well understood, however, and further study will be required to elucidate additional neuroblast-specific integrin expression and function.

2.4. Integrins in vascular system development

Similarly, the formation of the vascular system relies heavily on integrin function. During vasculogenesis, or *de novo* formation of blood vessels, and angiogenesis, the growth of new vessels from pre-existing vasculature, integrins play essential roles in endothelial cell migration, adhesion to basement membranes and cell survival. Endothelial cells are known to express a large number of β1 integrin heterodimers including the α1 through α6 subunits as well as integrins α6β4, αvβ5, and αvβ3. The expression of different subsets of these integrins is dependent on the activation state of the endothelial cells. For example, integrins αvβ3 and α4β1 are primarily expressed on activated or angiogenic endothelial cells [42]. Knockout of integrin αv leads to perinatal lethality due to vessel malformation [15] and studies on the αvβ3 heterodimer show that it is essential for the survival of angiogenic endothelial cells [43]. In addition, knock-out of integrin α4 in mice is embryonic lethal by day 14.5 due to placental and cardiac defects [11], likely due to a lack of binding to the α4 ligand, vascular cell adhesion molecule-1 (VCAM-1) which is present on endothelial and smooth muscle cells.

The formation of the vasculature, and angiogenesis in particular, is of interest to scientists who study neuroblastoma, which is typically a highly angiogenic disease. Although a focus has been placed on the roles of integrins in development of the neuronal and vascular systems, the ability of integrins to regulate such a large array of cellular functions renders them essential for most, if not all, developmental processes. Their roles may be directly associated with their adhesion and motility-related functions, or with the ability of integrins to indirectly enhance the efficiency of other signaling pathways [44].

3. Integrin expression during tumorigenesis and tumor progression

3.1. Tumors exploit integrins for local invasion

As cells are transformed from a normal to malignant state, their integrin expression is modulated to support pathologic behaviors. In primary tumors, integrin signaling can impact cell growth, differentiation, and vascular infiltration and continues to be important as the cancer progresses through the stages of metastasis (Figure 3). The initial steps of the metastatic process involve the degradation and remodeling of extracellular matrix adjacent to primary tumor cells, facilitating cancer cell migration into recruited blood vessels. This process is termed local invasion. Usually, for local invasion to begin, cells from the primary tumor shift from an epithelial or non-motile to a more mesenchymal phenotype. In addition, cells frequently create a pathway for themselves by inducing degradation of the matrix via enzymes such as matrix metalloproteases [45]. Integrins can regulate MMP expression and/or activity. For example, integrin $\alpha 2\beta 1$ is a positive regulator of MMP-1 expression [46, 47].

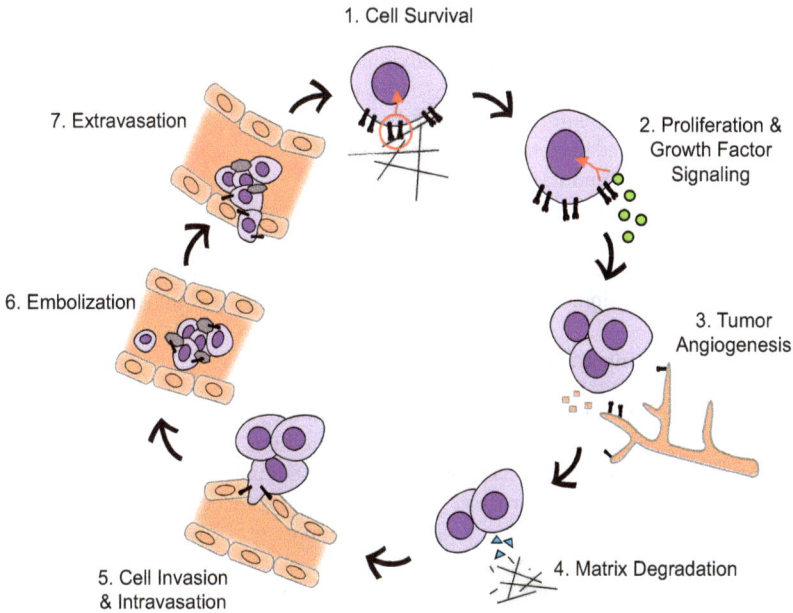

Figure 3. Roles Played by integrins in cancer progression Integrins play key roles in each phase of cancer progression. 1. Ligation of integrins promotes cell survival 2. Co-signaling with growth factor receptors impacts cell proliferation 3. Endothelial cell integrins are important for tumor angiogenesis 4. Integrins modulate the expression of proteolytic enzymes such as matrix metalloproteinases, which play a role in matrix degradation during tumor cell invasion 5. Integrins are required for migration during invasion and binding to endothelial cells during intravasation (entry into the vasculature) 6. In circulation, tumor cells interact with platelets and leukocytes via integrins and form cell emboli that can lodge in capillary beds of distant tissues 7. Binding of tumor cell integrins such as $\alpha 4\beta 1$ to endothelial VCAM-1 can then promote extravasation of tumor cells into surrounding tissues.

3.2. Integrins, tumor metastasis, and tissue tropism

For many types of cancer, metastasizing cells spread to a specific subset of secondary locations for establishment of metastatic nodules. This phenomenon, termed tissue tropism, has historically been explained by two major theories. The "seed and soil" hypothesis proposed by Stephen Paget in 1889 followed his observation of tissue-specific patterns of tumor metastasis in 735 breast cancer patients. Paget noted that the pattern of organs bearing metastases was not random, and suggested that certain tumor types preferentially metastasized to compatible environments [48]. He proposed that 'seeds' of tumors required compatible 'soil' to take root and grow. An alternative theory, by Ewing, suggests that tissue tropism is simply due to mechanical forces and circulatory patterns [49], and that tissue tropism results from this. These are not absolutely exclusive theories, and it is reasonable that blood flow patterns are important for the initial distribution of circulating tumor cells, while the propensity to invade, grow and survive may be dependent on the presence of the appropriate integrin ligands as well as other pro-survival factors.

Though there have been no studies specifically linking integrins to site-specific metastasis in neuroblastoma, integrins have been shown to play a role in tissue tropism. The primary sites of neuroblastoma metastasis are bone marrow, bone, lymph node and liver. In general, certain integrins have been linked to metastasis to these sites. For instance, integrin $\alpha 4\beta 1$ can promote homing to the bone [50] and has been shown to enhance bone metastasis in melanoma [51]. This effect may be due to expression of VCAM-1 on bone marrow stromal cells. Integrin $\alpha 4\beta 1$ may also promote lymphatic metastasis by enhancing binding to VCAM-1 present on lymphatic endothelial cells [52]. Integrin $\alpha 2\beta 1$ is associated with enhanced liver metastasis. This is potentially due to its binding to collagen type IV expressed in liver sinusoids [53].

3.3. Indirect roles for integrins in metastasis

Since the metastatic cascade involves several steps, including local tumor invasion, intravasation, survival in the lymphatics/blood stream, extravasation, invasion into the new tissue parenchyma and growth and establishment of metastatic nodules, there are many opportunities for integrins to facilitate this process. The role of integrins in local invasion is clear. Once cells gain entry into the vasculature, integrins are important for cell-cell and cell-platelet adhesion leading to increased formation of cell emboli [54] and subsequent lodging in capillary beds. Integrins are also important for the endothelial transmigration that follows. At the site of distant metastasis, the microenvironment and composition of the extracellular matrix may be different from that of the native tissue of the invading tumor cells. Here, the balance of ligated and unligated integrins impacts cell behavior and survival, as discussed in Section 4.

The shedding of gangliosides also impacts neuroblastoma metastasis. Gangliosides are glycosphingolipids with one or more sialic acids linked to them. In circulation, gangliosides are associated with lipoproteins. There are several different types of gangliosides that are classified based on the number of associated sialic acids. Some of these gangliosides, such as G_{M3}, are normally present in circulation. Conversely, elevated levels of circulating G_{D2}, a disialoganglioside, have been found in neuroblastoma patients and its concentration is inversely related to progression-free survival. Shedding of gangliosides enhances integrin $\alpha 2\beta 1$-dependent platelet activation, leading to platelet aggregation, and increased adhesion to vascular basement membranes [55]. These events can enhance tumor cell embolization impacting the occurrence of cells lodging in capillary beds and invading into surrounding tissue.

Finally, it is worth noting that at any phase of tumor progression, cancer cells must evade the immune system. Some T-cell lysis mechanisms are dependent on integrin expression. For instance, binding of T-cell integrin LFA-1 (αLβ2) to its ligands ICAM-1 on tumor cells is important in CD3-mediated T-cell lysis [56, 57]. Of note, ICAM expression on neuroblastoma cells is associated with increased susceptibility to lymphokine-activated killer (LAK) cell lysis following interferon gamma treatment [58].

3.4. Trends in integrin expression with neuroblastoma stage and grade

Since integrins impact cell differentiation and invasion, there has been an interest in linking the expression of subsets of integrins with a particular tumor stage, or more appropriately, with tumor 'risk.' Key risk predictors to date have been established by the Children's Oncology Group, and include status of the MYCN gene, the pathology of the tumor according to guidelines established by Shimada [59], and in some cases the relative ploidy of the tumor. Since integrins are associated with neuronal cell developmental stages and activities, it is reasonable that integrin expression could offer insights into tumor activities.

In pioneering studies, using 45 clinical samples, Favrot et al. showed that the α2 and α6 subunits were associated with low grade, well-differentiated neuroblastoma samples. The finding is consistent with observations of normal 'neural crest cell to neuronal' differentiation. The β1 subunit was expressed on all samples while the α5 subunit was not expressed on any samples examined. Samples expressing the α4, αv, β3, and β4 subunits revealed no N-Myc amplification, and were associated with a good prognosis. In addition, expression of α4 and β4 subunits was found selectively on Schwannian stromal cells [60].

Conversely, more recent studies have found that many neuroblastoma cell lines express integrin α4 and that α4 expression is associated with increased tumor stage (stages 3 and 4) in clinical samples [61]. At least on cell lines, integrin α5β1 also appears to be expressed [45] and integrin αvβ3 has been described to be present on some malignant neuroblastomas [62]. In addition, by flow cytometry, our lab consistently observes low levels of integrin αvβ5 on established neuroblastoma cell lines, although whether this is a tissue culture adaptation or reflects actual expression *in situ* remains unclear. Indeed, neuroblasts exhibit significant plasticity, and although integrins may be associated with specific stages of neuroblastoma, or specific developmental states where transformation of the neuroblast initially occurred, an alternative hypothesis is that neuroblastoma may retain the capacity to alter their relative integrin expression, and that this type of plasticity may itself be a malignancy factor.

Neuroblastomas fall into three common morphological/adhesive categories when grown *in vitro*: S (Substrate adherent), N (Neuroblastic), and I (Intermediate) types [63, 64]. These different types are sometimes ascribed to a particular cell line, though in many cases a cell line may contain cells of all three types. Studies using tissue culture cell lines have shown that, relative to S-type, N-type neuroblastomas exhibit decreased expression of β1 integrin and greater expression of αvβ3, and are more migratory *in vitro*. However, the expression of αvβ3 on these cells is still relatively low, at least when one compares with tissues well known to express αvβ3, such as angiogenic endothelium or melanoma. N-type cells also form more colonies in soft agar and are more tumorigenic when implanted in mice than S-type, which are rarely able to form xenograft tumors [65]. S-type cells express fibronectin; it is therefore not surprising that they represent the group of neuroblastoma that express α5β1integrin, the fibronectin receptor [66].

The third type of cells is the 'intermediate cells.' Noted as potential 'cancer stem cells' as early as 1989 by Ross and colleagues, these cells look like an intermediate between the N and S types via diverse measures including phase contrast microscopy, intermediate filament expression, tyrosine hydroxylase activity, and norepinephrine uptake [64]. Consistent with being a tumor stem-like cell (or tumor initiating cell), I-type cells are by far the most tumorigenic in mice and in *in vitro* surrogate assays of tumor formation. Treatment with 13-cis retinoic acid or 5-bromo-2′-deoxyuridine can differentiate I-type cells into N-type or S-type, respectively. Retinoic acid has significant effects on integrins, consistent with changes seen during neuronal differentiation, and can differentiate some neuroblastomas into a benign growth-arrested state [67]. Clinically, retinoic acid has also been demonstrated to improve event free and overall survival in a long-term follow-up on a large cohort of neuroblastoma patients [68].

4. Signaling by integrins

In addition to key roles in cell anchorage and migration, integrin-mediated ligation of the extracellular matrix results in the initiation of signaling events exerting both local and cellular effects. Thus, the extracellular matrix encodes information via the local milieu of cell surface or diffusible factors presented to the cell (Figure 4). Most of these signals have been studied in rigorously defined systems *in vitro* with cell lines, rather than primary *in vivo* investigation.

4.1. Integrin ligation promotes the activation of the nonreceptor tyrosine kinases FAK and Src

Signaling that follows the ligation of integrins by extracellular matrix components can be studied by introducing suspended neuroblastoma cells to a surface coated with an extracellular matrix component, such as fibronectin. This results in cell attachment and spreading. Concurrent with these events, phosphorylation is observed on cytosolic nonreceptor tyrosine kinases like FAK (tyrosine residue 397) and Src (tyrosine residue 418), which indicate activation of the tyrosine kinases. At least some of this activity is physically present in the integrin associated focal adhesion complex, and these kinases can be co-purified with integrins from this complex.

FAK and Src can associate with each other and with an array of cytosolic adaptor proteins and other effectors. For example, FAK can associate with the cytoskeletal adaptor protein talin, which also binds to integrins. The adhesion of NB7 neuroblastoma cells to fibronectin or collagen has been shown to promote co-association of these molecules together in a complex with the protease calpain. Calpain in turn cleaves talin in a cell-adhesion dependent manner, which faciliates more rapid turn over of the focal adhesion, and promotes neuroblastoma cell migration. The same cleavage is observed in other neuroblastoma cells, including NB5 and NB16, suggesting it may be a conserved pathway [69].

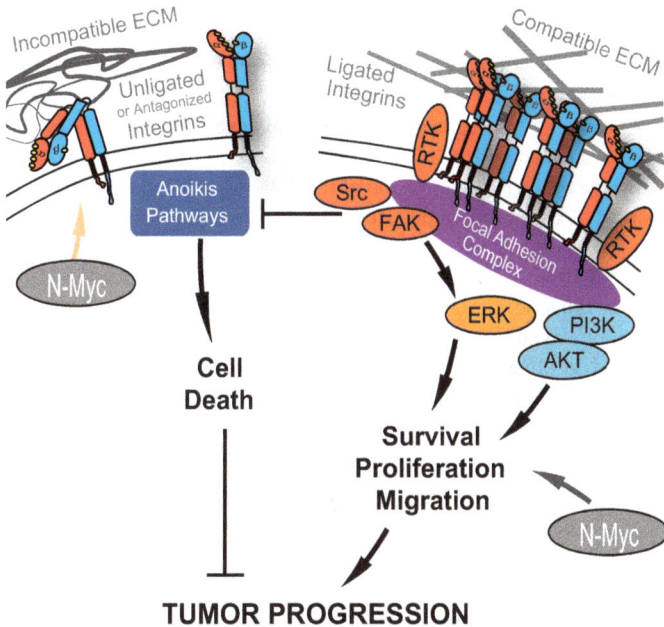

Figure 4. Signaling Pathways Downstream of Integrins The continued survival of a single cell and its progeny in the wrong environment can disrupt the homeostasis of the tissue that contains them. Thus, the impetus of individual cells to live or die is critical for the continued homeostasis of an organism. Recognition of compatible ECM promotes stable ligation and clustering of integrins, as well as assembly of the heterogeneous and dynamic focal adhesion complex. Signaling from integrins and focal adhesion-associated receptor tyrosine kinases (RTK) leads to downstream pro-survival signaling pathways such as the PI3K /AKT and Erk axes. By contrast, the presence of an incompatible ECM or of unligated or antagonized integrins promotes cell death via anoikis pathways, including integrin-mediated death. N-Myc exerts pleiotropic effects via transcription (or inhibition thereof) of many downstream genes, enhancing proliferation and survival, and attenuating the expression of integrins, and therefore decreasing anoikis signaling.

FAK also associates with Grb2 and SoS [70], key regulators of Ras-GTP mediated activation of the Raf/MEK/ERK pathway of MAP kinase signaling. This pathway helps to drive proliferation of the tumor cells, and may account for adhesion-based induction of cyclin E in neuroblastoma (and other) cells [71]. FAK is perhaps best known for its capacity to support and promote integrin-mediated cell migration on an ECM, and performs this function in neuroblastoma cells as well, although this appears to be integrin specific [61]. For example, integrin α5β1 activates FAK and uses this kinase for migration, while integrin α4β1 migration is dependent upon the non-receptor kinase Src. Both integrins can bind to a fibronectin substrate, thus the particular integrin ligated can have an impact on the cells' response. Other effects of specific integrin ligation have been reported in non-neuroblastoma cell lines, such as the FAK and α5β1-induced expression of the pro-survival gene Bcl-2 [72]. Thus, signals from FAK can play a role in regulating cell survival in an ECM and integrin-dependent manner.

4.2. Integrin activation of the phosphoinositide 3' kinase signaling axis

Integrins stabilized and ligated to correct ECM promote signaling via class I phosphoinisotol-3 kinases (PI3K). PI3K's are a family of lipid bound kinases found at the cell membrane or intracellular endosomes, and can promote cell motility, intracellular trafficking and survival. Among the four class I PI3K's, neuroblastoma tend to express P110α and p110β, with the latter more likely to be associated with N-Myc expressing tumors. Nonetheless, P110γ and p110δ are also sometimes detected [73]. Activation of the PI3K signaling axis promotes malignancy in numerous cancer cell lines and models of human cancer [74]. PI3K signaling also enhances turnover of pro-mitochondrial apoptotic proteins like Bad and promotes downstream pro-survival pathways, such as AKT and mTOR [75]. PTEN, a suppressor of PI3K, is frequently lost in cancer, although studies in neuroblastoma have shown a lesser degrees of loss, in the range of ~5% for homozygous deletion [76]. Mutations of PI3K that enhance kinase activity have been reported in other cancers [77], yet they have been proven to be infrequent in neuroblastoma [78]. Thus, the activity of PI3K appears to frequently depend upon extrinsic regulatory factors, mediated by receptor tyrosine kinases (eg., IGFR-1, ALK) and integrins.

Given the lack of effective therapies for malignant neuroblastoma, it is perhaps not surprising that the PI3K pathway is being pursued for pharmacological intervention [79]. In neuroblastoma, inhibition of PI3K has been demonstrated to decrease migration and survival of tumor cells *in vitro*, and inhibit tumor growth *in vivo* [80, 81]. The efficacy of pharmacological PI3K inhibition may be enhanced by combining a pro-drug with an RGDS peptide to target the agent to tumor sites [81]. The relative affinity for this linear peptide for integrin, however, is quite low, and it is improbable that enhanced efficacy is due to direct action on integrins, rather, it is likely due to improved pharmacokinetics associated with the targeting peptide.

4.3. Interplay between integrins and signature neuroblastoma signaling pathways

N-Myc is a transcription factor normally expressed during early lymphocyte development and in embryonic brain and kidney tissues [82], and is critical for survival of neural crest-derived neurons [83]. Amplification of greater than ten copies of the *MYCN* gene has long been recognized as a strong negative prognostic indicator of outcome in neuroblastoma [84]. N-Myc interacts with integrins in an antagonistic manner; while N-Myc seems to increase expression of FAK, it has also been shown to down-regulate the expression of integrins such as $\alpha3\beta1$ and $\alpha1\beta1$ [85-88]. Transcriptional analysis of the $\beta3$ and αv promoters have revealed negative transcriptional regulatory elements in their promoters by the closely related c-Myc [76], suggesting why $\alpha v\beta3$ is not highly expressed in neuroblastoma relative to other tumors. In fact, the loss of integrin expression may be important for survival in specific circumstances, particularly among tumors that retain intrinsic apoptotic capacity, as discussed below.

ALK is a tyrosine kinase that is expressed largely during development within the nervous system. ALK belongs to the 'insulin-like tyrosine kinase' family of receptors that is frequently upregulated or subject to oncogenic mutation in neuroblastoma [89]. Signaling by tyrosine kinases generally requires integrin ligation [5], activating downstream targets (such as FAK, Src, PI3K etc.). This suggests that there is an intrinsic requirement for ECM adhesion to permit a tumor to 'leverage' amplified ALK. However, mutant forms of ALK also exist, particularly a F1174 mutation that drives neuroblastoma malignancy cooperatively with MYCN. In this case, it is unclear whether integrin-mediated adhesion is actually required for cell proliferation, although it is likely to enhance signaling in keeping with the rationale described above. MYCN also leads to increased expression of a close ALK relative, insulin-like growth factor I receptor (IGF-IR). In this case, crosstalk between IGF-IR and integrins is also observed [90].

4.4. Integrins and cell survival signaling

Cells that lose anchorage for extended periods of time will typically undergo apoptosis. This phenomenon encompasses one aspect of anoikis (gr., homelessness), a phenomenon wherein a cell that finds itself in an inappropriate environment is signaled to undergo apoptosis. However, there is no 'central cell death pathway' associated with anoikis, and in fact many different pathways have been validated in the literature. This underscores the critical need for cell adhesion. One anoikis pathway is focused on the activation of caspase-9. Although many neuroblastomas lose expression of one copy of caspase-9 (as many are LOH1p21), this does not appear to impact the capacity of caspase-9 to activate [91]. Antagonism of b1 integrins on differentiated neuroblastoma, but not undifferentiated, promotes this apoptotic pathway [92].

Integrin-mediated death is an anoikis pathway in which the presence of unligated, or antagonized, integrins on the cell surface promote cell death via the activation of caspase-8. Neuroblastoma avoid this death pathway via several mechanisms. First, the amplification of MYCN can lead to an overall decrease in integrin expression, which lowers the capacity of the pathway to trigger. Secondly, stage III and IV neuroblastoma tend to methylate, delete, or disrupt the caspase-8 gene [93, 94], preventing the triggering of the apoptotic pathway, and this results in a survival advantage *in vitro* and a metastasis advantage *in vivo*. Finally, neuroblastoma that are seeded as individual cells in an 'inappropriate' three dimensional matrix will tend to either die or, within only a couple days, find each other and form small cell clusters. These islands of cells promote their own survival and can persist, although they are sometimes surrounded by apoptotic bodies as errant progeny try to migrate away from the original cell mass.

Opposing the induction of death by unligated or antagonized integrins, it is worth noting that a cell that has a robust interaction with the ECM is more resistant to certain insults than others, and integrin ligation has been linked to chemo and radiation resistance. Mechanistically, this is likely to result from remodeling of the ECM, combined with transcriptional alterations of survival promoting genes such as Bcl-2 family members, IAPs and others. However, direct effects, such as maturation-inhibiting phosphorylation of procaspase-8, cannot be excluded from contributing to this effect [95, 96].

5. Specific integrins in neuroblastoma progression

5.1. Integrin αvβ3

Integrin αvβ3 is the most 'promiscuous' member of the integrin family, in that it binds a variety of different RGD conformations, and thus binds to ligands that include vitronectin, fibronectin, fibrinogen, von Willebrand factor and others. Gladson et al. found that αv was present in all tumors they examined regardless of stage. While αvβ1 and αvβ5 heterodimers were found in normal adrenal tissues and ganglioneuroblastomas which exhibit lower levels of dissemination, the αvβ3 integrin was found to be expressed in highly metastatic, undifferentiated neuroblastomas [62]. By contrast, we observe only very low levels of integrin αvβ3 on our neuroblastoma specimens relative to melanoma or cultured endothelial cells, which express robust levels of αvβ3. However, it remains possible that the techniques originally used by Gladson were simply very sensitive and detected this modest but important level of integrin expression. Indeed, αvβ3 is, in some systems, a stem cell marker, and this may reflect the advanced stage and poor prognosis of her positive cohort.

In addition, on a variety of tumor cells, αvβ3 expression has been demonstrated to promote tumor progression by its ability to bind to a wide array of different ligands, facilitating anchorage and invasion. Integrin αvβ3 also stimulates MMP activity, promotes the activation of receptor and non-receptor tyrosine kinases including src, and the release of growth factors such as TGF that promote tumor response. This vascularization provides the growing tumor with the nutrients it needs and brings tumor cells proximal to vessels, which may facilitate invasion and metastasis. As previously mentioned, αvβ3 is also expressed on angiogenic endothelial cells where it promotes cell survival and migration. One study showed that there is higher β3 expression on invasive and metastatic melanomas than on noninvasive melanomas [97], although the levels demonstrated in these cases appear to be logarithmically higher than those seen on neuroblastoma cell lines [98].

5.2. Integrin α4β1 and tumor spread

Integrin α4β1 is primarily known as a trafficking integrin, as it is present on most leukocytes. Binding to its ligand VCAM-1, present on activated endothelial cells, enhances the transendothelial migration of white blood cells into surrounding tissues. Cancer cells that express α4β1 acquire this same enhanced trafficking potential and show increased tumor cell arrest in circulation and increased extravasation and colony formation. α4β1 may also enhance invasion and metastasis through promotion of angiogenesis and lymphangiogenesis [99, 100]. In [97], α4β1 expression was found on 40% of invasive and metastatic melanomas, although not on non-malignant melanocytes.

It is important to note that, though the expression of α4β1 can indeed promote extravasation, the overall role of integrin α4β1 in tumor progression and metastasis is highly controversial and is dependent on the level of expression and the phase of tumor progression. For example, high α4β1 expression in some primary tumors can enhance homotypic cell-cell adhesion [101], preventing cells from breaking away from the tumor and invading into surrounding tissues [102]. In addition, α4β1 expression can lead to a reduction in MMPs and impair the ability of the cells to degrade the matrix and create a pathway for invasion [103]. If cells do successfully metastasize to distant sites, α4β1 expression may promote or inhibit metastatic growth depending on the microenvironment.

6. Drugs that target integrins

The involvement of integrins in multiple stages of tumor progression makes them attractive therapeutic targets. Inhibition of integrin signaling can be achieved using several approaches including blocking ligand binding, preventing the formation of functional focal adhesion complexes and disrupting integrin association with the cytoskeleton. Because the structure of integrins has been extensively studied and because having an extracellular target eliminates the challenges of intracellular delivery, the most common approach has been to target the integrin ligand-binding site. This has been accomplished using blocking antibodies, cyclic and ligand-mimicking peptides, small molecule antagonists and disintegrins [104] (Table 2).

Target	Antagonist	Type	Clinical Development
αvβ3	Vitaxin	humanized antibody	Phase II trials
	CNTO 95	humanized antibody	Phase II trials
	c7E3 (Abciximab)	Chimeric mouse- human antibody	FDA approved (1994) for use in percutaneous coronary intervention (PCI)
	Cilengitide	cyclic peptide	Phase III trials for glioblastoma multiforme; Phase II trials for melanoma, glioma, and SCCHN; Phase I trials for NSCLC
	L000845704	Small molecule	Phase I trials
	SB273005	Small molecule	Pre-clinical animal studies
α4β1	Natalizumab	humanized antibody	FDA approved (1994) for treatment of multiple sclerosis and Crohn's disease
	MLN-00002	human antibody	Phase II trials
	Firategrast	small molecule	Phase II trials
αIIbβ3	c7E3 (Abciximab)	Chimeric mouse- human antibody	FDA approved (1994) for use in percutaneous coronary intervention (PCI)
	Eptifibatide	cyclic peptide	FDA approved (1998) for use in patients with acute coronary syndrome or undergoing PCI
	Tirofiban	small molecule	FDA approved in 1999
α5β1	Volociximab	chimeric human-mouse antibody	Phase II trials in melanoma, pancreatic cancer, and NSCLC
	JSM6427	small molecule	Phase I trials
α2β1	Rhodocetin	disintegrin	Pre-clinical

Table 2. Drugs that Target Integrins

6.1. Integrin αv

The primary rationale for targeting integrin αvβ3 in cancer is to reduce primary tumor growth and metastasis via nutrient deprivation due to inhibition of tumor angiogenesis. Several αvβ3 antagonists have gone to clinical trials with the most notable being cilengitide. Cilengitide is a cyclic peptide containing the RGD integrin-binding motif. It inhibits both αvβ3 and αvβ5. Cilengitide produces both anti-angiogenic and anti-tumor effects through inhibition of VEGF stimulation and FAK-Src and Erk signaling, respectively [105]. *In vitro*, cilengitide reduces cell growth and survival and inhibits endothelial and tumor cell migration. In clinical trials, cilengitide has been evaluated as a single agent and in combination with radiation, DNA-alkylating agents and gemcitibine. Importantly, cilengitide in combination with radiotherapy and temozolomide (a DNA-alkylating agent) has reached phase III trials in glioblastoma multiforme patients. Other small molecule antagonists are in development for noncancer indications.

6.2. Integrin α4

The integrin α4 subunit is predominantly expressed in lymphocytes and leukocytes and supports endothelial transmigration of these cells via binding to VCAM-1. Consequently, α4 is important for immune function and has been targeted in diseases such as multiple sclerosis (MS), Crohn's disease and asthma that are characterized by excessive inflammation or an improper immune response. Natalizumab, the only FDA approved α4 antagonist, is a humanized mouse monoclonal antibody that binds both α4 heterodimers. The use of natalizumab was successful in clinical trials in MS [106, 107] and Crohn's disease [108] with the exception of rare cases of progressive multi-focal leukoencephalopathy (PML) caused by reactivation of latent JC virus associated with immunosuppression [109]. Unfortunately, this side effect was detrimental enough to lead to limitation of the use of natalizumab to patients who are unresponsive to other treatments. Other α4 antagonists under clinical evaluation include MLN-00002 (human α4β7 antibody), firategrast and IVL745 (small molecules: [104]). Though the rationale for the use of most α4 antagonists is to reduce excessive infiltration of immune cells, these therapies have the potential for use against cancer cells that exploit α4 for tumor cell extravasation. The success of targeting α4 in cancer will depend on the ability to minimize immunosuppression or to indirectly impair α4 function via downstream targets.

6.3. Integrin αIIbβ3

Integrin αIIbβ3 is also a frequently targeted integrin. This heterodimer is expressed selectively on platelets and megakaryocytes and is mostly known for its role in blood coagulation. Antagonists of this receptor are primarily employed in diseases such as stroke, sickle cell anemia and acute coronary syndromes [104].

7. Summary and considerations

Integrins are a unique group of receptors that provide anchorage, mediate cell migration and invasion, and signal via cell survival and proliferation pathways. Aptly named, integrins integrate extracellular cues with intracellular signaling and serve to regulate many cellular processes that are mediated by other receptors, such as receptor tyrosine kinases. The importance of integrins in cancer development of the nervous system is well established; it seems inevitable therefore that they play a major role in neuroblastoma progression. In fact, integrin expression has been linked to malignancy in neuroblastoma, possibly due to alterations in invasiveness and the ability to evade cell death in foreign tissue environments. Aggressive disease may modulate integrin expression (i.e. N-Myc).

Targeting integrins has shown great clinical promise. By inhibiting ligand binding, many antagonists successfully disrupt cellular connections to the extracellular environment and pro-survival pathways that are necessary for tumor progression. As we continue to learn more about the downstream signaling activity of integrin receptors, we can also explore more therapeutic avenues against these targets, attacking the problem from both sides. However, the logical use of integrin antagonists in complex, multi-agent regimens is lacking. Given the synergy of integrins with signaling through receptor tyrosine kinases and in the induction of susceptibility to apoptosis, this is where one would suspect that these relatively non-toxic agents would have their greatest impact.

Though clinical studies of integrin-targeted drugs in neuroblastoma have not been performed, *in vitro* antagonism has been shown to decrease cell survival, migration and invasion. Despite these characteristics, integrin-targeted drugs are well tolerated. Given that current treatment for neuroblastoma still has a significant failure rate, the addition of new, low toxicity adjuncts to current treatment regimens seems a logical step forward. In the future, an increased understanding of the roles of specific integrins in neuroblastoma has the potential to provide better prognostic information regarding disease course, while targeting integrins, perhaps in combination with other targeted therapies as a cocktail addition to standard chemotherapy approaches, may lead to increased effectiveness in managing this disease.

Author details

Shanique A. Young, Ryon Graf and Dwayne G. Stupack*

*Address all correspondence to: dstupack@ucsd.edu

Reproductive Medicine Department, UCSD Moores Cancer Center, La Jolla, California, USA

References

[1] Hynes RO. The extracellular matrix: not just pretty fibrils. Science. 2009;326(5957): 1216-9. PubMed PMID: 19965464. eng.

[2]   Ingber D. Integrins as mechanochemical transducers. Curr Opin Cell Biol. 1991 Oct; 3(5):841-8. PubMed PMID: 1931084. eng.

[3]   Hynes RO. Integrins: a family of cell surface receptors. Cell. 1987 Feb;48(4):549-54. PubMed PMID: 3028640. eng.

[4]   Stepp MA, Spurr-Michaud S, Tisdale A, Elwell J, Gipson IK. Alpha 6 beta 4 integrin heterodimer is a component of hemidesmosomes. Proc Natl Acad Sci U S A. 1990 Nov;87(22):8970-4. PubMed PMID: 2247472. Pubmed Central PMCID: PMC55082. Epub 1990/11/01. eng.

[5]   Schlaepfer DD, Hunter T. Integrin signalling and tyrosine phosphorylation: just the FAKs? Trends Cell Biol. 1998 Apr;8(4):151-7. PubMed PMID: 9695829. eng.

[6]   Juliano RL, Reddig P, Alahari S, Edin M, Howe A, Aplin A. Integrin regulation of cell signalling and motility. Biochem Soc Trans. 2004 Jun;32(Pt3):443-6. PubMed PMID: 15157156. eng.

[7]   Beauvais-Jouneau A, Thiery JP. Multiple roles for integrins during development. Biol Cell. 1997 Mar;89(1):5-11. PubMed PMID: 9297778. eng.

[8]   Gardner H, Kreidberg J, Koteliansky V, Jaenisch R. Deletion of integrin alpha 1 by homologous recombination permits normal murine development but gives rise to a specific deficit in cell adhesion. Dev Biol. 1996 May;175(2):301-13. PubMed PMID: 8626034. eng.

[9]   Chen J, Diacovo TG, Grenache DG, Santoro SA, Zutter MM. The alpha(2) integrin subunit-deficient mouse: a multifaceted phenotype including defects of branching morphogenesis and hemostasis. Am J Pathol. 2002;161(1):337-44. PubMed PMID: 12107118. eng.

[10] Kreidberg JA, Donovan MJ, Goldstein SL, Rennke H, Shepherd K, Jones RC, et al. Alpha 3 beta 1 integrin has a crucial role in kidney and lung organogenesis. Development. 1996 Nov;122(11):3537-47. PubMed PMID: 8951069. eng.

[11] Yang JT, Rayburn H, Hynes RO. Cell adhesion events mediated by alpha 4 integrins are essential in placental and cardiac development. Development. 1995 Feb;121(2): 549-60. PubMed PMID: 7539359. eng.

[12] Yang JT, Rayburn H, Hynes RO. Embryonic mesodermal defects in alpha 5 integrin-deficient mice. Development. 1993 Dec;119(4):1093-105. PubMed PMID: 7508365. eng.

[13] Georges-Labouesse E, Messaddeq N, Yehia G, Cadalbert L, Dierich A, Le Meur M. Absence of integrin alpha 6 leads to epidermolysis bullosa and neonatal death in mice. Nat Genet. 1996 Jul;13(3):370-3. PubMed PMID: 8673141. eng.

[14] Mayer U, Saher G, Fässler R, Bornemann A, Echtermeyer F, von der Mark H, et al. Absence of integrin alpha 7 causes a novel form of muscular dystrophy. Nat Genet. 1997 Nov;17(3):318-23. PubMed PMID: 9354797. eng.

[15] Fässler R, Georges-Labouesse E, Hirsch E. Genetic analyses of integrin function in mice. Curr Opin Cell Biol. 1996 Oct;8(5):641-6. PubMed PMID: 8939651. eng.

[16] Hartner A, Haas C, Amann K, Sterzel RB. Aspects of the renal phenotype of adult alpha8 integrin-deficient mice. Nephrol Dial Transplant. 2002;17 Suppl 9:71-2. PubMed PMID: 12386295. Epub 2002/10/19. eng.

[17] Huang XZ, Wu JF, Ferrando R, Lee JH, Wang YL, Farese RV, Jr., et al. Fatal bilateral chylothorax in mice lacking the integrin alpha9beta1. Mol Cell Biol. 2000 Jul;20(14): 5208-15. PubMed PMID: 10866676. Pubmed Central PMCID: PMC85969. Epub 2000/06/24. eng.

[18] Srichai MB, Zent R. Integrin Structure and Function. In: Zent R, Pozzi A, editors. Cell-Extracellular Matrix Interactions in Cancer. 1st Edition ed. New York: Springer; 2009.

[19] McCarty JH, Monahan-Earley RA, Brown LF, Keller M, Gerhardt H, Rubin K, et al. Defective associations between blood vessels and brain parenchyma lead to cerebral hemorrhage in mice lacking alphav integrins. Mol Cell Biol. 2002 Nov;22(21):7667-77. PubMed PMID: 12370313. Pubmed Central PMCID: PMC135679. Epub 2002/10/09. eng.

[20] Fässler R, Meyer M. Consequences of lack of beta 1 integrin gene expression in mice. Genes Dev. 1995 Aug;9(15):1896-908. PubMed PMID: 7544313. eng.

[21] Wilson RW, Ballantyne CM, Smith CW, Montgomery C, Bradley A, O'Brien WE, et al. Gene targeting yields a CD18-mutant mouse for study of inflammation. J Immunol. 1993 Aug;151(3):1571-8. PubMed PMID: 8101543. eng.

[22] McHugh KP, Hodivala-Dilke K, Zheng MH, Namba N, Lam J, Novack D, et al. Mice lacking beta3 integrins are osteosclerotic because of dysfunctional osteoclasts. J Clin Invest. 2000 Feb;105(4):433-40. PubMed PMID: 10683372. Pubmed Central PMCID: PMC289172. eng.

[23] Dowling J, Yu QC, Fuchs E. Beta4 integrin is required for hemidesmosome formation, cell adhesion and cell survival. J Cell Biol. 1996 Jul;134(2):559-72. PubMed PMID: 8707838. Pubmed Central PMCID: PMC2120864. eng.

[24] Huang X, Griffiths M, Wu J, Farese Jr. RV, Sheppard D. Normal Development, Wound Healing, and Adenovirus Susceptibility in β5-Deficient Mice. 2000 2000-02-01. en.

[25] Huang XZ, Wu JF, Cass D, Erle DJ, Corry D, Young SG, et al. Inactivation of the integrin beta 6 subunit gene reveals a role of epithelial integrins in regulating inflammation in the lung and skin. J Cell Biol. 1996 May;133(4):921-8. PubMed PMID: 8666675. Pubmed Central PMCID: PMC2120829. eng.

[26] Wagner N, Löhler J, Kunkel EJ, Ley K, Leung E, Krissansen G, et al. Critical role for beta7 integrins in formation of the gut-associated lymphoid tissue. Nature. 1996 Jul; 382(6589):366-70. PubMed PMID: 8684468. eng.

[27] Mobley AK, Tchaicha JH, Shin J, Hossain MG, McCarty JH. Beta8 integrin regulates neurogenesis and neurovascular homeostasis in the adult brain. J Cell Sci. 2009;122(Pt 11):1842-51. PubMed PMID: 19461074. eng.

[28] Erickson CA, Perris R. The role of cell-cell and cell-matrix interactions in the morphogenesis of the neural crest. Dev Biol. 1993 Sep;159(1):60-74. PubMed PMID: 8365575. eng.

[29] Bartlett Bungee M. Schwann cell regulation of extracellular matrix biosynthesis and assembly. In: Dyck PJ, Thomas PK, Griffin J, Low P, Poduslo J, editors. Peripheral Neuropathy. Philadelphia, PA: Saunders; 1993.

[30] Kuhn TB, Schmidt MF, Kater SB. Laminin and fibronectin guideposts signal sustained but opposite effects to passing growth cones. Neuron. 1995 Feb;14(2):275-85. PubMed PMID: 7531986. eng.

[31] Luckenbill-Edds L, Kaiser CA, Rodgers TR, Powell DD. Localization of the 110 kDa receptor for laminin in brains of embryonic and postnatal mice. Cell Tissue Res. 1995 Feb;279(2):371-7. PubMed PMID: 7895274. eng.

[32] Fernandez-Valle C, Gwynn L, Wood PM, Carbonetto S, Bunge MB. Anti-beta 1 integrin antibody inhibits Schwann cell myelination. J Neurobiol. 1994 Oct;25(10):1207-26. PubMed PMID: 7529296. eng.

[33] Georges-Labouesse E, Mark M, Messaddeq N, Gansmüller A. Essential role of alpha 6 integrins in cortical and retinal lamination. Curr Biol. 1998 Aug;8(17):983-6. PubMed PMID: 9742403. eng.

[34] Graus-Porta D, Blaess S, Senften M, Littlewood-Evans A, Damsky C, Huang Z, et al. Beta1-class integrins regulate the development of laminae and folia in the cerebral and cerebellar cortex. Neuron. 2001 Aug;31(3):367-79. PubMed PMID: 11516395. eng.

[35] Delannet M, Martin F, Bossy B, Cheresh DA, Reichardt LF, Duband JL. Specific roles of the alpha V beta 1, alpha V beta 3 and alpha V beta 5 integrins in avian neural crest cell adhesion and migration on vitronectin. Development. 1994 Sep;120(9): 2687-702. PubMed PMID: 7525179. Pubmed Central PMCID: PMC2710119. eng.

[36] Duband JL, Belkin AM, Syfrig J, Thiery JP, Koteliansky VE. Expression of alpha 1 integrin, a laminin-collagen receptor, during myogenesis and neurogenesis in the avian embryo. Development. 1992 Nov;116(3):585-600. PubMed PMID: 1337741. eng.

[37] Kil SH, Krull CE, Cann G, Clegg D, Bronner-Fraser M. The alpha4 subunit of integrin is important for neural crest cell migration. Dev Biol. 1998 Oct;202(1):29-42. PubMed PMID: 9758701. eng.

[38] Testaz S, Delannet M, Duband J. Adhesion and migration of avian neural crest cells on fibronectin require the cooperating activities of multiple integrins of the (beta)1 and (beta)3 families. J Cell Sci. 1999 Dec;112 (Pt 24):4715-28. PubMed PMID: 10574719. eng.

[39] Bronner-Fraser M, Artinger M, Muschler J, Horwitz AF. Developmentally regulated expression of alpha 6 integrin in avian embryos. Development. 1992 May;115(1): 197-211. PubMed PMID: 1638980. eng.

[40] Perris R. The extracellular matrix in neural crest-cell migration. Trends Neurosci. 1997 Jan;20(1):23-31. PubMed PMID: 9004416. eng.

[41] Stewart HJ, Turner D, Jessen KR, Mirsky R. Expression and regulation of alpha1beta1 integrin in Schwann cells. J Neurobiol. 1997 Dec;33(7):914-28. PubMed PMID: 9407013. eng.

[42] Stupack DG, Cheresh DA. Integrins and angiogenesis. Current topics in developmental biology. 2004;64:207-38. PubMed PMID: 15563949. Epub 2004/11/27. eng.

[43] Brooks PC, Montgomery AM, Rosenfeld M, Reisfeld RA, Hu T, Klier G, et al. Integrin alpha v beta 3 antagonists promote tumor regression by inducing apoptosis of angiogenic blood vessels. Cell. 1994 Dec;79(7):1157-64. PubMed PMID: 7528107. eng.

[44] Bökel C, Brown NH. Integrins in development: moving on, responding to, and sticking to the extracellular matrix. Dev Cell. 2002 Sep;3(3):311-21. PubMed PMID: 12361595. eng.

[45] Kähäri NR. Matrix Metalloproteinases in Cancer Cell Invasion. 2000 2000. en.

[46] Znoyko I, Trojanowska M, Reuben A. Collagen binding alpha2beta1 and alpha1beta1 integrins play contrasting roles in regulation of Ets-1 expression in human liver myofibroblasts. Mol Cell Biochem. 2006 Jan;282(1-2):89-99. PubMed PMID: 16317516. Epub 2005/12/01. eng.

[47] Riikonen T, Westermarck J, Koivisto L, Broberg A, Kahari VM, Heino J. Integrin alpha 2 beta 1 is a positive regulator of collagenase (MMP-1) and collagen alpha 1(I) gene expression. J Biol Chem. 1995 Jun 2;270(22):13548-52. PubMed PMID: 7768957. Epub 1995/06/02. eng.

[48] Paget S. The distribution of secondary growths in cancer of the breast. 1889. Cancer Metastasis Rev. 1989 Aug;8(2):98-101. PubMed PMID: 2673568. eng.

[49] Ewing J. A treatise on tumors. Philadelphia, PA: W.B. Saunders Company; 1928.

[50] Kumar S, Ponnazhagan S. Bone homing of mesenchymal stem cells by ectopic alpha 4 integrin expression. FASEB J. 2007 Dec;21(14):3917-27. PubMed PMID: 17622670. eng.

[51] Matsuura N, Puzon-McLaughlin W, Irie A, Morikawa Y, Kakudo K, Takada Y. Induction of experimental bone metastasis in mice by transfection of integrin alpha 4

beta 1 into tumor cells. Am J Pathol. 1996 Jan;148(1):55-61. PubMed PMID: 8546226. Pubmed Central PMCID: PMC1861618. eng.

[52] Rebhun RB, Cheng H, Gershenwald JE, Fan D, Fidler IJ, Langley RR. Constitutive expression of the alpha4 integrin correlates with tumorigenicity and lymph node metastasis of the B16 murine melanoma. Neoplasia. 2010 Feb;12(2):173-82. PubMed PMID: 20126475. Pubmed Central PMCID: PMC2814355. eng.

[53] Yoshimura K, Meckel KF, Laird LS, Chia CY, Park JJ, Olino KL, et al. Integrin alpha2 mediates selective metastasis to the liver. Cancer Res. 2009 Sep;69(18):7320-8. PubMed PMID: 19738067. eng.

[54] Ruoslahti E, Giancotti FG. Integrins and tumor cell dissemination. Cancer Cells. 1989 Dec;1(4):119-26. PubMed PMID: 2701367. eng.

[55] Jabbar AA, Kazarian T, Hakobyan N, Valentino LA. Gangliosides promote platelet adhesion and facilitate neuroblastoma cell adhesion under dynamic conditions simulating blood flow. Pediatr Blood Cancer. 2006 Mar;46(3):292-9. PubMed PMID: 16317740. Epub 2005/12/01. eng.

[56] Anichini A, Mortarini R, Supino R, Parmiani G. Human melanoma cells with high susceptibility to cell-mediated lysis can be identified on the basis of ICAM-1 phenotype, VLA profile and invasive ability. Int J Cancer. 1990 Sep;46(3):508-15. PubMed PMID: 1975567. eng.

[57] Braakman E, Goedegebuure PS, Vreugdenhil RJ, Segal DM, Shaw S, Bolhuis RL. ICAM- melanoma cells are relatively resistant to CD3-mediated T-cell lysis. Int J Cancer. 1990 Sep;46(3):475-80. PubMed PMID: 1975566. eng.

[58] Naganuma H, Kiessling R, Patarroyo M, Hansson M, Handgretinger R, Gronberg A. Increased susceptibility of IFN-gamma-treated neuroblastoma cells to lysis by lymphokine-activated killer cells: participation of ICAM-1 induction on target cells. Int J Cancer. 1991 Feb 20;47(4):527-32. PubMed PMID: 1671670. Epub 1991/02/20. eng.

[59] Shimada H. The International Neuroblastoma Pathology Classification. Pathologica. 2003 Oct;95(5):240-1. PubMed PMID: 14988991. eng.

[60] Favrot MC, Combaret V, Goillot E, Lutz P, Frappaz D, Thiesse P, et al. Expression of integrin receptors on 45 clinical neuroblastoma specimens. Int J Cancer. 1991 Sep; 49(3):347-55. PubMed PMID: 1917132. eng.

[61] Wu L, Bernard-Trifilo JA, Lim Y, Lim ST, Mitra SK, Uryu S, et al. Distinct FAK-Src activation events promote alpha5beta1 and alpha4beta1 integrin-stimulated neuroblastoma cell motility. Oncogene. 2008 Feb 28;27(10):1439-48. PubMed PMID: 17828307. Pubmed Central PMCID: 2593630. Epub 2007/09/11. eng.

[62] Gladson CL, Hancock S, Arnold MM, Faye-Petersen OM, Castleberry RP, Kelly DR. Stage-specific expression of integrin alphaVbeta3 in neuroblastic tumors. Am J Path-

ol. 1996 May;148(5):1423-34. PubMed PMID: 8623914. Pubmed Central PMCID: PMC1861568. eng.

[63] Ross RA, Spengler BA. Human neuroblastoma stem cells. Semin Cancer Biol. 2007 Jun;17(3):241-7. PubMed PMID: 16839774. eng.

[64] Ciccarone V, Spengler BA, Meyers MB, Biedler JL, Ross RA. Phenotypic diversification in human neuroblastoma cells: expression of distinct neural crest lineages. Cancer Res. 1989 Jan;49(1):219-25. PubMed PMID: 2535691. eng.

[65] Spengler BA, Lazarova DL, Ross RA, Biedler JL. Cell lineage and differentiation state are primary determinants of MYCN gene expression and malignant potential in human neuroblastoma cells. Oncol Res. 1997;9(9):467-76. PubMed PMID: 9495452. eng.

[66] Meyer A, van Golen CM, Kim B, van Golen KL, Feldman EL. Integrin expression regulates neuroblastoma attachment and migration. Neoplasia. 2004 2004 Jul-Aug;6(4): 332-42. PubMed PMID: 15256055. Pubmed Central PMCID: PMC1502107. eng.

[67] Hadjidaniel MD, Reynolds CP. Antagonism of cytotoxic chemotherapy in neuroblastoma cell lines by 13-cis-retinoic acid is mediated by the antiapoptotic Bcl-2 family proteins. Mol Cancer Ther. 2010 Dec;9(12):3164-74. PubMed PMID: 21159604. Pubmed Central PMCID: PMC3182269. eng.

[68] Matthay KK, Reynolds CP, Seeger RC, Shimada H, Adkins ES, Haas-Kogan D, et al. Long-term results for children with high-risk neuroblastoma treated on a randomized trial of myeloablative therapy followed by 13-cis-retinoic acid: a children's oncology group study. J Clin Oncol. 2009 Mar;27(7):1007-13. PubMed PMID: 19171716. Pubmed Central PMCID: PMC2738615. eng.

[69] Barbero S, Mielgo A, Torres V, Teitz T, Shields DJ, Mikolon D, et al. Caspase-8 association with the focal adhesion complex promotes tumor cell migration and metastasis. Cancer research. 2009 May 1;69(9):3755-63. PubMed PMID: 19383910. Pubmed Central PMCID: 2684981. Epub 2009/04/23. eng.

[70] Schlaepfer DD, Hanks SK, Hunter T, van der Geer P. Integrin-mediated signal transduction linked to Ras pathway by GRB2 binding to focal adhesion kinase. Nature. 1994 1994 Dec 22-29;372(6508):786-91. PubMed PMID: 7997267. eng.

[71] Hulleman E, Bijvelt JJ, Verkleij AJ, Verrips CT, Boonstra J. Integrin signaling at the M/G1 transition induces expression of cyclin E. Exp Cell Res. 1999 Dec;253(2):422-31. PubMed PMID: 10585265. eng.

[72] Matter ML, Ruoslahti E. A signaling pathway from the alpha5beta1 and alpha(v)beta3 integrins that elevates bcl-2 transcription. J Biol Chem. 2001 Jul;276(30):27757-63. PubMed PMID: 11333270. eng.

[73] Spitzenberg V, König C, Ulm S, Marone R, Röpke L, Müller JP, et al. Targeting PI3K in neuroblastoma. J Cancer Res Clin Oncol. 2010 Dec;136(12):1881-90. PubMed PMID: 20224967. eng.

[74] Osaki M, Oshimura M, Ito H. PI3K-Akt pathway: its functions and alterations in human cancer. Apoptosis. 2004 Nov;9(6):667-76. PubMed PMID: 15505410. eng.

[75] Scott PH, Brunn GJ, Kohn AD, Roth RA, Lawrence JC. Evidence of insulin-stimulated phosphorylation and activation of the mammalian target of rapamycin mediated by a protein kinase B signaling pathway. Proc Natl Acad Sci U S A. 1998 Jun;95(13): 7772-7. PubMed PMID: 9636226. Pubmed Central PMCID: PMC22753. eng.

[76] Muñoz J, Lázcoz P, Inda MM, Nistal M, Pestaña A, Encío IJ, et al. Homozygous deletion and expression of PTEN and DMBT1 in human primary neuroblastoma and cell lines. Int J Cancer. 2004 May;109(5):673-9. PubMed PMID: 14999773. eng.

[77] Hafsi S, Pezzino FM, Candido S, Ligresti G, Spandidos DA, Soua Z, et al. Gene alterations in the PI3K/PTEN/AKT pathway as a mechanism of drug-resistance (review). Int J Oncol. 2012 Mar;40(3):639-44. PubMed PMID: 22200790. eng.

[78] Dam V, Morgan BT, Mazanek P, Hogarty MD. Mutations in PIK3CA are infrequent in neuroblastoma. BMC Cancer. 2006;6:177. PubMed PMID: 16822308. Pubmed Central PMCID: PMC1533846. eng.

[79] Fulda S. The PI3K/Akt/mTOR pathway as therapeutic target in neuroblastoma. Curr Cancer Drug Targets. 2009 Sep;9(6):729-37. PubMed PMID: 19754357. eng.

[80] Opel D, Naumann I, Schneider M, Bertele D, Debatin KM, Fulda S. Targeting aberrant PI3K/Akt activation by PI103 restores sensitivity to TRAIL-induced apoptosis in neuroblastoma. Clin Cancer Res. 2011 May;17(10):3233-47. PubMed PMID: 21355080. eng.

[81] Peirce SK, Findley HW, Prince C, Dasgupta A, Cooper T, Durden DL. The PI-3 kinase-Akt-MDM2-survivin signaling axis in high-risk neuroblastoma: a target for PI-3 kinase inhibitor intervention. Cancer chemotherapy and pharmacology. 2011 Aug; 68(2):325-35. PubMed PMID: 20972874. Pubmed Central PMCID: 3143317. Epub 2010/10/26. eng.

[82] Hurlin PJ. N-Myc functions in transcription and development. Birth Defects Res C Embryo Today. 2005 Dec;75(4):340-52. PubMed PMID: 16425253. eng.

[83] Sawai S, Shimono A, Wakamatsu Y, Palmes C, Hanaoka K, Kondoh H. Defects of embryonic organogenesis resulting from targeted disruption of the N-myc gene in the mouse. Development. 1993 Apr;117(4):1445-55. PubMed PMID: 8404543. eng.

[84] Brodeur GM, Seeger RC, Schwab M, Varmus HE, Bishop JM. Amplification of N-myc in untreated human neuroblastomas correlates with advanced disease stage. Science. 1984 Jun;224(4653):1121-4. PubMed PMID: 6719137. eng.

[85] Judware R, Lechner R, Culp LA. Inverse expressions of the N-myc oncogene and beta 1 integrin in human neuroblastoma: relationships to disease progression in a nude mouse model system. Clin Exp Metastasis. 1995 Mar;13(2):123-33. PubMed PMID: 7533687. eng.

[86] Judware R, Culp LA. Over-expression of transfected N-myc oncogene in human SKNSH neuroblastoma cells down-regulates expression of beta 1 integrin subunit. Oncogene. 1995 Dec;11(12):2599-607. PubMed PMID: 8545117. eng.

[87] Judware R, Culp LA. Concomitant down-regulation of expression of integrin subunits by N-myc in human neuroblastoma cells: differential regulation of alpha2, alpha3 and beta1. Oncogene. 1997 Mar;14(11):1341-50. PubMed PMID: 9178894. eng.

[88] Judware R, Culp LA. N-myc over-expression downregulates alpha3beta1 integrin expression in human Saos-2 osteosarcoma cells. Clin Exp Metastasis. 1997 May;15(3): 228-38. PubMed PMID: 9174124. eng.

[89] Azarova AM, Gautam G, George RE. Emerging importance of ALK in neuroblastoma. Semin Cancer Biol. 2011 Oct;21(4):267-75. PubMed PMID: 21945349. Pubmed Central PMCID: PMC3242371. eng.

[90] Zheng B, Clemmons DR. Blocking ligand occupancy of the alphaVbeta3 integrin inhibits insulin-like growth factor I signaling in vascular smooth muscle cells. Proc Natl Acad Sci U S A. 1998 Sep;95(19):11217-22. PubMed PMID: 9736716. Pubmed Central PMCID: PMC21622. eng.

[91] Teitz T, Lahti JM, Kidd VJ. Aggressive childhood neuroblastomas do not express caspase-8: an important component of programmed cell death. J Mol Med (Berl). 2001 Aug;79(8):428-36. PubMed PMID: 11511973. eng.

[92] Bonfoco E, Chen W, Paul R, Cheresh DA, Cooper NR. beta1 integrin antagonism on adherent, differentiated human neuroblastoma cells triggers an apoptotic signaling pathway. Neuroscience. 2000;101(4):1145-52. PubMed PMID: 11113363. eng.

[93] Teitz T, Wei T, Valentine MB, Vanin EF, Grenet J, Valentine VA, et al. Caspase 8 is deleted or silenced preferentially in childhood neuroblastomas with amplification of MYCN. Nat Med. 2000 May;6(5):529-35. PubMed PMID: 10802708. eng.

[94] Fulda S, Poremba C, Berwanger B, Häcker S, Eilers M, Christiansen H, et al. Loss of caspase-8 expression does not correlate with MYCN amplification, aggressive disease, or prognosis in neuroblastoma. Cancer Res. 2006 Oct;66(20):10016-23. PubMed PMID: 17047064. eng.

[95] Cursi S, Rufini A, Stagni V, Condo I, Matafora V, Bachi A, et al. Src kinase phosphorylates Caspase-8 on Tyr380: a novel mechanism of apoptosis suppression. The EMBO journal. 2006 May 3;25(9):1895-905. PubMed PMID: 16619028. Pubmed Central PMCID: 1456929. Epub 2006/04/19. eng.

[96] Keller N, Grütter MG, Zerbe O. Studies of the molecular mechanism of caspase-8 activation by solution NMR. Cell Death Differ. 2010 Apr;17(4):710-8. PubMed PMID: 19851329. eng.

[97]   Albelda SM, Mette SA, Elder DE, Stewart R, Damjanovich L, Herlyn M, et al. Integrin distribution in malignant melanoma: association of the beta 3 subunit with tumor progression. Cancer Res. 1990 Oct;50(20):6757-64. PubMed PMID: 2208139. eng.

[98]   Stupack DG, Teitz T, Potter MD, Mikolon D, Houghton PJ, Kidd VJ, et al. Potentiation of neuroblastoma metastasis by loss of caspase-8. Nature. 2006 Jan 5;439(7072): 95-9. PubMed PMID: 16397500. Epub 2006/01/07. eng.

[99]   Garmy-Susini B, Jin H, Zhu Y, Sung RJ, Hwang R, Varner J. Integrin alpha4beta1-VCAM-1-mediated adhesion between endothelial and mural cells is required for blood vessel maturation. J Clin Invest. 2005 Jun;115(6):1542-51. PubMed PMID: 15902308. Pubmed Central PMCID: PMC1088016. eng.

[100]   Garmy-Susini B, Varner JA. Roles of integrins in tumor angiogenesis and lymphangiogenesis. Lymphat Res Biol. 2008;6(3-4):155-63. PubMed PMID: 19093788. Pubmed Central PMCID: PMC2837754. eng.

[101]   Qian F, Vaux DL, Weissman IL. Expression of the integrin alpha 4 beta 1 on melanoma cells can inhibit the invasive stage of metastasis formation. Cell. 1994 May;77(3): 335-47. PubMed PMID: 8181055. eng.

[102]   Beauvais A, Erickson CA, Goins T, Craig SE, Humphries MJ, Thiery JP, et al. Changes in the fibronectin-specific integrin expression pattern modify the migratory behavior of sarcoma S180 cells in vitro and in the embryonic environment. J Cell Biol. 1995 Feb;128(4):699-713. PubMed PMID: 7532177. Pubmed Central PMCID: PMC2199886. eng.

[103]   Huhtala P, Humphries MJ, McCarthy JB, Tremble PM, Werb Z, Damsky CH. Cooperative signaling by alpha 5 beta 1 and alpha 4 beta 1 integrins regulates metalloproteinase gene expression in fibroblasts adhering to fibronectin. J Cell Biol. 1995 May; 129(3):867-79. PubMed PMID: 7537277. Pubmed Central PMCID: PMC2120442. eng.

[104]   Millard M, Odde S, Neamati N. Integrin targeted therapeutics. Theranostics. 2011;1:154-88. PubMed PMID: 21547158. Pubmed Central PMCID: PMC3086618. eng.

[105]   Oliveira-Ferrer L, Hauschild J, Fiedler W, Bokemeyer C, Nippgen J, Celik I, et al. Cilengitide induces cellular detachment and apoptosis in endothelial and glioma cells mediated by inhibition of FAK/src/AKT pathway. J Exp Clin Cancer Res. 2008;27:86. PubMed PMID: 19114005. Pubmed Central PMCID: PMC2648308. eng.

[106]   Dalton CM, Miszkiel KA, Barker GJ, MacManus DG, Pepple TI, Panzara M, et al. Effect of natalizumab on conversion of gadolinium enhancing lesions to T1 hypointense lesions in relapsing multiple sclerosis. J Neurol. 2004 Apr;251(4):407-13. PubMed PMID: 15083284. eng.

[107]   Havrdova E, Galetta S, Hutchinson M, Stefoski D, Bates D, Polman CH, et al. Effect of natalizumab on clinical and radiological disease activity in multiple sclerosis: a retrospective analysis of the Natalizumab Safety and Efficacy in Relapsing-Remitting

Multiple Sclerosis (AFFIRM) study. Lancet Neurol. 2009 Mar;8(3):254-60. PubMed PMID: 19201654. eng.

[108] Targan SR, Feagan BG, Fedorak RN, Lashner BA, Panaccione R, Present DH, et al. Natalizumab for the treatment of active Crohn's disease: results of the ENCORE Trial. Gastroenterology. 2007 May;132(5):1672-83. PubMed PMID: 17484865. eng.

[109] Lindå H, von Heijne A, Major EO, Ryschkewitsch C, Berg J, Olsson T, et al. Progressive multifocal leukoencephalopathy after natalizumab monotherapy. N Engl J Med. 2009 Sep;361(11):1081-7. PubMed PMID: 19741229. eng.

Chapter 9

Bone Marrow Infiltration in Neuroblastoma: Characteristics of Infiltrating Cells and Role of the Microenvironment

Fabio Morandi, Paola Scaruffi, Sara Stigliani,
Barbara Carlini and Maria Valeria Corrias

Additional information is available at the end of the chapter

1. Introduction

Neuroblastoma (NB) is a pediatric tumor that arises from peripheral nervous system. The clinical presentation of NB is highly heterogeneous, ranging from asymptomatic tumor masses requiring little, if any, treatment to metastatic disease requiring intensive multimodal therapies (see [1] for review). Also the outcome of NB patients is highly variable. The 5-years overall survival ranges from 98-100% for stage 1 infants without *MYCN* amplification to less than 20% for children with stage 4 *MYCN* amplified tumors [2]. The main prognostic factors are indeed stage, age at diagnosis and *MYCN* oncogene status [3].

At diagnosis, about 50% of cases present metastatic spread that mainly involves vascularized tissues, such as bone marrow (BM) and bone. According to the International Neuroblastoma Staging System (INSS [4]), patients with metastatic disease are categorized as stage 4, whereas in the absence of metastatic spread patients are categorized as stage 1, 2 and 3, depending on the extent of the primary tumor (within or across the midline), the involvement of ipsilateral or controlateral lymph nodes, and the surgical possibility of resection. Recently, the INSS has been replaced by the International Neuroblastoma Risk Group-Stage System (INRG-SS) based on image-defined surgical risk [5]. According to the INRG-SS criteria, patients with metastatic spread have stage M disease, while patients with localized disease have stage L1 or L2, depending on the level of surgical risk.

2. Role of bone marrow infiltration in staging of NB patients

Since the spread of tumor cells to the BM is a grim prognostic indicator for patients with NB, the search for BM infiltration is of utmost importance for both staging and therapeutic purposes. According to the INSS, presence of metastases is assessed by appropriate imaging, including ^{123}I-MIBG scintigraphy, and morphological examination of both BM smears and trephine biopsies [4]. In spite of the limited sensitivity of morphological analysis, alternative methods for NB cell detection, such as flow cytometry, immunocytology (IC) and reverse transcription-polymerase chain reaction (RT-PCR) for markers selectively expressed in NB cells, are not included into the staging system. The reason for this choice depends on the good survival rate of children with localized NB [2], suggesting that, even if present, few circulating tumor cells are not clinically relevant. Only few patients with localized NB, in fact, relapse or die of the disease. Therefore, the introduction of more sensitive methods for the detection of BM-infiltrating NB cells may cause inappropriate overtreatment of patients with localized NB, resulting in unnecessary toxicity and long term side effects. These sensitive methods, however, are currently evaluated in ongoing clinical protocols for patients with metastatic disease for their potential prognostic value.

3. Sensitive methods for detection of neuroblastoma cells in BM samples

3.1. Flow cytometry

Total cells from BM aspirates are incubated with a monoclonal antibody (mAb) directed against a neuroblastoma specific antigen, as the disialoganglioside GD2, and with a mAb specific for the hematopoietic cells, as the pan leukocyte CD45, each one labeled with a different fluorochrome. After removal of the unbound mAbs and erythrocyte lysis, samples are analyzed in a flow cytometer. The GD2-positive CD45-negative cells, shown in Figure 1, are considered BM-infiltrating NB cells and their number relative to the total hematopoietic cells can be determined.

3.2. Immunocytochemistry (IC)

Ficoll-purified mononuclear cells from BM aspirates are spotted onto slides that are fixed and then incubated with an anti-GD2 mAb. After stain development, the stained GD2-positive cells can be counted by light microscopy, relative to a given number of total mononuclear cells. Standardized conditions for IC analysis and reporting have been developed [6]. An example of a BM slide with GD2-positive cells is shown in Figure 2.

4. Molecular analysis (qualitative and quantitative RT-PCR)

BM aspirates from the iliac crests are stored in tubes containing RNA preservative. Total RNA is then extracted and reverse transcribed (RT). For qualitative PCR analysis, the cDNA is amplified for 35 cycles in a thermal cycler with primers specific for NB related markers, such as *Tyrosine hydroxylase (TH)* [7], *GD2 synthase* [8], *PHOX2B* [9], and for a housekeeping gene (*GAPDH, β2-microglobulin*). An aliquot of each PCR reaction is then loaded onto a 2% agarose gel and electrophoresed. The amplification products are visualized by staining with ethidium bromide. A sample is considered positive for the tested gene if an amplification product of the expected size is present, a sample is considered negative if product for the tested gene is absent and the product for the housekeeping gene is present, as shown in Figure 3.

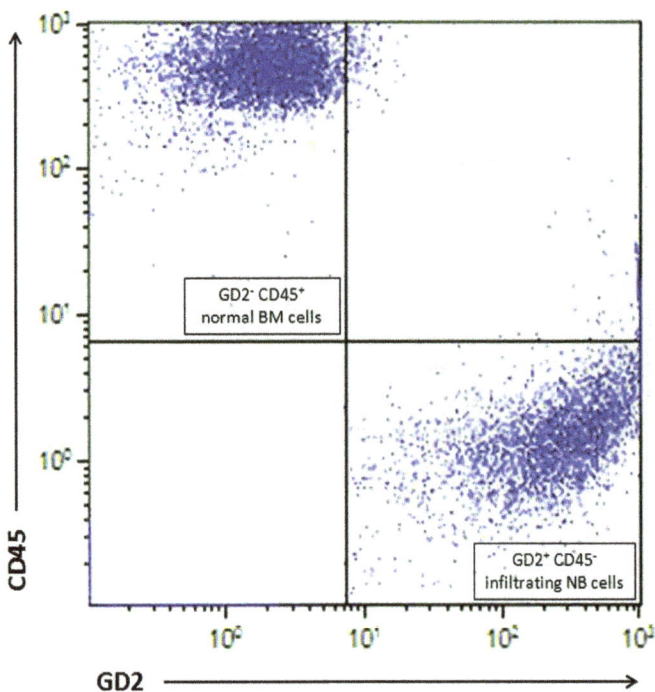

Figure 1. Cytofluorimetric analysis of BM cells from a patient with stage 4 NB, showing the presence of GD2-CD45+ normal hematopoietic cells (upper left panel 74% of total cells) and GD2+CD45- NB metastatic cells (right bottom panel 26% of total cells).

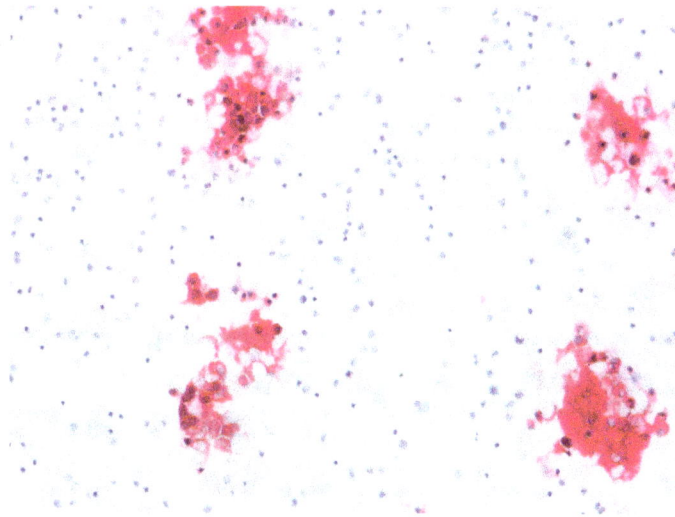

Figure 2. Immunocytological analysis of a BM smear from a patient with stage 4 NB, showing the presence of rosettes of NB cells stained in red and normal unstained hematopoietic cells (Magnification 20X).

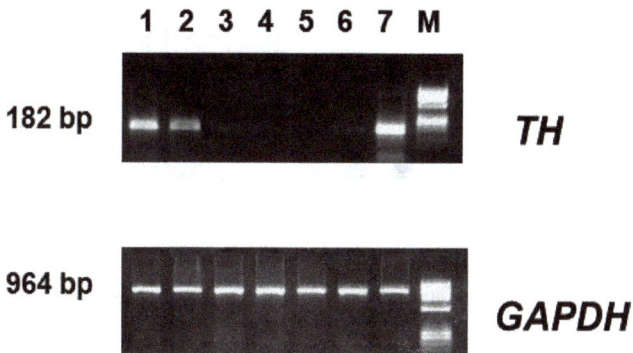

Figure 3. Representative agarose gel electrophoresis of PCR products. Samples 1, 2 and 7 are positive for TH expression, whereas samples 3, 4, 5 and 6 are negative. M: molecular weight DNA markers.

For quantitative analysis (qPCR), the cDNA is amplified for 40 cycles in triplicates in a real-time thermal cycler, using primers specific for a NB related marker and for a housekeeping gene, in the presence of specific probes labeled with different fluorochromes. If a cDNA specific for the NB marker is present, at each amplification cycle the probe-specific fluorescence is released and detected by the instrument. At the end of 40 cycles, the cycle at whom the released fluorescence overcomes the threshold is used to quantitate, through an algorithm [10], the relative amount of the NB-specific amplified product. An example of quantitative analysis is shown in Figure 4. Standardized conditions for RT-qPCR analysis and reporting have been developed [11].

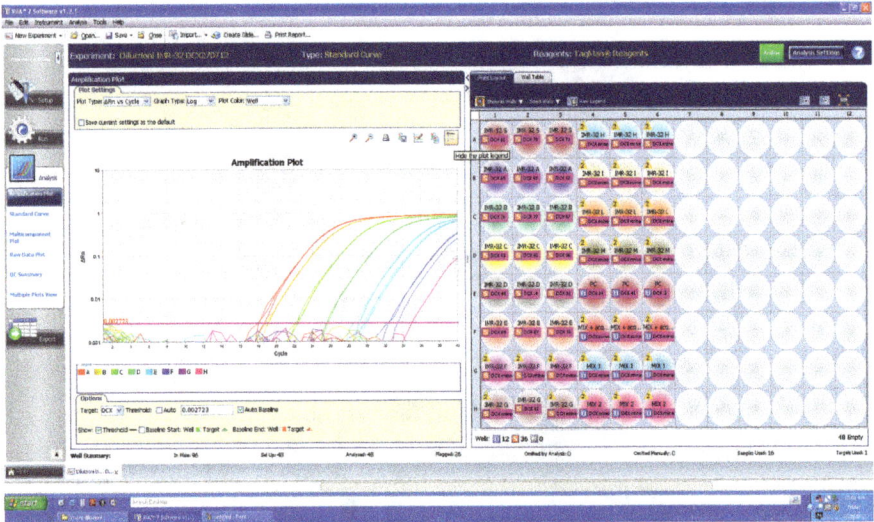

Figure 4. Representative amplification plots showing fluorescence amounts in relation to the number of cycles. Curves of the same color correspond to the replicates of the same sample. On the right side of the figure the plate layout is displayed.

4.1. Sensitivity, specificity, diagnostic accuracy and prognostic values of different detection methods

The sensitivity of morphological analysis is approximately 1 NB cell out of 10^3-10^4 for smear and bone trephine biopsy, respectively [12]. Sensitivity of flow cytometry, immunocytochemistry and molecular analysis is evaluated in spiking experiments by mixing logarithmic dilutions of a NB cell line with fixed amount of mononuclear cells from a healthy donor. Sensitivity of flow cytometry is 1 out of 10^4 cells [13], whereas that of both IC and RT-qPCR is 1 out of 10^6 cells [11, 12].

Specificity of flow cytometry and immunocytochemistry is assessed by negative results obtained in samples from healthy donors. For molecular analysis specificity is assessed by negative results in samples reverse transcribed without reverse transcriptase and in samples amplified without cDNAs.

4.2. Comparison of different techniques and markers

The sensitivity and specificity of different techniques and of different markers have been compared [12, 14-19]. Following the development of standardized conditions [6], GD2 is the marker of choice for IC analysis [20]. GD2-IC is currently evaluated for its prognostic significance in ongoing protocols for stage 4 NB patients, both in Europe and North America.

To overcome NB tumor heterogeneity and increase sensitivity and specificity of RT-PCR analysis, different panels of various NB-specific markers have been developed thanks to the microarray technology [9, 21, 22]. To date the panels have not been compared, but each panel is currently tested for its prognostic role in ongoing therapeutic protocols for stage 4 NB patients.

5. BM infiltration in patients with localized NB detected by sensitive methods

Patients with localized NB without *MYCN* amplification have good overall survival (OS) rates, following either surgery alone (stage 1 and 2, 95% and 86% OS, respectively), or standard-dose chemotherapy followed by surgery (stage 3, 65% OS) [23]. Both the histological features of the tumors [24] and the presence of no random genetic abnormalities [25] in the primary tumor are highly prognostic in patients with localized NB. Thus, these two parameters are presently evaluated at diagnosis to stratify the patients with localized disease into different therapeutic regimens. Some of the patients with favorable histology and genetics, however, relapse, making the search for new prognostic markers still necessary [3, 20].

Since conventional morphological methods have limited sensitivity, it has been suggested that some of the patients with localized NB could have a low number of metastatic cells that could be responsible for relapse. If such hypothesis was true, the use of sensitive methods, such as IC and RT-qPCR, may be helpful in identifying patients at risk of relapse and death. Indeed, we observed that in patients with localized NB the presence of GD2 positive cells in BM samples at diagnosis negatively associated with survival [12]. Since this finding was based on a small sample size with a relatively short follow-up, a further study performed in a larger cohort of patients confirmed the negative impact of BM GD2-positive cell infiltration on survival of patients with localized NB [26]. Moreover, the negative impact was demonstrated to be independent of *MYCN* amplification (Figure 5), the most important negative prognostic factor for these patients [3]. It is worth noting that *MYCN* amplification is a relatively rare event, occurring in about 10% of patients with localized NB [24, 27-29], making it inadequate to identify all the patients who will eventually relapse.

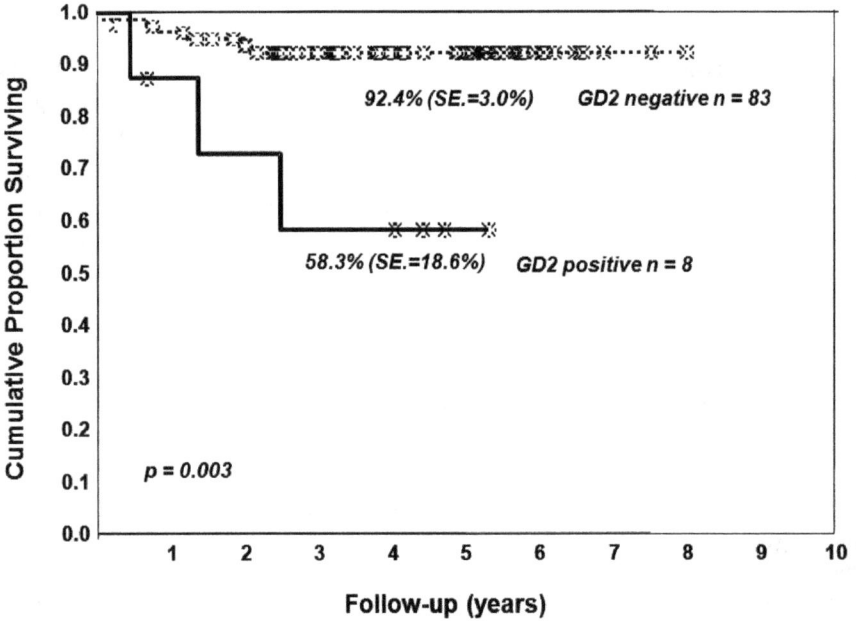

Figure 5. Overall survival of patients with localized disease without MYCN amplification stratified by GD2 immunocytochemistry status

Peripheral blood (PB) samples can be obtained without patient's sedation with evident advantages as compared to BM samples. Thus, we tested whether RT-qPCR analysis for NB-related markers in BM and PB samples from patients with localized NB had a prognostic impact on their survival [30]. The expression of seven different genes, previously shown to be specific for NB cells [7, 9, 13, 14, 18, 31-35], was evaluated and compared to those of healthy subjects. A high percentage of samples resulted positive for the various NB-related markers (Figure 6). Since the patients' cohort had a fairly good survival rate, in accordance with literature data [3, 36, 37], the positive results were likely related to low transcription levels by the PB hematopoietic cells [21, 22, 32, 38], or were due to the existence of so called dormant cells, i.e., tumor cells unable to proliferate [39].

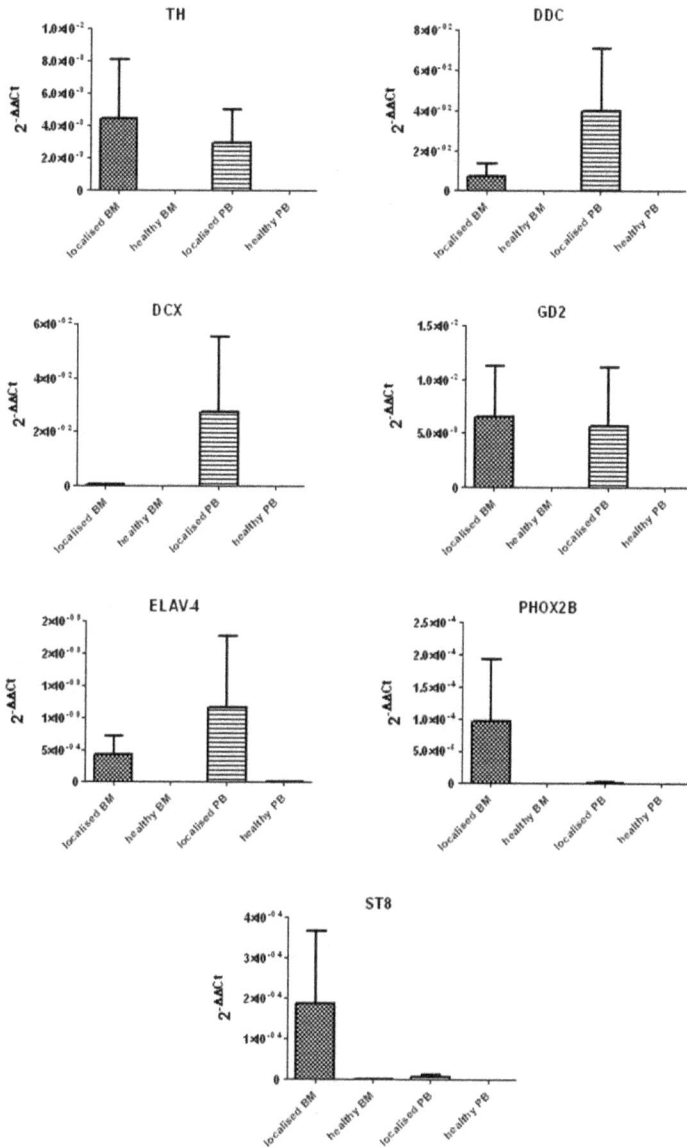

Figure 6. Expression of various NB-related markers in BM and PB samples from patients with localized disease and healthy children

In the attempt to discriminate between illegitimate transcription by hematopoietic cells and transcription by low numbers of NB cells, ROC analysis was applied to find cut-off levels able to discriminate patients with localized NB from healthy subjects. Although the use of cut-off levels for each NB-related marker in PB and BM samples increased their specificity, the percentage of positive results that did not correlate with clinical events remained high. Also a modified ROC analysis [40] failed to improve the prognostic value of RT-qPCR analysis for any of the tested marker. However, *TH* expression in PB samples significantly correlated with worse EFS of patients with localized NB (Figure 7).

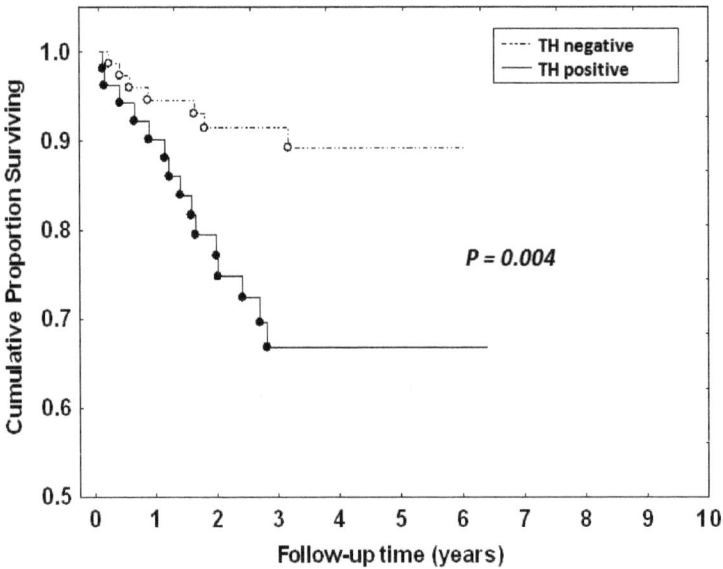

Figure 7. Event-free survival of patients with localized disease stratified by TH status in peripheral blood samples

Indeed, *TH* expression was significantly higher in relapsing patients than in patients that remained in complete remission. Similar results were reported by Yanez *et al.* [41] that tested BM and PB samples from patients with localized NB for *TH* and *DCX* mRNA expression. Although the use of multiple markers has been recommended [20], the results obtained in these studies indicated that, in the subset of patients with localized NB, molecular analysis should be limited to *TH* expression in PB samples, because multiple target analysis did not add useful information to that obtained by *TH* analysis alone.

In conclusion, in patients with localized NB, detection of metastatic cells in BM by means of GD2-IC analysis and detection of *TH* mRNA expression in PB samples significantly associated with a higher risk of relapse. Therefore, both analyses may help individuating patients at risk of relapse that may require a closer follow-up.

6. BM infiltration in patients with metastatic disease

Presence of metastasis at diagnosis in children over 18 months of age is a powerful prognostic factor for a poor outcome [2, 3]. In order to understand the mechanisms responsible for such aggressive behavior, an extensive characterization of primary tumor cells from stage 4 NB patients has been performed. DNA abnormalities [42, 43], gene expression profiles [44-46], and non-coding RNAs expression [47, 48] have been proposed as sensitive indicators of NB tumor aggressiveness. Unfortunately, all the gene classifiers, although validated on independent patient cohorts [46, 49], did not appear to be helpful in stratifying stage 4 patients into different risk groups. Moreover, whole genome sequencing of primary NB tumors [50] demonstrated that no specific mutations or chromosomal alterations were present in NB tumors, suggesting that the mechanisms responsible for invasiveness and metastasis should be searched elsewhere.

6.1. Role of the BM microenvironment for NB metastatic invasion

The processes of invasion, survival and proliferation at distant sites may be mediated in part by the microenvironment. In the BM, several cell types, such as adipocytes, stromal and endothelial cells are present together with cells of all hematopoietic lineages. Each cell type may secrete factors that affect several signaling pathways leading to modifications in BM structural organization and cell function. Among these factors, the CXCL12 chemokine has been proposed to play an important role in NB invasiveness [51-53], but conflicting results have been obtained [54, 55]. Thus, we decided to compare the gene expression profiles of resident BM cells from healthy children to those of BM cells from patients with localized and metastatic NB. The results indicated that the resident BM cells from patients with either localized or metastatic NB have a different genetic signature from healthy children. However, the deregulation of transcription was more evident in the BM microenvironment of patients with metastatic stage 4 disease (Figure 8) [56],

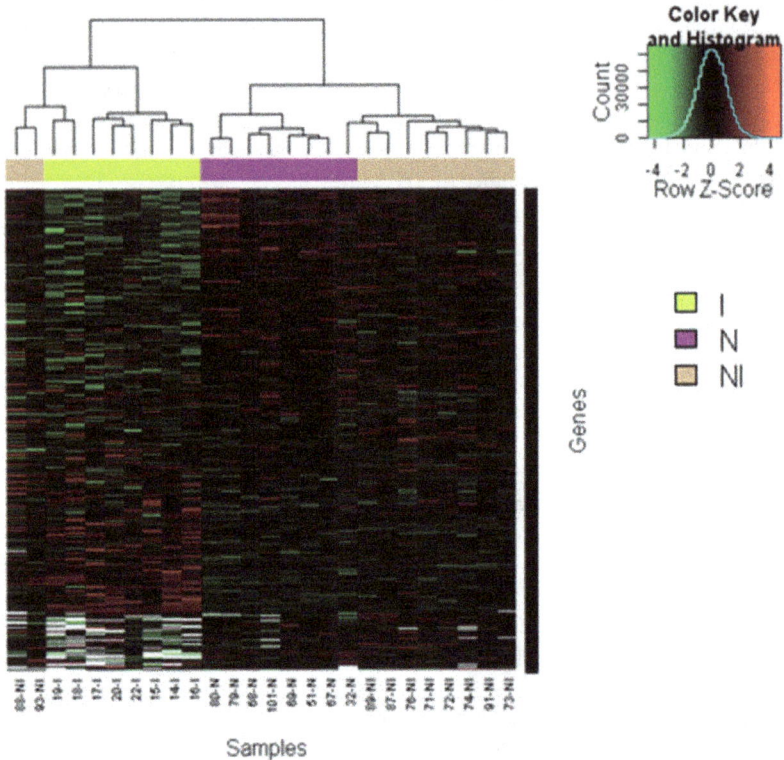

Figure 8. Hierarchically clustered heat maps of differentially expressed genes in BM cells from stage 4 patients (infiltrated BMs, I), normal BMs (N) from healthy children, and BM cells from localized NB patients (non-infiltrated BMs, NI). Each color patch represents the expression level of genes (row) in that sample (column), with a continuum of expression levels from bright green (lowest) to bright red (highest).

Precisely, BM samples from NB patients significantly overexpressed genes involved in the innate immune responses. In particular, all NB patients expressed an interferon (IFN) signature [57].

IFNs are pleiotropic cytokines involved in different biological processes [58], and IFN signatures have been associated with tumor progression of melanoma and colorectal cancer [59]. Moreover IFN signatures associated with the worse prognosis of African-American patients with prostate [60] and breast [61] cancer as compared to Caucasian patients. The IFN signature includes genes involved in the defense against bacterial and viral pathogens [62, 63]. Since all NB patients showed the IFN signature it was proposed that the NB primary tumor may release, or induce the release of, soluble factors as occurring during an infection. The BM microenvironment of NB patients up-regulated also the IFN related DNA damage resistance signature (IRDS), that was shown to be associated with resistance to radiation-induced DNA damage [64], as summarized in Table 1.

Gene Symbol	IFN-α and IFN-β (IFN type I)	IFN-γ (IFN type II)	IFN-λ (IFN type III)	BM subgroup	IRDS signature
EGR1		x		I_BM	
GALNT1		x		I_BM	
IFI44L		x	x	I_BM	
IFI6	x	x	x	I_BM	
IFIT1	x	x	x	I_BM	x
ISG15	x	x	x	I_BM	
MX1	x	x	x	I_BM	x
OAS2	x	x	x	I_BM	
OAS3	x	x	x	I_BM	x
OASL	x	x	x	I_BM	
PLEC1	x	x		I_BM	
PML		x	x	I_BM	
PPIB	x	x		I_BM	
TAP1		x	x	I_BM	
TNF		x		I_BM	
ADAMTSL4		x		I_BM, NI_BM	
B2M	x	x	x	I_BM, NI_BM	
CASP1		x	x	I_BM, NI_BM	
CASP8	x	x		I_BM, NI_BM	
CCL3	x			I_BM, NI_BM	
CCR3		x		I_BM, NI_BM	
CD69	x	x		I_BM, NI_BM	x
HLA-G	x	x		I_BM, NI_BM	x
IFI44		x	x	I_BM, NI_BM	
IFIT3	x	x	x	I_BM, NI_BM	x
PARP10		x		I_BM, NI_BM	
STAT3	x	x		I_BM, NI_BM	
STRN	x			I_BM, NI_BM	
STXBP3	x			I_BM, NI_BM	
TAGAP		x		I_BM, NI_BM	
TRA2A	x			I_BM, NI_BM	
TRIM14	x	x	x	I_BM, NI_BM	
UPP1	x	x		I_BM, NI_BM	
IFNG	x	x		NI_BM	
IL1R2	x			NI_BM	x

Table 1. List of the most relevant genes of the IFN and IRDS signatures overexpressed by resident BM cells from patients with metastatic (I_BM) and localized (NI_BM) neuroblastoma.

In conclusion, children with NB have evidence of chronic inflammation, more intense in the presence of infiltrating NB cells [56], that may reduce anti-tumor immune responses and promote tumor progression [65].

Furthermore, resident BM cells from patients with NB down-regulated genes involved in cell adhesion, in erythrocyte, myeloid and platelet differentiation, and most importantly, CXCL12 expression. The CXCL12 down-regulation reached near complete silencing in patients with metastatic disease (Figure 9), likely explaining the anemia and platelet dysfunctions observed in stage 4 patients.

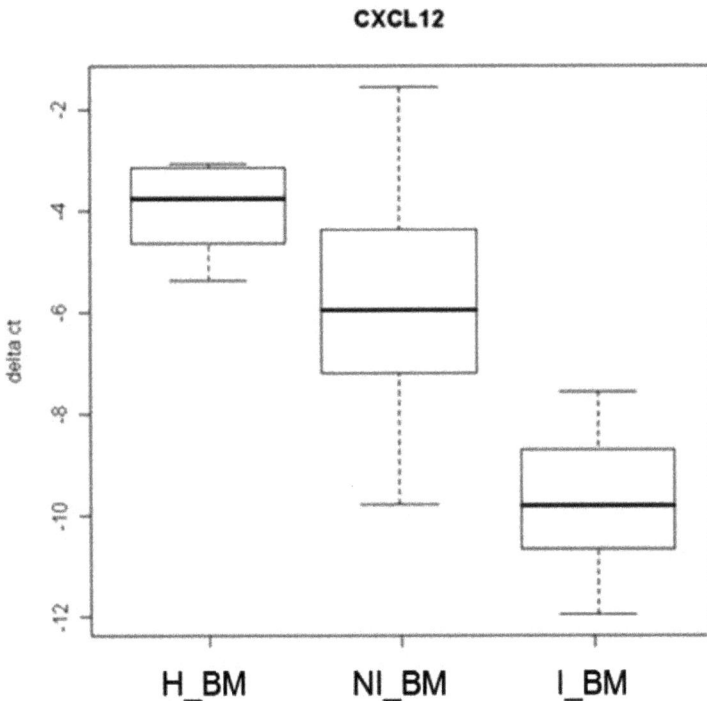

Figure 9. Expression of CXCL12 in BM samples from healthy children (H_BM), and children with localized (NI_BM) and metastatic (I_BM) neuroblastoma.

The CXCL12 mRNA down-regulation was independent of direct contact between neuroblasts and resident BM cells, as expected from the down-regulation observed in patients with localized NB. Since it is known that CXCL12 expression is regulated by the circadian secretion of noradrenaline [66], we speculated that CXCL12 down-regulation may be dependent on noradrenaline secretion by NB tumor cells [67]. Although, the CXCL12 chemokine has been proposed to play a pivotal role in promoting the homing of the CXCR4 positive NB cells in the

BM [51, 68], the absence of CXCL12 in the BM of NB patients makes highly unlikely that the axis CXCL12/CXCR4 play a role in the BM infiltration by NB cells. It is worth noting that we had previously shown that CXCR4 in freshly isolated human metastatic NB cells was not functional [54], and that Carlisle *et al.* [55] showed that CXCR4 expression was regulated independently of CXCL12.

In conclusion, NB tumor growth at the primary site can alter the BM microenvironment, and the presence of BM-infiltrating NB cells makes these alterations only more pronounced. Therefore, the BM microenvironment is unlikely to be responsible for the presence of NB cells in the BM.

6.2. Characteristics of the BM-infiltrating NB cells

After *in vitro* culture of BM samples from patients with metastatic disease, Hansford *et al.* [69] isolated cells endowed with high tumorigenic potential, suggesting that metastatic cells may be enriched in tumor initiating cells (TICs). A gene expression profiling of TICs has been reported [70]. However, it has been demonstrated that the isolated TICs were not NB cells [71], and Coulon *et al.* [72] had recently demonstrated that *in vitro* expanded stem-like NB cells were a dynamic and heterogeneous cell population, quite difficult to characterize because of the influence of external stimuli.

To avoid any modification or selection following *in vitro* culture, we thus decided to charac-terize freshly isolated BM-infiltrating NB cells. The metastatic cells expressed several co-stimulatory molecules [73] and were susceptible to NK cell-mediated lysis [74]. Moreover, as mentioned above, the CXCR4 expressed by these cells was not functional [54].

Since the proteins selectively over-expressed by the BM-infiltrating NB cells may represent novel prognostic markers and potential targets for biologically driven therapy for metastatic NB patients, we performed gene expression profiling of these cells, as compared to the cells in the primary tumors [75]. The results of the study showed that the BM-infiltrating GD2-positive cells were enriched in CD56-positive and NB84-positive mononuclear NB cells, had the same genetic aberration as the primary tumor cells, and expressed NB-specific genes as primary tumor cells. The BM-infiltrating GD2-positive cells up-regulated several genes normally expressed by different lineages of resident BM cells. Therefore, to ascribe the expression of the proteins encoded by these genes to the metastatic NB cells, we took advantage of multiple color cytofluorimetric analysis of unprocessed BM samples from stage 4 patients. While in unprocessed BM samples from healthy individuals the GD2 expression was absent [76], in BM samples from stage 4 NB patients the GD2-positive cells represented about 20-30% of mononuclear cells. These latter cells never express the pan-leukocyte CD45 antigen and always co-express the NB specific markers B7H3 and CD56 [77, 78] (Figure 10), thus confirming that the GD2-positive BM-infiltrating cells were indeed metastatic NB cells. All freshly isolated GD2-positive BM-infiltrating NB cells never expressed CD133, sometime co-expressed c-KIT, CD37 and CD177, but most importantly, they always expressed both HLA-G and calprotectin, as shown in Figure 10.

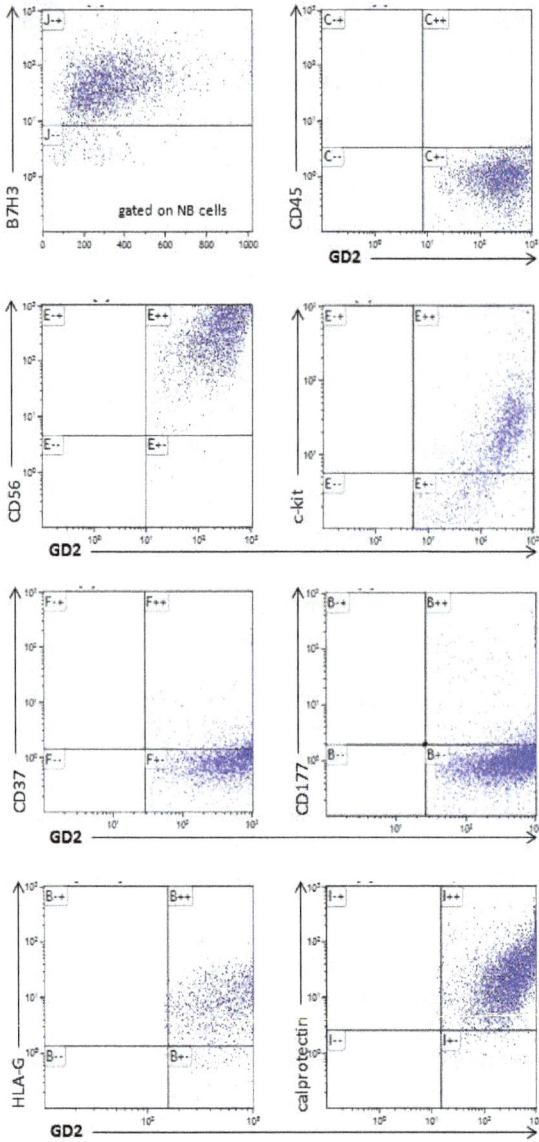

Figure 10. A representative two color cytofluorimetric analysis of a fresh BM sample from a patient with metastatic stage 4 NB, tested with anti-GD2 mAb and: anti-B7H3 (5B14), anti CD45, anti-CD56, anti-CD117 (c-kit), anti-CD37, anti-CD177, anti-HLA-G, and anti-calprotectin. Each plot shows specific mAb fluorescence intensity (Y axes) versus side-scatter (X axes), after gating on GD2 positive cells.

The heterodimer protein calprotectin, encoded by the *S100A8* and *S100A9* genes, is a member of the S100 family, composed of small (10–12 kDa) acidic calcium and zinc binding proteins. Calprotectin is normally expressed by phagocytes and polymorph nuclear leukocyte and it is released into biological fluids during inflammation. Calprotectin, in fact, is widely used as a biomarker of inflammation [79]. Calprotectin is a potent ligand of the Toll-like receptor 4 (TLR4) [80], which is responsible for specific response to endogenous danger signals. Thus, the expression of calprotectin by the BM-infiltrating metastatic cells may be responsible in part for the state of chronic inflammation of the BM microenvironment (see previous paragraph for details). Moreover, the calprotectin-TLR4 axis may also guide metastatic cell invasion, and facilitate the survival and proliferation of cancer cells at the metastatic site [79].

The GD2-positive BM-infiltrating cells also expressed HLA-G, a monomorphic HLA class Ib molecule, whose over-expression facilitate tumor escape from host immune response in a wide variety of human cancers [81]. Since primary NB tumors did not express HLA-G [82], it is conceivable that HLA-G may contribute to the high aggressiveness of BM-infiltrating NB cells throughout its immunosuppressive activity.

7. Conclusion

Presence of NB cells within the BM is the most powerful negative prognostic factor for patients with NB. Presently, sensitive methods of detection of metastatic cells have been standardized [20], and prospective studies are ongoing to demonstrate their relative or combined prognostic role. In the near future these methods will help stratification of stage 4 patients into different risk groups. Conversely, these sensitive methods are of limited use in patients with localized NB.

To date, information about the role of the BM microenvironment in driving infiltration by metastatic cells is few and still conflicting. However, the finding that the BM microenvironment of patients with localized disease is not so different from that of patients with metastatic disease [56], strongly support the hypothesis that the invasion of the BM mainly depends on the characteristics of the metastatic cells, rather than on the properties of the BM microenvironment. In this regard the findings that the BM-infiltrating NB cells expressed proteins not found in the primary tumor cells is intriguing [75]. In fact, both calprotectin and HLA-G favor tumor escape from anti-tumor immune responses, likely contributing to the survival and proliferation of the metastatic cells in the BM. These proteins may be also responsible for the state of intense chronic inflammation observed in patients with metastatic NB [56]. Future studies are needed to elucidate the mechanisms responsible for the acquisition of the different properties of metastatic cells as compared to primary tumor cells. However, the proteins specifically expressed by BM-infiltrating metastatic NB cells could be new prognostic markers and novel therapeutic targets for high risk NB patients.

Acknowledgements

The Authors wish to thank the parents and legal guardians that have allowed the use of their children's samples for research studies and all the physicians and pathologists that collected and centralized the samples.

The studies were supported in part by Fondazione Italiana per la Lotta al Neuroblastoma and by Ministero della Salute.

BC is recipient of Fondazione Italiana per la Lotta al Neuroblastoma fellowship.

Author details

Fabio Morandi[1], Paola Scaruffi[2], Sara Stigliani[2], Barbara Carlini[1] and Maria Valeria Corrias[1]

1 Laboratory of Oncology, IRCCS Giannina Gaslini Institute, Genoa, Italy

2 Center of Physiopathology of Human Reproduction, Obstetrics and Gynecology Unit, IRCCS San Martino Hospital-National Cancer Research Institute, Genoa, Italy

References

[1] Maris, J. M. Recent advances in neuroblastoma. New England Journal of Medicine (2010). , 362(23), 2202-2211.

[2] Spix, C, Pastore, G, Sankila, R, Stiller, C. A, & Steliarova-foucher, E. Neuroblastoma incidence and survival in European children (1978-1997): report from the Automated Childhood Cancer Information System project. European Journal of Cancer (2006). , 42(13), 2081-2091.

[3] Cohn, S. L, Pearson, A. D, London, W. B, Monclair, T, Ambros, P. F, Brodeur, G. M, et al. The International Neuroblastoma Risk Group (INRG) classification system: an INRG Task Force report. Journal of Clinical Oncology (2009). , 27(2), 289-297.

[4] Brodeur, G. M, Pritchard, J, Berthold, F, Carlsen, N. L, Castel, V, Castelberry, R. P, et al. Revisions of the international criteria for neuroblastoma diagnosis, staging, and response to treatment. Journal of Clinical Oncology (1993). , 11(8), 1466-1477.

[5] Monclair, T, Brodeur, G. M, Ambros, P. F, Brisse, H. J, Cecchetto, G, Holmes, K, et al. The International Neuroblastoma Risk Group (INRG) staging system: an INRG Task Force report. Journal of Clinical Oncology (2009). , 27(2), 298-303.

[6] Swerts, K, Ambros, P. F, Brouzes, C, Navarro, J. M, Gross, N, Rampling, D, et al. Standardization of the immunocytochemical detection of neuroblastoma cells in bone marrow. Journal of Histochemistry and Cytochemistry (2005). , 53(12), 1433-1440.

[7] Burchill, S. A, Lewis, I. J, Abrams, K. R, Riley, R, Imeson, J, Pearson, A. D, et al. Circulating neuroblastoma cells detected by reverse transcriptase polymerase chain reaction for tyrosine hydroxylase mRNA are an independent poor prognostic indicator in stage 4 neuroblastoma in children over 1 year. Journal of Clinical Oncology (2001). , 19(6), 1795-1801.

[8] Cheung, I. Y, & Cheung, N. K. Quantitation of marrow disease in neuroblastoma by real-time reverse transcription-PCR. Clinical Cancer Research (2001). , 7(6), 1698-1705.

[9] Stutterheim, J, Gerritsen, A, Zappeij-kannegieter, L, Kleijn, I, Dee, R, Hooft, L, et al. PHOX2B is a novel and specific marker for minimal residual disease testing in neuroblastoma. Journal of Clinical Oncology (2008). , 26(33), 5443-5449.

[10] Livak, K. J, & Schmittgen, T. D. Analysis of relative gene expression data using real-time quantitative PCR and the 2(-Delta Delta C(T)) Method. Methods (2001). , 25(4), 402-408.

[11] Viprey, V, Corrias, M, Kagedal, B, Oltra, S, Swerts, K, Vicha, A, et al. Standardisation of operating procedures for the detection of minimal disease by QRT-PCR in children with neuroblastoma: quality assurance on behalf of SIOPEN-R-NET. European Journal of Cancer (2007). , 43(2), 341-350.

[12] Corrias, M. V, Faulkner, L. B, Pistorio, A, Rosanda, C, Callea, F, Piccolo, M. S, et al. Detection of neuroblastoma cells in bone marrow and peripheral blood by different techniques: accuracy and relationship with clinical features of patients. Clinical Cancer Research (2004). , 10(23), 7978-7985.

[13] Swerts, K, De Moerloose, B, Dhooge, C, Vandesompele, J, Hoyoux, C, Beiske, K, et al. Potential application of ELAVL4 real-time quantitative reverse transcription-PCR for detection of disseminated neuroblastoma cells. Clinical Chemistry (2006). , 52(3), 438-445.

[14] Cheung, I. Y, & Cheung, N. K. Detection of microscopic disease: comparing histology, immunocytology, and RT-PCR of tyrosine hydroxylase, GAGE, and MAGE. Medical Pediatric Oncology (2001). , 36(1), 210-212.

[15] Swerts, K, De Moerloose, B, Dhooge, C, Brichard, B, Benoit, Y, Laureys, G, et al. Detection of residual neuroblastoma cells in bone marrow: comparison of flow cytometry with immunocytochemistry. Cytometry and Clinical Cytomorphology (2004). , 61(1), 9-19.

[16] Tsang, K. S, Li, C. K, Tsoi, W. C, Leung, Y, Shing, M. M, Chik, K. W, et al. Detection of micrometastasis of neuroblastoma to bone marrow and tumor dissemination to

hematopoietic autografts using flow cytometry and reverse transcriptase-polymerase chain reaction. Cancer (2003). , 97(11), 2887-2897.

[17] Mehes, G, Luegmayr, A, Kornmuller, R, Ambros, I. M, Ladenstein, R, Gadner, H, et al. Detection of disseminated tumor cells in neuroblastoma: 3 log improvement in sensitivity by automatic immunofluorescence plus FISH (AIPF) analysis compared with classical bone marrow cytology. American Journal of Pathology (2003). , 163(2), 393-399.

[18] Ifversen, M. R, Kagedal, B, Christensen, L. D, Rechnitzer, C, Petersen, B. L, & Heilmann, C. Comparison of immunocytochemistry, real-time quantitative RT-PCR and flow cytometry for detection of minimal residual disease in neuroblastoma. International Journal of Cancer (2005). , 27(1), 121-129.

[19] Trager, C, Vernby, A, Kullman, A, Ora, I, Kogner, P, & Kagedal, B. mRNAs of tyrosine hydroxylase and dopa decarboxylase but not of GD2 synthase are specific for neuroblastoma minimal disease and predicts outcome for children with high-risk disease when measured at diagnosis. International Journal of Cancer (2008). , 123(12), 2849-2855.

[20] Beiske, K, Burchill, S. A, Cheung, I. Y, Hiyama, E, Seeger, R. C, Cohn, S. L, et al. Consensus criteria for sensitive detection of minimal neuroblastoma cells in bone marrow, blood and stem cell preparations by immunocytology and QRT-PCR: recommendations by the International Neuroblastoma Risk Group Task Force. British Journal of Cancer (2009). , 100(10), 1627-1637.

[21] Cheung, I. Y, Feng, Y, Gerald, W, & Cheung, N. K. Exploiting gene expression profiling to identify novel minimal residual disease markers of neuroblastoma. Clinical Cancer Research (2008). , 14(21), 7020-7027.

[22] Viprey, V. F, Lastowska, M. A, Corrias, M. V, Swerts, K, Jackson, M. S, & Burchill, S. A. Minimal disease monitoring by QRT-PCR: guidelines for identification and systematic validation of molecular markers prior to evaluation in prospective clinical trials. Journal of Pathology (2008). , 216(2), 245-252.

[23] Spitz, R, Betts, D. R, Simon, T, Boensch, M, Oestreich, J, Niggli, F. K, et al. Favorable outcome of triploid neuroblastomas: a contribution to the special oncogenesis of neuroblastoma. Cancer Genetics and Cytogenetics (2006). , 167(1), 51-56.

[24] Perez, C. A, Matthay, K. K, Atkinson, J. B, Seeger, R. C, Shimada, H, Haase, G. M, et al. Biologic variables in the outcome of stages I and II neuroblastoma treated with surgery as primary therapy: a children's cancer group study. Journal of Clinical Oncology (2000). , 18(1), 18-26.

[25] Schleiermacher, G, Michon, J, Huon, I, Enghien, d, Klijanienko, C. D, & Brisse, J. H, et al. Chromosomal CGH identifies patients with a higher risk of relapse in neuroblastoma without MYCN amplification. British Journal of Cancer (2007). , 97(2), 238-246.

[26] Corrias, M. V, Parodi, S, Haupt, R, Lacitignola, L, Negri, F, Sementa, A. R, et al. Detection of GD2-positive cells in bone marrow samples and survival of patients with localised neuroblastoma. British Journal of Cancer (2008). , 98(2), 263-269.

[27] Haase, G. M, Perez, C, & Atkinson, J. B. Current aspects of biology, risk assessment, and treatment of neuroblastoma. Seminars in Surgical Oncology (1999). , 16(2), 91-104.

[28] Maris, J. M. The biologic basis for neuroblastoma heterogeneity and risk stratification. Current Opinion in Pediatrics (2005). , 17(1), 7-13.

[29] Henry, M. C, Tashjian, D. B, & Breuer, C. K. Neuroblastoma update. Current Opinion in Oncology (2005). , 17(1), 19-23.

[30] Corrias, M. V, Haupt, R, Carlini, B, Cappelli, E, Giardino, S, Tripodi, G, et al. Multiple target molecular monitoring of bone marrow and peripheral blood samples from patients with localized neuroblastoma and healthy donors. Pediatric Blood and Cancer (2012). , 58(1), 43-49.

[31] Trager, C, Kogner, P, Lindskog, M, Ponthan, F, Kullman, A, & Kagedal, B. Quantitative analysis of tyrosine hydroxylase mRNA for sensitive detection of neuroblastoma cells in blood and bone marrow. Clinical Chemistry (2003). , 49(1), 104-112.

[32] Kuci, Z, Seitz, G, Kuci, S, Kreyenberg, H, Schumm, M, Lang, P, et al. Pitfalls in detection of contaminating neuroblastoma cells by tyrosine hydroxylase RT-PCR due to catecholamine-producing hematopoietic cells. Anticancer Research (2006). A):, 2075-2080.

[33] Bozzi, F, Luksch, R, Collini, P, Gambirasio, F, Barzano, E, Polastri, D, et al. Molecular detection of dopamine decarboxylase expression by means of reverse transcriptase and polymerase chain reaction in bone marrow and peripheral blood: utility as a tumor marker for neuroblastoma. Diagnostic and Molecular Pathology (2004). , 13(3), 135-143.

[34] Oltra, S, Martinez, F, Orellana, C, Grau, E, Fernandez, J. M, Canete, A, et al. The doublecortin gene, a new molecular marker to detect minimal residual disease in neuroblastoma. Diagnostic and Molecular Pathology (2005). , 14(1), 53-57.

[35] Cheung, I. Y, Vickers, A, & Cheung, N. K. Sialyltransferase STX (ST8SiaII): a novel molecular marker of metastatic neuroblastoma. International Journal of Cancer (2006). , 119(1), 152-156.

[36] Navarro, S, Amann, G, Beiske, K, Cullinane, C. J, Amore, d, & Gambini, E. S. C, et al. Prognostic value of International Neuroblastoma Pathology Classification in localized resectable peripheral neuroblastic tumors: a histopathologic study of localized neuroblastoma European Study Group 94.01 Trial and Protocol. Journal of Clinical Oncology (2006). , 24(4), 695-699.

[37] De Bernardi, B, Mosseri, V, Rubie, H, Castel, V, Foot, A, Ladenstein, R, et al. Treatment of localised resectable neuroblastoma. Results of the LNESG1 study by the

SIOP Europe Neuroblastoma Group. British Jornal of Cancer (2008). , 99(7), 1027-1033.

[38] Stutterheim, J, Gerritsen, A, Zappeij-kannegieter, L, Yalcin, B, Dee, R, Van Noesel, M. M, et al. Detecting minimal residual disease in neuroblastoma: the superiority of a panel of real-time quantitative PCR markers. Clinical Chemistry (2009). , 55(7), 1316-1326.

[39] Vessella, R. L, Pantel, K, & Mohla, S. Tumor cell dormancy: an NCI workshop report. Cancer Biology and Therapy (2007). , 6(9), 1496-1504.

[40] Parodi, S, Muselli, M, Carlini, B, Fontana, V, Haupt, R, Pistoia, V, et al. Restricted ROC curves are useful tools to evaluate the performance of tumour markers. Statistical Methods in Medical Research (2012). Jun 26. E-pub ahead of print.

[41] Yanez, Y, Grau, E, Oltra, S, Canete, A, Martinez, F, Orellana, C, et al. Minimal disease detection in peripheral blood and bone marrow from patients with non-metastatic neuroblastoma. Journal of Cancer Research and Clinical Oncology (2011). , 137(8), 1263-1272.

[42] Bilke, S, Chen, Q. R, Wei, J. S, & Khan, J. Whole chromosome alterations predict survival in high-risk neuroblastoma without MYCN amplification. Clinical Cancer Research (2008). , 14(17), 5540-5547.

[43] Stigliani, S, Coco, S, Moretti, S, Oberthuer, A, Fischer, M, Theissen, J, et al. High genomic instability predicts survival in metastatic high-risk neuroblastoma. Neoplasia (2012). , 14(9), 823-832.

[44] Asgharzadeh, S, Pique-regi, R, Sposto, R, Wang, H, Yang, Y, Shimada, H, et al. Prognostic significance of gene expression profiles of metastatic neuroblastomas lacking MYCN gene amplification. Journal of the National Cancer Institute (2006). , 98(17), 1193-1203.

[45] Coco, S, Defferrari, R, Scaruffi, P, & Cavazzana, A. Di Cristofano C, Longo L, et al. Genome analysis and gene expression profiling of neuroblastoma and ganglioneuroblastoma reveal differences between neuroblastic and Schwannian stromal cells. Journal of Pathology (2005). , 207(3), 346-357.

[46] Oberthuer, A, Hero, B, Berthold, F, Juraeva, D, Faldum, A, Kahlert, Y, et al. Prognostic impact of gene expression-based classification for neuroblastoma. Journal of Clinical Oncology (2010). , 28(21), 3506-3515.

[47] Chen, Y, & Stallings, R. L. Differential patterns of microRNA expression in neuroblastoma are correlated with prognosis, differentiation, and apoptosis. Cancer Research (2007). , 67(3), 976-983.

[48] Scaruffi, P, Stigliani, S, Moretti, S, Coco, S, De Vecchi, C, Valdora, F, et al. Transcribed-Ultra Conserved Region expression is associated with outcome in high-risk neuroblastoma. BMC Cancer (2009).

[49] Vermeulen, J, De Preter, K, Naranjo, A, Vercruysse, L, Van Roy, N, Hellemans, J, et al. Predicting outcomes for children with neuroblastoma using a multigene-expression signature: a retrospective SIOPEN/COG/GPOH study. Lancet Oncology (2009). , 10(7), 663-671.

[50] Molenaar, J. J, Koster, J, Zwijnenburg, D. A, Van Sluis, P, Valentijn, L. J, Van Der Ploeg, I, et al. Sequencing of neuroblastoma identifies chromothripsis and defects in neuritogenesis genes. Nature (2012). , 483(7391), 589-593.

[51] Geminder, H, Sagi-assif, O, Goldberg, L, Meshel, T, Rechavi, G, Witz, I. P, et al. A possible role for CXCR4 and its ligand, the CXC chemokine stromal cell-derived factor-1, in the development of bone marrow metastases in neuroblastoma. Journal of Immunology (2001). , 167(8), 4747-4757.

[52] Nevo, I, Sagi-assif, O, Meshel, T, Geminder, H, Goldberg-bittman, L, Ben-menachem, S, et al. The tumor microenvironment: CXCR4 is associated with distinct protein expression patterns in neuroblastoma cells. Immunology Letters (2004).

[53] Russell, H. V, Hicks, J, Okcu, M. F, & Nuchtern, J. G. CXCR4 expression in neuroblastoma primary tumors is associated with clinical presentation of bone and bone marrow metastases. Journal of Pediatric Surgery (2004). , 39(10), 1506-1511.

[54] Airoldi, I, Raffaghello, L, Piovan, E, Cocco, C, Carlini, B, Amadori, A, et al. CXCL12 does not attract CXCR4+ human metastatic neuroblastoma cells: clinical implications. Clinical Cancer Research (2006). , 12(1), 77-82.

[55] Carlisle, A. J, Lyttle, C. A, Carlisle, R. Y, & Maris, J. M. CXCR4 expression heterogeneity in neuroblastoma cells due to ligand-independent regulation. Molecular Cancer (2009). , 8, 126-131.

[56] Scaruffi, P, Morandi, F, Gallo, F, Stigliani, S, Parodi, S, Moretti, S, et al. Bone marrow of neuroblastoma patients shows downregulation of CXCL12 expression and presence of IFN signature. Pediatric Blood and Cancer (2012). , 59(1), 44-51.

[57] Der SDZhou A, Williams BR, Silverman RH. Identification of genes differentially regulated by interferon alpha, beta, or gamma using oligonucleotide arrays. Proceeding National Academy of Science USA (1998). , 95(26), 15623-15628.

[58] Stark, G. R, Kerr, I. M, Williams, B. R, Silverman, R. H, & Schreiber, R. D. How cells respond to interferons. Annual Review of Biochemistry (1998). , 67, 227-264.

[59] Kim, S. H, Gunnery, S, Choe, J. K, & Mathews, M. B. Neoplastic progression in melanoma and colon cancer is associated with increased expression and activity of the interferon-inducible protein kinase, PKR. Oncogene (2002). , 21(57), 8741-8748.

[60] Wallace, T. A, Prueitt, R. L, Yi, M, Howe, T. M, Gillespie, J. W, Yfantis, H. G, et al. Tumor immunobiological differences in prostate cancer between African-American and European-American men. Cancer Research (2008). , 68(3), 927-936.

[61] Martin, D. N, Boersma, B. J, Yi, M, Reimers, M, Howe, T. M, Yfantis, H. G, et al. Dif-
      ferences in the tumor microenvironment between African-American and European-
      American breast cancer patients. Plos One (2009). e4531.

[62] Degols, G, Eldin, P, & Mechti, N. ISG20, an actor of the innate immune response. Bio-
      chimie (2007).

[63] Brodsky, L. I, Wahed, A. S, Li, J, Tavis, J. E, Tsukahara, T, & Taylor, M. W. A novel
      unsupervised method to identify genes important in the anti-viral response: applica-
      tion to interferon/ribavirin in hepatitis C patients. Plos One (2007). e584.

[64] Khodarev, N. N, Beckett, M, Labay, E, Darga, T, Roizman, B, & Weichselbaum, R. R.
      STAT1 is overexpressed in tumors selected for radioresistance and confers protection
      from radiation in transduced sensitive cells. Proceeding National Academy of Sci-
      ence USA (2004). , 101(6), 1714-1719.

[65] Rook, G. A, & Dalgleish, A. Infection, immunoregulation, and cancer. Immunology
      Reviews (2011). , 240(1), 141-159.

[66] Mendez-ferrer, S, Lucas, D, Battista, M, & Frenette, P. S. Haematopoietic stem cell re-
      lease is regulated by circadian oscillations. Nature (2008). , 452(7186), 442-447.

[67] Goodall, A. R, Danks, K, Walker, J. H, Ball, S. G, & Vaughan, P. F. Occurrence of two
      types of secretory vesicles in the human neuroblastoma SH-SY5Y. Journal of Neuro-
      chemistry (1997). , 68(4), 1542-1552.

[68] Meier, R, Muhlethaler-mottet, A, Flahaut, M, Coulon, A, Fusco, C, Louache, F, et al.
      The chemokine receptor CXCR4 strongly promotes neuroblastoma primary tumour
      and metastatic growth, but not invasion. Plos One (2007). e1016.

[69] Hansford, L. M, Mckee, A. E, Zhang, L, George, R. E, Gerstle, J. T, Thorner, P. S, et al.
      Neuroblastoma cells isolated from bone marrow metastases contain a naturally en-
      riched tumor-initiating cell. Cancer Research (2007). , 67(23), 11234-11243.

[70] Morozova, O, Vojvodic, M, Grinshtein, N, Hansford, L. M, Blakely, K. M, Maslova,
      A, et al. System-level analysis of neuroblastoma tumor-initiating cells implicates
      AURKB as a novel drug target for neuroblastoma. Clinical Cancer Research (2010). ,
      16(18), 4572-4582.

[71] Mohlin, S, Pietras, A, Wigerup, C, Ora, I, Andang, M, Nilsson, K, et al. Tumor-initiat-
      ing cells in childhood neuroblastoma--letter. Cancer Research (2012). author reply 3.,
      72(3), 821-2.

[72] Coulon, A, Flahaut, M, Muhlethaler-mottet, A, Meier, R, Liberman, J, Balmas-bour-
      loud, K, et al. Functional sphere profiling reveals the complexity of neuroblastoma
      tumor-initiating cell model. Neoplasia (2011). , 13(10), 991-1004.

[73] Airoldi, I, Lualdi, S, Bruno, S, Raffaghello, L, Occhino, M, Gambini, C, et al. Expres-
      sion of costimulatory molecules in human neuroblastoma. Evidence that CD40+ neu-

roblastoma cells undergo apoptosis following interaction with CD40L. British Journal of Cancer (2003). , 88(10), 1527-1536.

[74] Castriconi, R, Dondero, A, Corrias, M. V, Lanino, E, Pende, D, Moretta, L, et al. Natural killer cell-mediated killing of freshly isolated neuroblastoma cells: critical role of DNAX accessory molecule-1-poliovirus receptor interaction. Cancer Research (2004). , 64(24), 9180-9184.

[75] Morandi, F, Scaruffi, P, Gallo, F, Stigliani, S, Moretti, S, Bonassi, S, et al. Bone marrow-infiltrating human neuroblastoma cells express high levels of calprotectin and HLA-G proteins. Plos One. (2012). e29922.

[76] Martinez, C, Hofmann, T. J, Marino, R, Dominici, M, & Horwitz, E. M. Human bone marrow mesenchymal stromal cells express the neural ganglioside GD2: a novel surface marker for the identification of MSCs. Blood (2007). , 109(10), 4245-4248.

[77] Bassili, M, Birman, E, Schor, N. F, & Saragovi, H. U. Differential roles of Trk and neurotrophin receptors in tumorigenesis and chemoresistance ex vivo and in vivo. Cancer Chemotherapy and Pharmacology. (2010). , 75.

[78] Castriconi, R, Dondero, A, Augugliaro, R, Cantoni, C, Carnemolla, B, Sementa, A. R, et al. Identification of 4Ig-B7-H3 as a neuroblastoma-associated molecule that exerts a protective role from an NK cell-mediated lysis. Proceeding National Academy of Science USA (2004). , 101(34), 12640-12645.

[79] Ghavami, S, Rashedi, I, Dattilo, B. M, Eshraghi, M, Chazin, W. J, Hashemi, M, et al. S100A8/A9 at low concentration promotes tumor cell growth via RAGE ligation and MAP kinase-dependent pathway. Journal of Leukocyte Biology (2008). , 83(6), 1484-1492.

[80] Vogl, T, Tenbrock, K, Ludwig, S, Leukert, N, Ehrhardt, C, Van Zoelen, M. A, et al. Mrp8 and Mrp14 are endogenous activators of Toll-like receptor 4, promoting lethal, endotoxin-induced shock. Nature Medicine (2007). , 13(9), 1042-1049.

[81] Rouas-freiss, N, Moreau, P, & Menier, C. LeMaoult J, Carosella ED. Expression of tolerogenic HLA-G molecules in cancer prevents antitumor responses. Seminars in Cancer Biology (2007). , 17(6), 413-421.

[82] Morandi, F, Levreri, I, Bocca, P, Galleni, B, Raffaghello, L, Ferrone, S, et al. Human neuroblastoma cells trigger an immunosuppressive program in monocytes by stimulating soluble HLA-G release. Cancer Research (2007). , 67(13), 6433-6441.

Neuroblastoma, Biology - 3

Chapter 10

Clinical Implications of Neuroblastoma Stem Cells

Xao X. Tang and Hiroyuki Shimada

Additional information is available at the end of the chapter

1. Introduction

Neuroblastoma (NB) is a childhood neoplasm and the cause of ~15% of cancer deaths in children. The clinical behavior of NB is highly variable. While some tumors are easily treatable, nearly 50% of the tumors exhibit very aggressive behavior. The latter tumors are classified as high-risk NB and are characterized by widespread tumor dissemination and poor long-term survival. Determining the prognosis of NBs at the time of diagnosis is important because of the clinical heterogeneity of the disease. Current prognostic factors used by the COG (Children's Oncology Group) Neuroblastoma Study for patient stratification and protocol assignment include: Age (<18 months *vs* >18 months), Stage (1, 2, 4S *vs* 3, 4), *MYCN* status (amplification *vs* non-amplification), Ploidy (diploid *vs* hyperdiploid), International Neuroblastoma Pathology Classification (Shimada system: Favorable *vs* Unfavorable Histology), 1pLOH (present *vs* absent), and 11qLOH (present *vs* absent) [1-3]. About half of high-risk NBs exhibit *MYCN* amplification, which is associated with older age, rapid tumor progression, and the worst prognosis [4]. According to the International Neuroblastoma Pathology Classification, NBs exhibiting *MYCN* amplification have unique histologic features, namely, an undifferentiated/poorly differentiated appearance and a high mitosis-karyorrhexis index. Nonetheless, certain NB with these histologic characteristics do not show *MYCN* amplification [5]. A previous report suggests that in non-*MYCN*-amplified unfavorable NB tumors, MYC rather than MYCN expression is responsible for the aggressive phenotype [6].

Current treatment for high-risk NB includes high dosage cytotoxic chemotherapy or myeloablative cytotoxic therapy with autologous hematopoietic stem cell transplantation [7]. Late relapse is often seen in patients with high-risk NB despite achieving a complete clinical remission. A subset of high-risk NBs, which is refractory to current front-line therapy designed for high-risk NB, is termed ultra high-risk NB [8, 9]. These tumors are totally unresponsive to current therapies, and thus reliable diagnostic tools to identify ultra high-risk NB prior to treatment and innovative and effective therapeutic agents against these NBs are in need of development.

In this article, we will discuss our recent study on neuroblastoma stem cells, histopathological characteristics of these cells, and why the knowledge gained would help improve diagnosis and treatment of children with the most malignant NBs. We have recently reported the establishment of phenotypically stabilized stem cell-like NB cells (refer to as iCSC, see below) by short-term treatments of conventional monolayer NB cell lines with epigenetic modifiers [10]. The study addresses a fundamental problem that has affected a complete success in treating patients with cancers. Cancer stem cells (CSCs) are plastic in nature, a characteristic that hampers cancer therapeutics. To date, two models have been proposed to explain the existence of cancer stem cells in a tumor mass: the stochastic model and the hierarchical model. According to the stochastic model, transformed single cells develop unlimited proliferative capability to cause a tumor. Initially, a single or few transformed cells result in uncontrolled growth. Accumulations of different mutations then occur driving additional tumor growth and resulting in heterogeneous subpopulations within the tumor. These cancer cells are believed to participate in tumor growth, develop resistance, and cause recurrence. Hence, all cells are considered tumorigenic and are targets for treatment. In contrast, the hierarchical or current CSC model states that in a given tumor, there exists a population of cancer cells that have characteristics similar to stem cells. Cancer stem cells have the capacity to renew indefinitely, to initiate tumor formation, and to give rise to multiple non-tumorigenic progenies via asymmetric cell division. As a result of this phenotypic drift, an established tumor would always consist of a mixture of CSC and non-CSC. Current anti-cancer therapies are believed to target the more differentiated tumor cells, but not the CSC component, which is ultimately responsible for tumor recurrence. Based on the most current thinking, the two models are not mutually exclusive.

To create phenotypically stabilized stem cell-like NB cells, our approach includes a short-term treatment (i.e., five days) of NB monolayer cell lines (SKNAS, SKNBE(2)C, CHP134, SY5Y) with either an inhibitor of DNA methylation and/or an HDAC inhibitor followed by cell culturing in the sphere-forming medium without the epigenetic modifiers. This strategy not only significantly augments the expression of the Yamanaka reprogramming factors and stem cell markers in the NB spheres generated, but it also captures these spheres in the "totally undifferentiated status" over a long period of time *in vitro* and *in vivo*. To date, known stemness/reprogramming factors include MYC/MYCN, SOX2, OCT4, NANOG, LIN28, and KLF4. These factors were shown to initiate reverse differentiation or reprogramming of somatic cells [11-13]. In addition, several stem cells markers (CD133, CXCR4, ABCG2) [14-16] and neural crest stem cell markers (p75^{NTR}, SOX9, SOX10, SLUG, Musashi-1, CD24, and HES1) have been reported [17-22].

The stem cell-like NB cells that are created in our recent study are characterized by their high expression of stemness factors, stem cell markers, and their open chromatin structure. We referred to these cells as induced CSC (iCSC) [10]. Our *in vivo* studies show that the NB iCSCs possess a high tumor-initiating ability and a high metastatic potential. SKNAS iCSC and SKNBE(2)C iCSC clones (as few as 100 cells) injected subcutaneously into SCID/Beige mice

SKNAS Xenografts

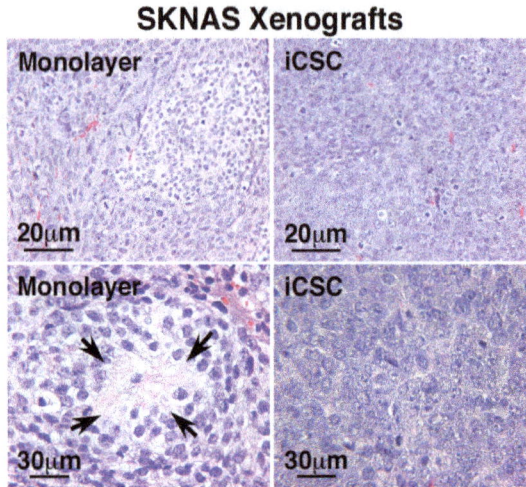

Figure 1. Histopathological examinations of SKNAS monolayer cell and iCSC xenografts. The monolayer cell xenografts were composed of two distinct components having different cellular morphologies. Tumor cells in the first component were larger cells. Tumor cells in the other component were smaller in both cellular and nuclear size and had smaller nucleoli. These small tumor cells often produced neurites or neuropils (indicated by the arrows). The monolayer cell xenografts were thus classified as poorly differentiated NB. In contrast, iCSC xenografts were composed of uniformly large cells with vesicular nuclei and one or more prominent nucleoli, and thus were classified as totally undifferentiated "large-cell" NB. Adapted from Fig. 4 of Ikegaki et al., [10].

formed tumors, and in one case, SKNBE(2)C iCSC metastasized to the adrenal gland, suggesting their increased metastatic potential [10]. Important histopathological observations were also made on the NB iCSC xenografts, and highlights of these findings are described in below.

The NB iCSC xenografts resemble human totally undifferentiated "Large-Cell" NB, the most aggressive and deadly form of NB. Histologically, NBs are classically divided into undifferentiated (UD), poorly differentiated (PD) and differentiating (D) subtypes. However, a unique histological subset of NBs within the UD and PD subtypes has been identified in the past years [5, 23]. These tumors are uniformly composed of large cells with sharply outlined nuclear membranes and one to four prominent nucleoli, and are referred to as "Large-Cell Neuroblastomas" or LCNs. Most importantly, the LCNs are the most aggressive and deadly tumors among the unfavorable NBs. Patients with the UD neuroblastoma and with the LCN appearance had a very poor prognosis regardless of age at diagnosis, clinical stage, and DNA index. Surprisingly, non-*MYCN* amplified UDs behaved significantly worse than *MYCN* amplified UDs [24]. As described below, our recent study demonstrates that NB iCSC xenografts do in fact resemble human LCN. In addition, there are histological differences between NB monolayer cell xenografts and iCSC xenografts.

As shown in Fig. 1, the SKNAS monolayer cell xenografts presented a mosaic pattern and were composed of at least two distinct components having different cellular morphologies. Tumor cells in the first component were larger cells. Tumor cells in the other component were smaller

SKNAS Monolayer Cell Xenograft

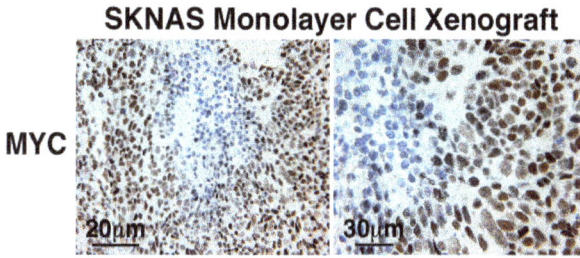

MYC

Figure 2. Immunohistochemical examination of SKNAS monolayer cell xenografts for MYC expression. As shown in Fig. 1, the SKNAS monolayer cell xenografts were composed of two distinct components having different cellular morphologies. The smaller tumor cells had reduced activities of mitosis and karyorrhexis (see also text). Accordingly, immunohistochemical examination of SKNAS monolayer cell xenografts with the anti-MYC antibody showed that the smaller tumor cells lacked MYC expression.

SKNAS iCSC Xenograft   Human Large-Cell Neuroblastoma

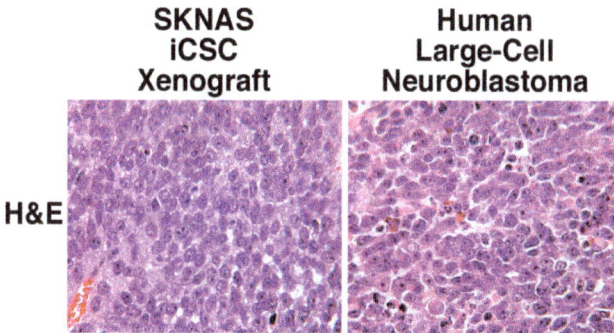

H&E

Figure 3. Histopathological examinations of SKNAS iCSC xenografts and the human large-cell" NBs. H&E stained sections showed that the SKNAS iCSC xenografts resembled human undifferentiated "large-cell" NBs histologically. Adapted from Fig. 5 of Ikegaki et al., [10].

in both cellular and nuclear size, and had smaller nucleoli (Fig. 1, upper left panel). Furthermore, these small tumor cells in the second component had reduced activities of mitosis and karyorrhexis (either intermediate MKI of 100~200/5,000 cells or low MKI of <100/5,000 cells) and often produced neurites or neuropils (Fig. 1, lower left panel). In addition, these smaller cells do not express MYC (Fig. 2). The monolayer cell xenografts were thus classified as poorly differentiated NB. In contrast, the SKNAS iCSC xenografts were composed of a diffuse and solid growth of medium-sized, rather uniform cells with a large vesicular nucleus and one or few prominent nucleoli (Fig. 1 right panel). Mitotic and karyorrhectic activities were frequently encountered (either intermediate MKI of 100~200/5,000 cells or high MKI of >200/5,000 cells). The iCSC xenografts were thus classified as totally undifferentiated "large-cell" NB, according to the International Neuroblastoma Pathology Classification [2, 3, 23, 25]. In fact, as reported in our study, all of the other iCSC xenografts from SKNBE(2)C, CHP134, and SY5Y have the

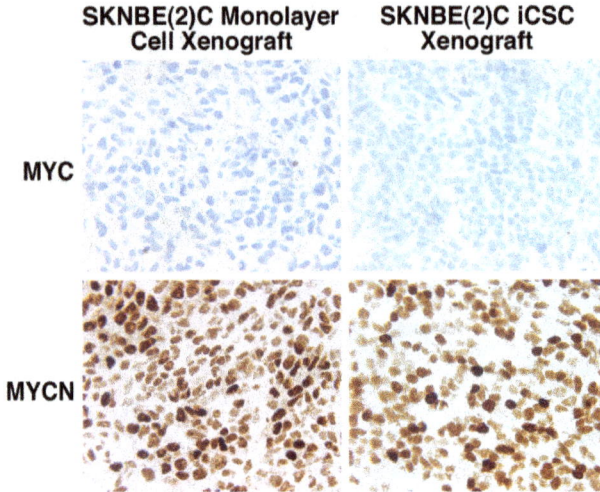

Figure 4. MYCN expression in SKNBE(2)C monolayer cell and iCSC xenografts. SKNBE(2)C are *MYCN*-amplified cells and uniformly expressed high-levels of MYCN in both monolayer cell and iCSC xenografts. MYC expression was examined for comparison. Microscopic magnification of 400X was used for all pictures. Adapted from Fig. 7 of Ikegaki et al., [10].

LCN phenotype [10]. Fig. 3 shows a remarkable resemblance of SKNAS iCSC xenografts and human LCN histologically.

MYC/MYCN expression and CXCR4 expression in NB monolayer cell xenografts and iCSC xenografts. Monolayer NB cell lines in culture express high levels of MYC (non-MYCN amplified cells) or MYCN (MYCN amplified cells). In consistent with this, our immunohistochemical analysis demonstrate that all NB monolayer cell xenografts and iCSC xenografts express high levels of MYC (SKNAS, SY5Y) or MYCN (SKNBE(2)C, CHP134)[10]. Fig. 4 shows a representative data of SKNBE(2)C.

In contrast to the consistently high MYC/MYCN expression, among the NB xenografts examined, there is a differential expression of CXCR4 in the SKNAS iCSC xenografts over monolayer cell counterparts (Fig. 5). It should be mentioned that both the larger and smaller cells of the SKNAS monolayer cell xenografts described in Fig. 1 were negative for CXCR4 staining, except some rare cases where a few cells were focally positive for CXCR4 staining (Fig. 5). These observations suggest that the large cells in SKNAS iCSC xenografts had different molecular and biological characteristics from the larger cells in the monolayer cell xenografts. However, the pattern of CXCR4 expression observed among the SKNAS xenografts was not always seen among the other iCSCs. Xenografts from both iCSC and monolayer cells of SKNBE(2)C, CHP134, SY5Y were all positive for CXCR4, but the staining in these cases was not intense and uniform [10].

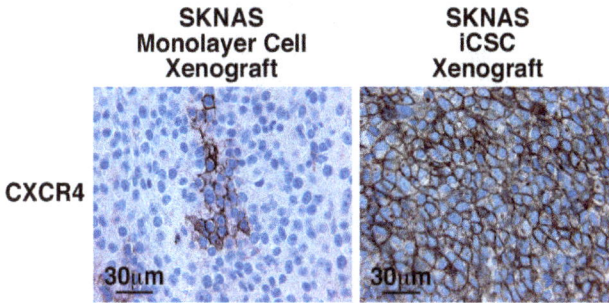

Figure 5. Differential expression of CXCR4 in SKNAS iCSC and monolayer cell xenografts. Immunohistochemical analysis showed that SKNAS iCSC xenografts were uniformly positive for CXCR4. In contrast, SKNAS monolayer cell xenografts were negative for CXCR4 with the exception of some rare cases where a few cells were focally positive for CXCR4 staining. Adapted from Fig. 3 of Ikegaki et al., [10].

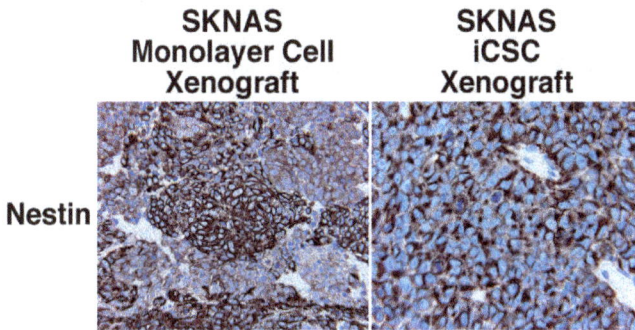

Figure 6. Immunohistochemical examination of SKNAS iCSC and monolayer cell xenografts for nestin expression. Nestin expression was examined with the anti-nestin antibody to determine whether or not nestin could serve as a marker of NB CSCs. Nestin was expressed In both SKNAS iCSC and monolayer cell xenografts. Notably, the smaller tumor cells of the monolayer cell xenograft expressed higher levels of nestin than the larger cells. These smaller cells were in fact negative for MYC expression (see Fig. 2). These observations indicate that nestin expression may not be a specific marker of NB stem cells.

Nestin expression in NB monolayer cell xenografts and iCSC xenografts. Nestin is a type VI intermediate filament protein, and nestin expression has been suggested to be a NB stem cell marker [26, 27]. Nonetheless, our data showed that nestin is expressed in SKNAS iCSC xenografts, and in both the smaller cells and larger cells of SKNAS monolayer cell-xenografts (Fig. 6). This pattern of nestin expression together with the fact that the smaller cells of SKNAS monolayer cell-xenografts are MYC negative (Fig. 2), nestin expression may therefore not serve for a specific marker of NB stem cells.

p75^{NTR} expression in NB monolayer cell xenografts and iCSC xenografts. p75^{NTR} is the low-affinity nerve growth factor receptor and a neural crest stem cell marker [18]. Our in vitro study show

p75^NTR

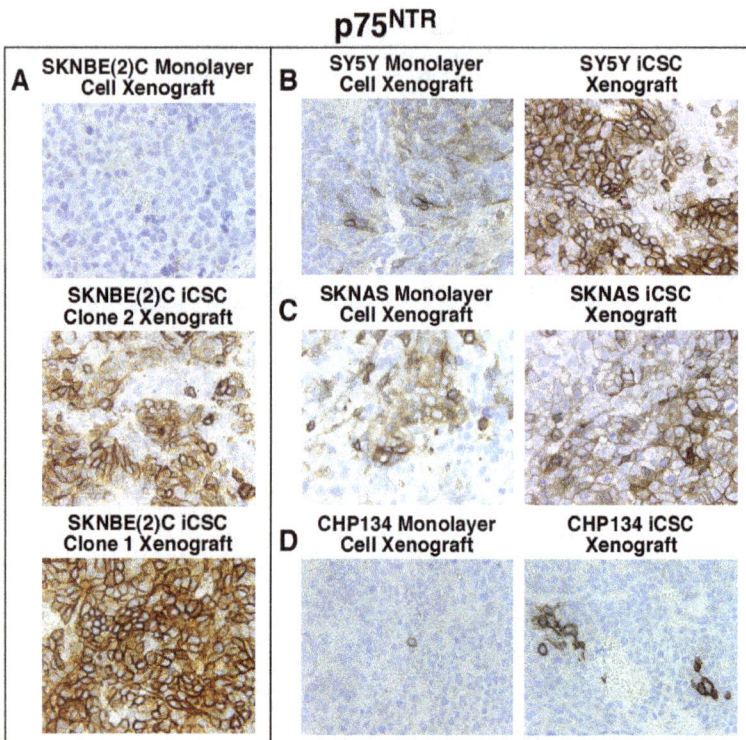

Figure 7. (A) The expression of p75^{NTR} in xenografts derived from iCSC clones and monolayer cells of SKNBE(2)C. Immunohistochemical examination was performed to assess p75^{NTR} expression in SKNBE(2)C iCSC clones and monolayer cell xenografts. The SKNBE(2)C monolayer cell xenografts rarely and faintly expressed p75^{NTR}. In contrast, subcutaneous xenografts of both Clone 1 and Clone 2 expressed high levels of p75^{NTR}, though Clone 2 xenografts contained cells with positive for p75^{NTR} and those devoid of p75^{NTR} staining. Subcutaneous xenografts of Clone 1 are consistently positive for p75^{NTR}. The expression of p75^{NTR} in xenografts derived from iCSCs and monolayer cells of (B) SY5Y, (C) SKNAS and (D) CHP134. Immunohistochemical examination was performed to assess p75^{NTR} expression in xenografts of SY5Y, SKNAS, and CHP134 iCSCs and monolayer cells. SY5Y monolayer cell xenografts expressed low level of p75^{NTR}, whereas SY5Y iCSC xenografts contained the majority of cells highly positive for p75^{NTR} and the minority of cells with low p75^{NTR} expression. The xenografts of SKNAS iCSC contained larger clusters of cells strongly positive for p75^{NTR} with the surrounding cells of weak p75^{NTR} staining, whereas the xenografts of SKNAS monolayer cells had medium size clusters of p75^{NTR} positive cells that were surrounded by p75^{NTR} negative cells. Only rare and faintly positive cells for p75^{NTR} were detected in CHP134 monolayer cell xenografts, while CHP134 iCSC xenografts contained small islands of positive cells for p75^{NTR}. Microscopic magnification of 400X was used for all pictures. Adapted from Fig. S8 of Ikegaki et al., [10].

that SKNAS iCSC, SKNBE(2)C iCSC, and SY5Y iCSC express high levels of p75^{NTR} [10], and these observations are confirmed by the xenograft data shown in Fig. 7. As described in our study, the expression of p75^{NTR} in CHP 134 iCSC xenograft was minimal [10]. Interestingly, the pattern of p75^{NTR} expression in the SKNAS monolayer cell xenografts suggests that p75^{NTR} expression is not related to neuronal differentiation in NB (Fig. 8).

SKNAS iCSC Xenograft

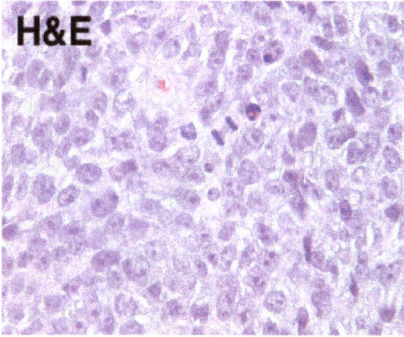

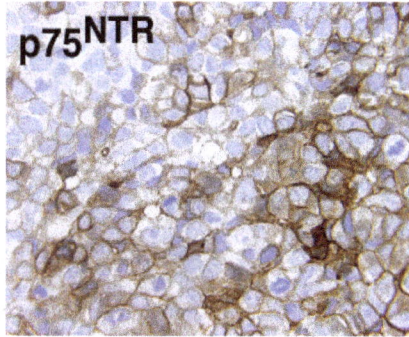

SKNAS Monolayer Cell Xenograft

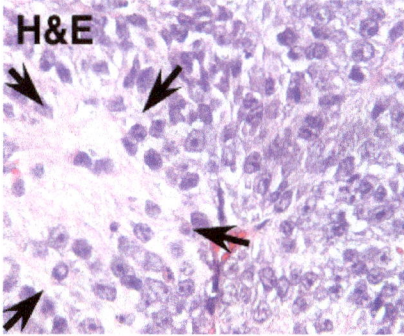

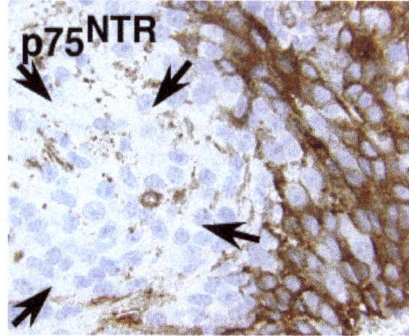

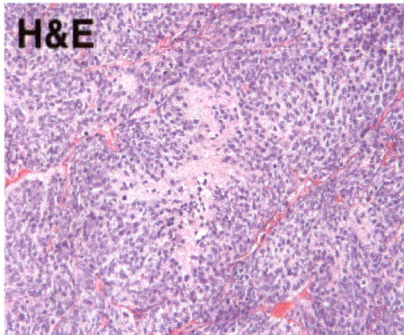

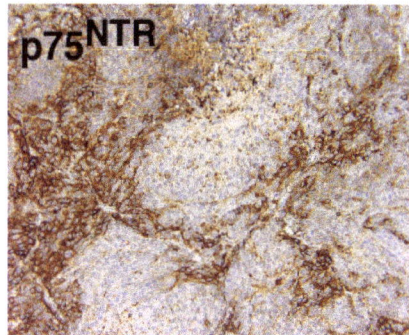

Figure 8. The expression of p75^{NTR} is not related to neuronal differentiation in NB. Varying numbers of cells were positive for p75^{NTR} in SKNAS monolayer cell xenografts. However, in the SKNAS monolayer cell xenografts, the cells with active neuropil formations were negative for p75^{NTR} staining as indicated by arrows. Microscopic magnification of 400X was used for four pictures in the first and second rows, and 100X was used for two pictures in the bottom row. Adapted from Fig. 8 of Ikegaki et al., [10].

2. Conclusion

In conclusion, the xenografts established from the NB iCSCs shared two consistent and common features: the LCN phenotype and high-level MYC/MYCN expression. In addition, our observations suggest that NB cells with large and vesicular nuclei, representing their open chromatin structure, are indicative of stem cell-like tumor cells, and that epigenetic changes may have contributed to the development of these most malignant NB cells. These observations have significant clinical implications. Specifically, one may identify the most malignant and aggressive type of NBs that require immediate innovative therapeutic intervention by examining histological/cytological appearance of the tumor, namely totally undifferentiated large-cell NB with prominent nuclei and high-level expression of MYC and/or MYCN by immunohistochemical analysis. Finally, the availability of the NB iCSCs will serve as useful tools to develop effective anti-CSC agents for NB in vivo and will help improve treatment and cure for children with neuroblastoma.

Acknowledgements

Dr. Xao Tang is supported by grants from NIH CA97255, CA127571, and a grant from the St. Baldrick Foundation. We would like to acknowledge Dr. Naohiko Ikegaki for his significant contribution in the development and establishment of the iCSCs described in this study and Jonathan Harbert for his technical assistance with the immunohistochemistry analyses.

Author details

Xao X. Tang[1] and Hiroyuki Shimada[2]

1 Department of Anatomy and Cell Biology, College of Medicine, University of Illinois at Chicago, Chicago, Illinois, USA

2 Department of Pathology & Laboratory Medicine, Children's Hospital Los Angeles and University of Southern California Keck School of Medicine, Los Angeles, California, USA

References

[1] Cohn SL, Pearson AD, London WB, Monclair T, Ambros PF, Brodeur GM, Faldum A, Hero B, Iehara T, Machin D, Mosseri V, Simon T, Garaventa A, Castel V, Matthay KK; INRG Task Force. The International Neuroblastoma Risk Group (INRG) classification system: an INRG Task Force report. J Clin Oncol 2009;27(2) 289-297.

[2] Shimada H, Ambros IM, Dehner LP, Hata J, Joshi VV, Roald B. Terminology and morphologic criteria of neuroblastic tumors: recommendations by the International Neuroblastoma Pathology Committee. Cancer 1999;86(2) 349-363.

[3] Shimada H, Ambros IM, Dehner LP, Hata J, Joshi VV, Roald B, Stram DO, Gerbing RB, Lukens JN, Matthay KK, Castleberry RP. The International Neuroblastoma Pathology Classification (the Shimada system). Cancer 1999;86(2) 364-372.

[4] Seeger RC, Brodeur GM, Sather H, Dalton A, Siegel SE, Wong KY, Hammond D. Association of multiple copies of the N-myc oncogene with rapid progression of neuroblastomas. New England Journal of Medicine 1985;313(18) 1111-1116.

[5] Kobayashi C, Monforte-Munoz HL, Gerbing RB, Stram DO, Matthay KK, Lukens JN, Seeger RC, Shimada H. Enlarged and prominent nucleoli may be indicative of MYCN amplification: a study of neuroblastoma (Schwannian stroma-poor), undifferentiated/poorly differentiated subtype with high mitosis-karyorrhexis index. Cancer 2005;103(1) 174-180.

[6] Fredlund E, Ringner M, Maris JM, Pahlman S. High Myc pathway activity and low stage of neuronal differentiation associate with poor outcome in neuroblastoma. Proc Natl Acad Sci U S A 2008;105(37) 14094-14099.

[7] Matthay KK, Villablanca JG, Seeger RC, Stram DO, Harris RE, Ramsay NK, Swift P, Shimada H, Black CT, Brodeur GM, Gerbing RB, Reynolds CP. Treatment of high-risk neuroblastoma with intensive chemotherapy, radiotherapy, autologous bone marrow transplantation, and 13-cis- retinoic acid. Children's Cancer Group. N Engl J Med 1999;341(16) 1165-1173.

[8] Katzenstein HM, Cohn SL, Shore RM, Bardo DM, Haut PR, Olszewski M, Schmoldt J, Liu D, Rademaker AW, Kletzel M. Scintigraphic response by 123I-metaiodobenzylguanidine scan correlates with event-free survival in high-risk neuroblastoma. J Clin Oncol 2004;22(19) 3909-3915.

[9] Naranjo A, Parisi MT, Shulkin BL, London WB, Matthay KK, Kreissman SG, Yanik GA. Comparison of (1)(2)(3)I-metaiodobenzylguanidine (MIBG) and (1)(3)(1)I-MIBG semi-quantitative scores in predicting survival in patients with stage 4 neuroblastoma: a report from the Children's Oncology Group. Pediatr Blood Cancer 2011;56(7) 1041-1045.

[10] Ikegaki N, Shimada H, Fox AM, Regan PL, Jacobs JR, Hicks SL, Rappaport EF, Tang XX. Transient treatment with epigenetic modifiers yields stable neuroblastoma stem cells resembling aggressive large-cell neuroblastomas. Proc Natl Acad Sci U S A 2013;in press.

[11] Takahashi K, Tanabe K, Ohnuki M, Narita M, Ichisaka T, Tomoda K, Yamanaka S. Induction of pluripotent stem cells from adult human fibroblasts by defined factors. Cell 2007;131(5) 861-872.

[12] Takahashi K, Yamanaka S. Induction of pluripotent stem cells from mouse embryonic and adult fibroblast cultures by defined factors. Cell 2006;126(4) 663-676.

[13] Yu J, Vodyanik MA, Smuga-Otto K, Antosiewicz-Bourget J, Frane JL, Tian S, Nie J, Jonsdottir GA, Ruotti V, Stewart R, Slukvin II, Thomson JA. Induced pluripotent stem cell lines derived from human somatic cells. Science 2007;318(5858) 1917-1920.

[14] Hermann PC, Huber SL, Herrler T, Aicher A, Ellwart JW, Guba M, Bruns CJ, Heeschen C. Distinct populations of cancer stem cells determine tumor growth and metastatic activity in human pancreatic cancer. Cell Stem Cell 2007;1(3) 313-323.

[15] Ho MM, Ng AV, Lam S, Hung JY. Side population in human lung cancer cell lines and tumors is enriched with stem-like cancer cells. Cancer Res 2007;67(10) 4827-4833.

[16] Singh SK, Clarke ID, Terasaki M, Bonn VE, Hawkins C, Squire J, Dirks PB. Identification of a cancer stem cell in human brain tumors. Cancer Res 2003;63(18) 5821-5828.

[17] Kim J, Lo L, Dormand E, Anderson DJ. SOX10 maintains multipotency and inhibits neuronal differentiation of neural crest stem cells. Neuron 2003;38(1) 17-31.

[18] Morrison SJ, White PM, Zock C, Anderson DJ. Prospective identification, isolation by flow cytometry, and in vivo self-renewal of multipotent mammalian neural crest stem cells. Cell 1999;96(5) 737-749.

[19] Nieto MA, Sargent MG, Wilkinson DG, Cooke J. Control of cell behavior during vertebrate development by Slug, a zinc finger gene. Science 1994;264(5160) 835-839.

[20] Sakakibara S, Imai T, Hamaguchi K, Okabe M, Aruga J, Nakajima K, Yasutomi D, Nagata T, Kurihara Y, Uesugi S, Miyata T, Ogawa M, Mikoshiba K, Okano H. Mouse-Musashi-1, a neural RNA-binding protein highly enriched in the mammalian CNS stem cell. Dev Biol 1996;176(2) 230-242.

[21] Scott CE, Wynn SL, Sesay A, Cruz C, Cheung M, Gomez Gaviro MV, Booth S, Gao B, Cheah KS, Lovell-Badge R, Briscoe J. SOX9 induces and maintains neural stem cells. Nat Neurosci 2010;13(10) 1181-1189.

[22] Ohtsuka T, Ishibashi M, Gradwohl G, Nakanishi S, Guillemot F, Kageyama R. Hes1 and Hes5 as notch effectors in mammalian neuronal differentiation. EMBO J 1999;18(8) 2196-2207.

[23] Tornoczky T, Kalman E, Kajtar PG, Nyari T, Pearson AD, Tweddle DA, Board J, Shimada H. Large cell neuroblastoma: a distinct phenotype of neuroblastoma with aggressive clinical behavior. Cancer 2004;100(2) 390-397.

[24] Wang LL, Suganuma R, Tovar JP, Naranjo A, London WB, Hogarty MD, Gastire-Foster JM, Look AT, Park JR, Maris JM, Cohn SL, Shimada H. Neuroblastoma, Undifferentiated subtype: A report from the Children's Oncology Group. Pediatric Dev Pathol 2012;in press.

[25] Tornoczky T, Semjen D, Shimada H, Ambros IM. Pathology of peripheral neuroblastic tumors: significance of prominent nucleoli in undifferentiated/poorly differentiated neuroblastoma. Pathol Oncol Res 2007;13(4) 269-275.

[26] Mahller YY, Williams JP, Baird WH, Mitton B, Grossheim J, Saeki Y, Cancelas JA, Ratner N, Cripe TP. Neuroblastoma cell lines contain pluripotent tumor initiating cells that are susceptible to a targeted oncolytic virus. PLoS ONE 2009;4(1) e4235.

[27] Thomas SK, Messam CA, Spengler BA, Biedler JL, Ross RA. Nestin is a potential mediator of malignancy in human neuroblastoma cells. J Biol Chem 2004;279(27) 27994-27999.

Chapter 11

Copper as a Target for Treatment of Neuroblastoma: Molecular and Cellular Mechanisms

Emanuela Urso and Michele Maffia

Additional information is available at the end of the chapter

1. Introduction

1.1. Copper and carcinogenesis, a double-edged sword

Copper is a trace metal essential to the catalysis of a wide range of enzymatic activities, including those involved in the process of energy production (cytochrome c oxidase), the cell response to oxidant injuries (Cu,Zn-superoxide dismutase), the catecholamine (dopamine β-monooxygenase) and melanin (tyrosinase) production, the remodelling of extracellular matrix (lysyl oxidase), blood clotting processes (Factors V and VIII) and iron metabolism (ceruloplasmin and hephaestin) [1]. The catalytic properties of copper are linked to its ability to easily assume the oxidized (Cu^{2+}) and reduced (Cu^{+}) states, but just the metal reactive behaviour can trigger severe cell alterations through the generation of hydroxyl radicals in Fenton-like reactions [2,3]. When the cytosolic copper concentration is above the optimal level, the newly formed reactive oxygen species (ROS) rapidly bind to DNA, thus inducing the breaking of the nucleic acid strands and initiating a series of cascade events that can lead to significant damage to cell structures and function [4].

Considerable intrinsic oxidative stress and enhanced serum and tissue copper levels depict a disease condition that often accompanies the progression of several tumour forms, in turn resulting from a perturbed energy metabolism, mitochondrial dysfunction, release of cytokines and inflammation [5]. Copper is intimately involved in all these cell functions, thus targeting the elevated copper levels would be an ideal therapeutic strategy to effectively counteract the tumour development [5].

This issue is anyway highly debated. In fact, the topical delivery of copper complexes to tumour tissues has been demonstrated to kill the cancer cells through a "therapeutic" induction of oxidative stress [6]. At the same time, especially in the case of solid tumours, as *neuroblas-*

toma, copper is directly involved in the spread of the primary tumour, mainly through the stimulation of tumour angiogenesis [6]. It follows that targeting the tumour copper content to limit the cancer aggressiveness requires a comprehensive knowledge of the cell metal management under the disease state. Here, the multifaceted contribution of copper to the pathophysiology of neuroblastoma will be dissected, with special attention paid to the regulation of membrane copper transporters and their role in sustaining the cancer spread. To make the reader familiar with the main copper transport systems in mammalian cells, a short description has been provided in Box 1.

2. Neuroblastoma and Copper: A complex relationship

Neuroblastoma is the most common pediatric extra-cranial neoplasm [7], whose malignant form accounts for about a 50% of cancer mortality in chemoradiotherapy-treated subjects [8]. The aggressiveness of advanced-staged neuroblastomas is notoriously associated with the N-*myc* oncogene amplification, which translates in a strong expression of a pleiotropic transcription factor, responsible for the rich tumour vasculature, the metastatic behaviour, and the chemotherapy resistance [9-11]. Thus, N-*myc* overexpression is a well-known adverse prognostic factor [12]. Interestingly, the degree of N-*myc* oncogene amplification in neuroblastoma cells has been put in relation to the trace metal cell content (iron, copper, zinc) in both cultured neuroblasts and murine xenografts [13-15]. In particular, the number of N-*myc* oncogene copies has been demonstrated to proportionally correlate with the neuroblastoma copper content. This finding, together with evidences from the literature, lets us suppose that copper accumulation strictly determines the neuroblastoma invasiveness. Plausible mechanisms underlining the copper dependence of neuroblastoma metastasis are both direct/specific, and mediated by the metal-induced accumulation of ROS.

Referring to the latter category of mechanisms, an *in vitro* study in 31 subjects affected by advanced neuroblastoma revealed an elevated activation of specific tissue matrix metallo proteinases (MMP-2 isoform) and the reduced expression of their specific inhibitors (TIMP-2) [16], that can be associated with copper-induced oxidative stress [17]. In this regard, we observe that metallo proteinases are secreted by tumour cells and facilitate the cancer dissemination by the degradation of the extracellular matrix.

The high copper levels detected in neuroblastoma can at least partly confer a growth advantage to the tumour cells by metal specific pathways. Significantly, copper acts as a cofactor for the cytochrome c oxidase enzyme that allows the conversion of cytosolic ferric ion into the ferrous form, subsequently incorporated into ferritin, the most important iron storage protein. Iron-complexed ferritin is then secreted by cancer cells, so enriching the serum protein pool. The importance of this copper/iron antagonism is evident if we consider that neuroblastoma patients with high ferritin levels undergo a bad prognosis [18].

Given the complexity of the copper-neuroblastoma relationship, in order to guide the reader through the text, we observe that the lines of copper intervention in neuroblastoma progression can be substantially subdivided as follows:

i.   cancer energy metabolism

ii.   tumour vascularization

Copper transport systems are gaining growing importance in the studies about the various aspects of the metal role in neuroblastoma, so the peculiar expression pattern will be described before discussing the pathological topics.

3. Copper transport systems in neuroblastoma cells: Regulation and physiopathological implications

Copper critically regulates the degree of neuroblastoma growth and microvascularization, which determines the tumour aggressive phenotype [19,20]. The importance of this metal is emphasized by the strong presence of specific transport proteins in neuroblastoma cells, that testifies to a lively management of tumour copper stores. Highly variegated mechanisms of regulation of copper homeostasis have been specifically reported for neuroblastoma (some of them reviewed here), that make it difficult to establish the nature of copper involvement: is the ion metabolic disruption a cause or an effect?

Copper import. It is widely believed that copper import in neuroblastoma cells is mediated by hCtr1 [21]. However, recent work from our laboratory in an *in vitro* neuroblastoma cell model has enlightened a role for the cellular prion protein PrP^C in mediating the high affinity copper intake, upon normal metal availability [22]. In addition, we demonstrated that copper shortness induces an up-regulation of PrP^C expression in a neuroblastoma cell model, a cell adaptive strategy aimed at restoring the standard copper status [23].

In support of its involvement in tumorigenesis, the PrP^C expression is up-regulated in nervous tissues affected by hypoxia, a condition typically occurring during the growth of a solid tumour [24]. The reader is referred to paragraphs 4.2 and 6.2 for a detailed account of the PrP^C functions in the tumour spread.

Copper efflux. The ATP7A copper ATPase (full length 170 KDa protein) is strongly expressed by neuroblastoma cell lines [21,23] and subjected to an articulated copper-dependent regulation.

In many cell types this efflux pump delivers copper to the secretory compartments and, when copper should accumulate inside the cytosol, it traffics toward the cell periphery to export the ion excess [25]. However, peculiar regulative mechanisms have been documented in neuroblastoma models.

In fact, it has been demonstrated in the M17 neuroblastoma cell line that fluctuating copper levels (excess/starvation) in the cell microenvironment can favour the interaction of ATP7A proteins with clusterins (apolipoprotein J), the last ones targeting the pumps toward degradation through the lysosomal pathway [26]. This copper-regulated clusterin function may have multiple implications, if we consider that a recent study on neuroblastoma cell lines, mouse models, and human specimens evidenced that this molecular chaperon behaves as a tumour and metastasis suppressor, negatively regulated by N-*myc* in the most aggressive forms [27].

In our opinion, the copper-clusterin link deserves further exploration in the light of the reported elevation in copper neuroblastoma content observed in N-*myc* amplified tumours.

If N-*myc* really down-regulates clusterin (still controversial aspect), one would expect an increase in copper export function and so an overall reduction of the ion cancerogenic action. This evidently contradicts the N-*myc* - tumour malignancy binomial association (where copper should exert a prominent role) and minimizes the contribution of clusterin to the copper-dependent tumour progression. In fact, considering that N-*myc* elevates the neuroblastoma copper content, one can suppose that the cytosolic copper lowering due to a down-regulated expression of clusterin is overridden by other cell mechanisms causing the increase of cancer copper levels.

Copper uptake

Ctr1 (Copper transporter 1). High-affinity Cu^+ importer, composed of three main domains: an extracellular N-terminal tail containing multiple copper-binding methionine residues; a trans-membrane segment consisting of three α-helical regions; an intracellular C-terminal domain. Three subunits assemble to form a homo-trimeric channel (9 Å pore diameter) within the plasma membrane (see [118] for a review).

Ctr2 (Copper transporter 2). Copper permease, whose structure resembles that of Ctr1. Predominantly localized to endosomes and lysosomes, it seems to provide a mechanism of copper recycling from degraded cuproenzymes [119].

PrP[C] (Cellular Prion protein). Endogenous copper-binding glycoprotein, mainly expressed in the central nervous system. The protein structure includes an unstructured N-terminal domain and a C-terminal globular region composed of three α -helices and two short beta-strands. When Cu^{2+} ions bind to the N-terminal octapeptide repeats (residues 51–90), the protein undergoes endocytosis, that providing a route for cell copper entry [58,59].

Cytosolic transport

CCS. Metallo chaperone required for copper delivery to Cu,Zn Superoxide dismutases 1; up-regulated in response to copper deficiency [120].

Cox17. Metallo chaperone delivering copper to Sco1 and Cox11 proteins in order to catalyse the cytochrome c oxidase copper loading [121].

Atox1. Metallo chaperone that delivers copper to ATP7A and ATP7B Cu^+ efflux pumps [122].

Metallothioneins. Small cysteine-rich proteins tightly binding copper ions and buffering the ion excess [123].

Copper efflux

ATP7A. Cu^+-transporting P-type ATPase expressed by all cell types, with the exception of liver. Structural features include eight membrane-spanning domains and six N-terminal cysteine-rich metal binding motifs (MXCXXC) [25].

Box 1. Main proteins involved in cell copper homeostasis

Coming back to main focus of this paragraph, multiple ATP7A spliced variants can be retrieved in human cells, not necessarily related to disease states, with a cell type-specific expression pattern. The expression of a 11.2 KDa splicing product (103 amino acids) has been reported in SY5Y neuroblastoma cells, harbouring a sequence able to bind copper ions [28]. It has been proposed that such spliced product can work as a copper chaperon to direct the cytosolic copper toward the nuclear compartment.

Intracellular copper distribution. Among copper chaperons, the contribution of COMMD1 (Copper Metabolism MURR1 Domain containing 1) to the copper status in neuroblastoma cells is an unexplored issue so far. However, some inputs from the recent scientific literature let us hypothesize an involvement.

Endogenous COMMD1 expression has been reported in the SH-SY5Y neuroblastoma cell line, together with the isoform 3. A punctate cytoplasmic distribution, denser in the perinuclear region, has been shown for COMMD1, while COMMD3 appears more diffused [29]. The role of COMMD1 in neuroblastoma progression is potentially articulated on multiple levels of action, even if direct demonstrations are missing and the following dissertation aims at enlightening some aspects of copper-dependent regulation of the protein fate.

A role in preventing tumour growth and metastasis has been proposed for COMMD1, based on its ability to repress the NF-KB pathway and the HIF1α/β dimerization and so inhibit the expression of genes involved in tumour angiogenesis [30]. However, as documented in N2a neuroblastoma cell line, upon copper excess, COMMD1 can form a hetero-complex with CCS and SOD1, leading to decreased levels of SOD1 dimers and subsequently reduced anti-oxidant activity [31]. In other words, in the presence of high copper, the COMMD1 cell fate can potentially assume a negative connotation.

COMMD1 is also an interacting partner of ATP7A proteins and, analogously to clusterin, can drive their degradation through a proteasomal pathway [32], this indicating a further contribution of this chaperon to the neuroblastoma copper content. However, knowledge about these aspects is still limited.

The COMMD1 involvement in determining the neuroblastoma copper condition is strictly linked to the protein XIAP (X-linked inhibitor of apoptosis). XIAP protective action is due to the prevention of the activation of a subset of cell death proteases (caspases 3, 7 and 9) [33,34], and inhibiton of Fas- [35] and Bax-induced apoptosis [33].

During the last decade, a role for XIAP in controlling the cell copper homeostasis has been described [36]. In fact, the overexpression of XIAP protein (not transcript) selectively reported in chemotherapy-resistant neuroblastomas, but no other tissues [37], may indicate the occurrence of a particular copper status. XIAP is a copper-binding protein that, in the olo-form, favours the ubiquitination and degradation of COMMD1, that in turn interacts with ATP7A to support copper excretion [36]. Where overexpressed, it is reasonable to presume a subsequent consistent reduction of COMMD1 cytosolic protein levels, and so an increase of the cellular copper content.

However, the binding of copper to XIAP negatively impacts the protein stability, so a negative feedback exists [38]. In the case of chemotherapy-resistant neuroblastomas, the protein overexpression probably overcomes the effects deriving from copper-driven XIAP inactivation.

Preclinical evidences of the importance of XIAP as a target to treat neuroblastoma have been recently collected, all based on the lowering of the threshold for the induction of apoptosis through the depression of XIAP expression. The use of Thymoquinone, a bioactive compound from *nigella sativa*, has been shown to selectively down-regulate XIAP in neuroblastoma cells, but not in normal neuronal cells, with an expected higher copper efflux [39]. Smac (Second mitochondria-derived activator of caspase) mimetics (e.g. LBW242) have been reported to sensitize chemotherapy resistant and XIAP-overexpressing neuroblastomas, by favouring the degradation of XIAP and TNF-α expression [37].

4. Copper-dependence of neuroblastoma metabolic changes

The oxygen partial pressure within a solid tumour ranges from 5-10 mmHg in highly vascularized regions to absence (anoxia) around the necrotic areas [40,41]. Most cancer cells tend to adapt to the intra-tumour hypoxic microenvironment by activating a pro-survival signalling, a pro-angiogenic pattern of gene expression and through the metabolic switching from the oxidative phosphorylation to the glycolytic pathways (Warburg effect) [42].

Currently, there is not a homogeneous view on the causative events, but two major factors are usually indicated as responsible, the Hypoxia-Inducible Factors 1 and 2 (HIF1,2), and p53 transcription factor.

HIF1 and 2 are heterodimeric basic helix-loop-helix-PAS domain transcription factors, composed of a constitutively expressed β subunit and a α regulatory subunit (HIF1α/2α), whose expression is induced by hypoxia, cancer-associated mutations, or inflammatory cytokines [43,44].

HIF-1α and HIF-2α are major actors in the cell adaptive response to hypoxic conditions and control the expression of distinct, but functionally converging genes [45]. Each cell type exhibits a peculiar profile of HIF-1α and 2α expression and their functions may also differ. In the case of *neuroblastoma*, at a careful analysis of the expression pattern, tumour stage, and copper status, it can be observed that copper heavily influences the response to hypoxia and that the tumour progression and the evolution of copper metabolism go hand in hand.

4.1. HIF-1α

HIF-1α, but not HIF-2α, is preferentially expressed and up-regulated by moderate hypoxia in N-*myc* amplified neuroblastoma cell lines and primary tumours, correlating with a poor prognosis [41,46]. In the light of the linear increase of copper neuroblastoma levels with the degree of N-*myc* gene amplification and the proven role of Cu^{2+} ions in stabilizing the structure of the HIF-1α subunit [47], it can be deduced that copper plays in key role in inducing the neuroblastoma metabolic changes.

Cu^{2+} ions determine the structural stabilization of the HIF-1α subunit (oxygen-sensitive) through the inhibition of prolyl-4-hydroxilases, which allow the subsequent ubiquitination and degradation of such factor [47].

Interestingly, by this way Cu^{2+} indirectly promotes the synthesis of ceruloplasmin, a plasma and liquor copper chaperon with a ferroxidase activity, whose expression is typically under HIF-1 control [48]. Being ceruloplasmin a major copper vehicle, such mechanism can be interpreted as cancer "self-nourishing". It must be added that HIF-1 target genes also include VEGF (Vascular Endothelial Growth Factor), a recognized chemotactic and mitogen factor [49], and VEGFR-1 (VEGF Receptor-1) [50], both involved in the positive regulation of the sprouting of blood vessels within the primary tumour.

Further, White et al. (2009) demonstrated that the up-regulation of the hypoxia inducible factor HIF-1α causes the selective distribution of copper ions to the secretory pathway. They observed in tumour-associated macrophages that the hypoxic stress can influence the intracellular distribution of copper ions, determining an increased ion entry through the high affinity channel Ctr1 and then an elevated efflux through the ATP7A pump [51].

All these experimental evidences underline the prominent role of copper in sustaining the HIF-1α-dependent adaptation to hypoxia in N-*myc* amplified neuroblastomas, as well as the hypoxia-stimulated activation of copper transport activities.

4.2. HIF-2α

HIF-2α, but not HIF-1α, has been shown to be highly expressed in neuroblastoma vascularized areas, and this pattern seems to be associated with an unfavourable patient outcome, due to the occurrence of distal metastasis [41]. In addition, a small subset of neuroblastoma cells strongly HIF-2α-positive has been described, which could represent the cancer stem cells [52]. To our knowledge, no precise data are available about the copper-dependent activity/ activation of HIF-2α, however some molecular evidences collected in other cell models strongly point at a potential existence of such a link.

As an example, Menkes copper ATPase (Atp7a) gene expression has been demonstrated to be strongly induced by HIF-2α in mammalian intestine [53]. HIF-2α has been also demonstrated to induce the expression of DMT1 and Ctr1 (by about 25%) copper importers in human intestinal cells, so determining a parallel increase (fivefold) in the processes of cellular copper uptake [54].

These findings confirm that, independently on the involvement of HIF-1α or HIF-2α, tumour hypoxia activates a series of processes functional to distribute copper toward the secretory pathway (enzyme-complexed) or make it available in the extracellular medium. Here, copper may function as a signalling molecule and sustain the angiogenic processes, essential to the neuroblastoma growth.

The scientific literature also suggests that the HIF-2α prolonged response to hypoxia can be alternatively mediated by a high affinity copper-binding protein, namely the cellular prion protein PrP^C [55] (Box 1). Accordingly, the PrP^C expression degree is elevated in hypoxic nervous tissues [56], and its overexpression has been shown to confer a highly invasive phenotype to tumour cells [55,57].

By virtue of a direct involvement of PrP^C in the cell copper import [22,58,59], an elevated protein expression under hypoxia could represent a cancer cell strategy to assure the neuroblastoma growth through the enhanced copper intake [23]. In fact, copper stimulates neuroblastoma cell proliferation [60].

Interestingly, although it has been demonstrated that the up-regulation of PrP^C in human colorectal carcinoma cells induces the glucose transporter-1 (Glut-1) expression and a subsequent increase in the glycolytic rate via Fyn-HIF-2α pathway [55], the transfection of a plasmid expressing wild-type HIF-2α in N-*myc* amplified neuroblastoma cells has been demonstrated to be marginally involved in the regulation of glycolytic genes [46]. Surprisingly, notwithstanding a rise in Glut-1 expression, the glucose influx was not increased [46].

Conclusively, to reinforce the concept of an autonomous cancerogenic role of copper, it can be observed that elevated HIF levels have been observed even under normoxic conditions, meaning that other factors than hypoxia, e.g. copper, can sustain the aerobic glycolysis and induce the expression of HIF-targeted genes.

4.3. p53

p53 transcription factor is a key tumour suppressor protein, whose functions contribute to prevent cancer progression. Mutated p53 gene products or defects in the integration of proteins with which p53 is connected, are associated with the malignant progression of the majority of human tumours [61]. Neuroblastoma rarely shows mutated p53 at diagnosis, thus therapies result effective at first. However, gene mutations, p53 cytosolic sequestration, or deregulated p53/MDM2 (ubiquitin protein ligase -E3- for p53) pathways have been reported during neuroblastoma relapses or therapies, thus conferring high-level multidrug resistance [62-65].

Loss of p53 function seems to impair the efficiency of mitochondrial respiration by hampering the insertion of copper ions as cofactors into the cytochrome c oxidase enzymatic complex [66]. That would cause the switching from cell respiration to *aerobic glycolysis* (Warburg effect), typical metabolic change observed in cancer cells.

In detail, p53 directly regulates the expression of the SCO2 (Synthesis of Cytochrome c Oxidase) gene, coding for a protein that facilitates the copper delivery to the subunit II of cytochrome c oxidase, determining the assembly of the enzymatic complex [66].

As suggested in [67], given the essential role of copper in determining the Warburg effect in cancer cells, it cannot be excluded that deregulated p53 pathways may affect the expression or function of other proteins involved in cell copper acquisition and utilization.

5. Copper promotes the neuroblastoma survival and growth by sustaining the anti-oxidant enzyme activities

Cutting copper supply can represent a valuable therapeutic strategy for neuroblastoma, as the induced mitochondrial impairment and oxidative stress can make neuroblastoma cells vulnerable. Accordingly, even under unstressed environment, mitochondria in this cell type exhibit a high rate of protein oxidation, this indicating a consistent susceptibility to the oxidative injury [68,69]. The positive connotation of a drop in the neuroblastoma cell copper content has been demonstrated and emphasized by a rich literature showing that copper chelation (triethylene tetramine tetrahydrochloride) can effectively promote the apoptosis of neuroblastoma cells [70,71].

Here follow some argumentations from the literature around the negative impact of copper starvation on neuroblastoma cell survival, extrapolated from *in vitro* preclinical studies.

SH-SY5Y neuroblastoma cells have been widely used as a model to dissect the molecular basis of the tumour sensitivity to copper.

In particular, the continuous exposure (up to three passages) of SH-SY5Y neuroblastoma cells to the copper-chelating agent Trien has been demonstrated to induce the expression of antioxidants and a 40% apoptotic cell loss at the end of the third passage [70]. Copper has been shown to be important in keeping a critical level of ATP. In fact, the relevant Cu,Zn SOD and cytochrome c oxidase activities were reduced by, respectively, 80 and 68% [70]. Another report has confirmed these findings, indicating that copper starvation by Trien impairs the antioxidant defences of neuroblastoma cells, with obvious implications with respect to the therapeutic inhibition of the tumour growth [71].

Arciello et al. (2011) further characterized the effects of Trien treatment in SH-SY5Y neuroblastoma cells [72]. SOD1 (cuproenzyme) expression decline was associated with a reduction of the enzyme activity, mainly due to copper shortness rather than to a decreased protein expression. In fact, copper replenishment was able to reactivate the apo-form of the enzyme, in agreement with previous observations [73]. Copper depletion also favoured the entrance of the SOD1 apo-form (not metallated) into the mitochondria [72], where it was retained due to a partial unfolded and obviously inactive configuration. The authors also observed an increased expression of CCS (Box 1), finalized to optimize the copper intracellular distribution [72].

It the light of these findings, it can be observed that the neuroblastoma commitment to the apoptotic death was not due to an irreversible mitochondrial damage, even considering that the loss of the mitochondria-associated SOD1 was much less evident than observed for the cytosolic one [72]. However, it is plausible that the absence of copper prevented SOD1 from counteracting the oxidative-mediated damage to mitochondrial proteins [74]. Accordingly, it has been shown that brain tissues exhibit a SOD1 localization inside the mitochondrial matrix with an antioxidant function [75].

In our laboratory we analysed the anti-oxidant response to copper starvation in a rat neuroblastoma model (B104), investigating in parallel the expression of copper membrane transporters [23]. A significant increase of caspase-3 activity was detected in copper-starved cells, indicating the activation of a cell death program through the induction of oxidative stress. In agreement, the total Cu,Zn SOD activity resulted half-reduced with respect to normal conditions, as expected in consideration of the role of copper as a cofactor [23]. Interestingly, the cellular prion protein expression in copper-starved neuroblastoma cells was heavily induced. This finding was reconsidered in the light of a rich literature showing that the ^{64}Cu loading and the enzymatic activity of Cu,Zn SOD from the brain of *P-rnp* $^{0/0}$ mice result 10-50% reduced with respect to the wild-type genotype [76-78].

A special attention has been dedicated to the adaptive response actuated by PrP^C, that is physiologically and consistently localized on the outer surface of neurons at synapses and gliocytes [79,80]. Under normal conditions, PrP^C binds copper ions with high specificity and affinity (femto- to nanomolar range), by the repeated sequences present on its N-terminal region. By virtue of this property and the ability to undergo endocytosis upon copper binding, PrP^C is believed to drive the cellular copper intake [22,58,59].

The up-regulation of PrP^C upon copper limitation has been interpreted as a compensatory mechanism to re-establish the standard cell copper status through a direct transport activity. It has been also demonstrated to be responsible for the ability of copper-starved cells to almost completely recover the SOD enzyme function upon re-exposure to standard growth conditions. The authors conclusively demonstrated that the PrP^C neuroprotective action in neuroblastoma cells is due to its ability to translocate copper ions into the cytosol. Here, they can act as cofactors in Cu,Zn SOD activation [23].

6. Critical role of copper transporters in neuroblastoma vascularization and spread

Most pro-angiogenic factors implicated in neuroblastoma progression need copper to properly work or exert their own functions by activating copper-dependent pathways and enzymes.

The best known pro-angiogenic mediator, namely the Vascular Endothelial Growth Factor (VEGF), has been demonstrated to be overexpressed in high-risk neuroblastomas at the time of diagnosis and to be a bad prognostic marker [81]. The elevated copper levels detected in malignant neuroblastoma are expected to heavily sustain the VEGF tumour angiogenesis, since this metal is a potent inducer of VEGF expression and reinforces the stimulating effect exerted by hydrogen peroxide [82].

The growth of neuroblastoma is anyway sustained by multiple pro-angiogenic factors other than VEGF [10], including Platelet Derived Growth Factor-A (PDGF-A), Fibroblast Growth Factor-2 (FGF-2), and Angiopoietin-2 (Ang-2), as documented in 22 neuroblastoma cell lines and 37 tumour samples [10]. Many among these factors share an intimate relationship with copper, known to variously enhance their angiogenic action through direct (physical interaction) or indirect (expression/release) ways.

As an example, the specific binding of copper to angiogenin, a major angiogenic factor, is able to largely increase its efficiency of interaction with endothelial cells [83,84]. This metal is also fundamental for the release of another pro-angiogenic factor involved in angiogenesis, Fibroblast Growth Factor (FGF) 1, as a part of a multiprotein aggregate (FGF1-p40 Syt1-S100A13) [85].

If on one hand high copper levels can facilitate the tumour development, on the other the stimulation of copper uptake and egress has been associated with the sprouting of new blood vessels within solid tumours, this depicting a high complex picture. A prominent role of copper transport systems emerges.

6.1. Potential role of ATP7A and Ctr1 copper transporters

Several experimental evidences point to a crucial role of copper in tumour angiogenesis [86]. Its ability to stimulate the endothelial cell proliferation, migration and sprouting mainly grounds on its role as a powerful inducer/enhancer of the expression of several angiogenic mediators, including $VEGF_{165}$ and interleukins [82,87], and a stabilizer of the angiogenin interaction with its receptor [83]. Surprisingly, well-characterized pro-angiogenic factors as $VEGF_{165}$ and bFGF, if administered to microvascular endothelial cell cultures, have been shown to rapidly promote the relocalization of the intracellular copper stores (about 80-90%) toward the cell periphery, where the ion efflux occurs, presumably by the ATP7A transport activity [88]. Such process may result contradictory in the light of the discussed role of copper as a powerful pro-angiogenic mediator. Nevertheless, this mechanism may be considered "cancer self-sustaining", making copper available in the tumour microenvironment (paracrine loop).

In addition, it must be observed that the vascular remodelling and the stimulation of cell migration depend on the activity of copper-dependent secreted enzymes (Lysil Oxidase, LOX), so the released metal is probably mostly carried by proteins.

In support of such hypothesis, a report from Ashino et al. (2010) illustrated how the pro-angiogenic Platelet Derived Growth Factor (PDGF) determines in vascular smooth muscle cells the translocation of the ATP7A copper transporter from the Trans Golgi Network toward special membrane domains (lipid rafts), where the pump is essential for the correct release of copper bound pro-LOX [89]. The authors also demonstrated that the membrane recruitment of Rac-1, a GTPase involved in the extension of lamellipodia, is dependent on copper and on the expression of the high affinity importer Ctr1 (Copper Transporter 1), this further confirming the existence of a solid link between the tumour metastasis and copper homeostasis.

6.2. Potential role of the cellular prion protein PrP^C

To our knowledge, a few data are reported in the literature around the prion protein role in defining the neuroblastoma aggressiveness. Nevertheless, the substantial expression level observed within the nervous system, which is further elevated by pathological conditions, testifies to a possible involvement of prion protein in the nervous response to cell injuries. In detail, this particular protein may have major implications in modulating the biological cascade leading to metastasis in patients with cancer, mainly by virtue of its presumed ability to sustain cell survival and exert a pro-angiogenic action.

A modest literature discusses a likely role of prion proteins in influencing the angiogenic processes, given a large disagreement about its actual expression in endothelial cells. In fact, although prion protein has been detected in the capillaries of the intestinal mucosa and kidney [90], normal endothelial cells derived from the umbilical cord and other vessels in the adults do not show detectable prion protein amounts *in vivo* [91]. However, prion protein seems to be up regulated in some pathological circumstances, such as in advanced carotid plaques, in association with the endothelial marker CD105, increasingly expressed in activated endothelia [92], and in brain tissues affected by ischemia [93,94]. By virtue of the latter studies, prion protein could reasonably play a key role in brain tumour progression, being the related gene responsive to the ischemic/hypoxic injury [94]. Accordingly, a neuroprotective action has been described for prion proteins in this context, based on the following evidences: i. prion protein is bound to caveolin-1 and, by recruiting Fyn tyrosine kinase, it can activate the signalling promoting cell survival and angiogenesis events [95]; ii. prion protein co-localizes with the VEGF receptor 2 (KDR), that indicating that prion protein may have a role in VEGF-driven angiogenesis [96].

7. Anti-angiogenic therapies target the neuroblastoma copper status: two examples

7.1. TNP-470

The administration of angiogenic inhibitors has been introduced as a complement to traditional therapies, in order to hinder the tumour spread.

Several anti-angiogenic therapeutics have been incorporated into clinical trials. Among them, in the '90s, TNP-470, an angiogenesis inhibitor, has emerged as a promising adjuvant in dormancy therapies for high-risk neuroblastoma. In particular, its effectiveness in arresting hepatic metastasis of neuroblastoma has been documented in [97] and [98]. In the light of [99], the anti-angiogenic activity of TNP-470 is reasonably linked to its interference with the hepatic copper metabolism. In fact, the continuous administration of TNP-470 in both normal and tumour-bearing rats has been shown to increase the serum copper levels, as a consequence of a limited hepatic retention [99]. This feature has been associated with a reduced density of hepatic tumour capillaries [99]. Accordingly, when the administration of TNP-470 was interrupted, angiogenesis was activated and at the same time the serum copper levels fell down [99].

7.2. Retinoids target the ATP7A gene expression

Among the most promising possibilities, retinoids (Vitamin A derivatives) may be of help in arresting the cancer growth and delaying the occurrence of recurrences, because of their proven ability to induce cell differentiation and inhibit the VEGF and FGF-2-induced endothelial activation [100]. Interestingly, a recent report from Bohlken et al. (2009) demonstrated that retinoids are able to starve neuroblastoma cells of copper through a significant increase in the ion efflux processes [60]. In fact, the retinoic acid receptor β (RARβ) up-regulates the expression of ATP7A copper efflux pump in BE(2)-C and SH-SY5Y human neuroblastoma cell models, but not in other cell types.

8. Cell copper transporters modulate the neuroblastoma sensitivity to chemotherapy

Cisplatin-based chemotherapy is commonly employed for neuroblastoma treatment at an advanced stage [101], but the development of resistance to the drug can affect the therapeutic efficacy. Highly diversified mechanisms have been proposed to explain this behaviour, although a definitive understanding has not been achieved. It has been demonstrated that Cisplatin-resistant neuroblastoma cells undergo an increase in the DNA methyltransferase activities that would depress the transcription of specific and widely undefined genes [102]. In fact, it is known that an acute Cisplatin administration can alter the genome methylation status in neuroblastoma cells [103].

Increasing evidences point out a central role of (broad substrate spectrum/specific) drug transporters to explain the onset of Cisplatin resistance. In detail, Haber et al. (1999) observed that malignant neuroblastoma forms, carrying the N-*myc* oncogene amplification, show an up regulation of the Multidrug Resistance-associated Protein (MRP) gene, associated with a poor sensitivity to low affinity substrates, including Cisplatin [104].

Interestingly, it has been widely demonstrated that Cisplatin shares with copper the pathways of cellular efflux and entry [105,106]. In particular, the cellular uptake of cisplatin (water soluble) is mediated by a member of the SLC (Solute Carrier) group, namely the copper transporter 1 (SLC31A1) [105-107], by mechanisms that partially overlap with those copper-specific [105,108]. Candidate Cisplatin-binding sequences have been identified in the extrac-ellular region of hCtr1, this providing further evidence of the Cisplatin transport activity by this channel [109].

Further, the copper efflux transporters, ATP7A and ATP7B, are known to regulate the efflux of cisplatin, and so their expression may be also predictive of drug sensitivity [110].

Neuroblastoma cells are known to express both hCtr1 import and ATP7A export proteins, this suggesting that copper transport systems may participate in determining the development of cisplatin resistance. In support of such hypothesis, a recent study on microRNAs expression pattern in variously N-*myc* amplified and cisplatin resistant neuroblastoma cells, led to the identification of eight microRNAs, each one targeting at least one of the two cited copper transporters [111]. Furthermore, it has been demonstrated that ATP7A expression may be a target to sensitize cancer cells to Cisplatin [112].

In the light of these findings, it has been argued that an increased cisplatin sensitivity may arise from the upregulation of Ctr1 transporter or by downregulation of the copper/cisplatin efflux transporter ATP7A. In this sense, a therapeutic regimen combining a preconditioning by a copper chelating agent (i.e. Tetrathiomolybdate) and platinum-containing drugs has been proven to enhance the Cisplatin efficacy in a mouse model of cervical cancer, without affecting the integrity of healthy tissues [113].

Another copper-dependent mechanism of resistance to cisplatin involves metallothioneins, a family of low molecular weight copper-binding proteins, whose expression is metal-induced in neuroblastoma cell models [114] and elevated in cisplatin-resistant cell lines [115]. When cisplatin enters a cancer cell, it is vulnerable to metallothionein-inactivation [116]. This mechanism assumes a prioritary connotation if we consider that N-*myc* amplified neuroblastomas show an increased copper content, that translates in a remarkable induction of metallothioneins and reduced efficacy of Cisplatin-based therapies.

9. Conclusion

Multifaceted pathophysiological features determine the progression of neuroblastoma malignancies. Mainly on the basis of *in vitro* and pre-clinical studies, copper, playing a key role within the human nervous system, is candidate to be the actual target of novel therapies. Accordingly, high copper levels seem to underline the development of tumour malignancies, even if we honestly observe that the scientific literature does not offer so many clear cues about the nature of *in vivo* copper involvement in neuroblastoma. The conclusive impression is that copper interacts with the neuroblastoma microenvironment at various levels, and the effects may be profoundly different, depending on the interested cell type (e.g. endothelial, neuroblast). The overall effects arise from the sum of specific and sometimes discordant copper-driven processes.

If few clinical data are currently available in this regard, the challenge toward the development of a copper-targeting therapy has anyway been launched. On the other hand, recent studies have recognized for neuroblastoma patients the benefits of preconditioning therapies based on the use of copper chelating agents (i.e. tetrathiomolibdate). Such intriguing approach would modulate the expression and/or subcellular localization of copper transport systems, and so both the cancer metal levels and chemoresistance. However, caution is needed in this sense, since the comprehension of copper metabolism in neuroblastoma cancer cells is still preliminary and the routes of copper transport are currently partially known. Significantly, it is only recently that an anion exchanger has been proposed as an additional copper importer in mammalian cells [117].

Acknowledgements

The authors gratefully acknowledge funding from the Italian Ministry of Education, University and Research (MIUR) through the project PRIN 2008 200875WHMR, for allowing a part of the experimental activities discussed in this chapter.

Author details

Emanuela Urso and Michele Maffia*

Department of Biological and Environmental Sciences and Technology, University of Salento, Lecce, Italy

References

[1] Tapiero H, Townsend DM, Tew KD. Trace elements in human physiology and pathology. Copper. Biomedicine & Pharmacotherapy 2003;57(9) 386-398.

[2] Halliwell B, Gutteridge JM. Oxygen toxicity, oxygen radicals, transition metals and diseases. Biochemical Journal 1984;219 1-4.

[3] Halliwell B, Gutteridge JM. Role of free radicals and catalytic metal ions in human disease: an overview. Methods in Enzymology 1990;186 1-85.

[4] Theophanides T, Anastassopoulou J. Copper and carcinogenesis. Critical reviews in oncology/hematology 2002;42(1) 57-64.

[5] Gupte A, Mumper RJ. Elevated copper and oxidative stress in cancer cells as a target for cancer treatment. Cancer Treatment Reviews 2009;35(1) 32-46.

[6] Tardito S, Marchiò L. Copper compounds in anticancer strategies. Current Medicinal Chemistry 2009;16(11) 1325-1348.

[7] Brodeur GM. Neuroblastoma: biological insights into a clinical enigma. Nature Reviews. Cancer 2003;3(3) 203-216.

[8] Matthay KK, Villablanca JG, Seeger RC, Stram DO, Harris RE, Ramsay NK, Swift P, Shimada H, Black CT, Brodeur GM, Gerbing RB, Reynolds CP. Treatment of high-risk neuroblastoma with intensive chemotherapy, radiotherapy, autologous bone marrow transplantation, and 13-cis-retinoic acid. Children's Cancer Group. The New England journal of medicine 1999;341(16) 1165-1173.

[9] Shusterman S, Maris JM. Prospects for therapeutic inhibition of neuroblastoma angiogenesis. Cancer Letters 2005;228(1-2) 171-179.

[10] Eggert A, Ikegaki N, Kwiatkowski J, Zhao H, Brodeur GM, Himelstein BP. High-level expression of angiogenic factors is associated with advanced tumor stage in human neuroblastomas. Clinical Cancer Research 2000;6(5) 1900-1908.

[11] Ferrandis E, Da Silva J, Riou G, Bénard I. Coactivation of the MDR1 and MYCN genes in human neuroblastoma cells during the metastatic process in the nude mouse. Cancer Research 1994;54(8) 2256-2261.

[12] Rubie H, Hartmann O, Michon J, Frappaz D, Coze C, Chastagner P, Baranzelli MC, Plantaz D, Avet-Loiseau H, Bénard J, Delattre O, Favrot M, Peyroulet MC, Thyss A, Perel Y, Bergeron C, Courbon-Collet B, Vannier JP, Lemerle J, Sommelet D. N-Myc gene amplification is a major prognostic factor in localized neuroblastoma: results of the French NBL 90 study. Neuroblastoma Study Group of the Société Francaise d'Oncologie Pédiatrique. Journal of Clinical Oncology 1997;15(3) 1171-1182.

[13] Gouget B, Sergeant C, Llabador Y, Deves G, Vesvres M, Simonoff M, Benard J. Trace metals and cancer: The case of neuroblastoma. Nuclear Instruments and Methods in Physics Research Section B 2001;181(1-4) 465-469.

[14] Gouget B, Sergeant C, Benard J, Llabador Y, Simonoff M. N-myc oncogene amplification is correlated to trace metal concentrations in neuroblastoma cultured cells. Nuclear Instruments and Methods in Physics Research Section B 2000;170(3-4) 432-442.

[15] Ortega R, Gouget B, Moretto P, Michelet C, Sergeant C, Llabador Y et al. Trace metal content in distinct genotypes of human neuroblasma cells: preliminary results. Nuclear Instruments and Methods in Physics Research Research Section B: Beam Interactions with Materials and Atoms 1997:130(1-4) 449-453.

[16] Ara T, Fukuzawa M, Kusafuka T, Komoto Y, Oue T, Inoue M, Okada A. Immunohistochemical expression of MMP-2, MMP-9, and TIMP-2 in neuroblastoma: association with tumor progression and clinical outcome. Journal of Pediatric Surgery 1998;33(8) 1272–1278.

[17] Szatrowski TP, Nathan CF. Production of large amounts of hydrogen peroxide by human tumor cells. Cancer Research 1991;51(3) 794-798.

[18] Mills CF. Interactions between elements in tissues: Studies in animal models. Federation Proceedings 1981;40(8) 2138-2143.

[19] Meitar D, Crawford SE, Rademaker AW, Cohn SL. Tumor angiogenesis correlates with metastatic disease, N-Myc amplification, and poor outcome in human neuroblastoma. Journal of Clinical Oncology 1996;14(2) 405-414.

[20] Ribatti D, Vacca A, Nico B, De Falco G, Giuseppe Montaldo P, Ponzoni M. Angiogenesis and anti-angiogenesis in neuroblastoma. European Journal of Cancer 2002;38(6) 750-757.

[21] Qian Y, Zheng Y, Abraham L, Ramos KS, Tiffany-Castiglioni E. Differential profiles of copper-induced ROS generation in human neuroblastoma and astrocytoma cells. Brain Research. Molecular Brain Research 2005;134(2) 323-332.

[22] Urso E, Rizzello A, Acierno R, Lionetto MG, Salvato B, Storelli C, Maffia M (2010) Fluorimetric analysis of copper transport mechanisms in the B104 neuroblastoma cell model: a contribution from cellular prion protein to copper supplying. Journal of Membrane Biology 233(1–3) 13–21.

[23] Urso E, Manno D, Serra A, Buccolieri A, Rizzello A, Danieli A, Acierno R, Salvato B, Maffia M. Role of the cellular prion protein in the neuron adaptation strategy to copper deficiency. Cellular and Molecular Neurobiology 2012;32(6) 989-1001.

[24] McLennan NF, Brennan PM, McNeill A, Davies I, Fotheringham A, Rennison KA, Ritchie D, Brannan F, Head MW, Ironside JW, Williams A, Bell JE. Prion protein accumulation and neuroprotection in hypoxic brain damage. The American Journal of Pathology 2004;165(1) 227-235.

[25] Lutsenko S, Petris MJ (2002) Function and regulation of the mammalian copper-transporting ATPases: insights from biochemical and cell biological approaches. Journal of Membrane Biology 2003;191(1) 1-12.

[26] Materia S, Cater MA, Klomp LW, Mercer JF, La Fontaine S. Clusterin (apolipoprotein J), a molecular chaperone that facilitates degradation of the copper-ATPases ATP7A and ATP7B. The Journal of Biological Chemistry 2011;286(12) 10073-10083.

[27] Chayka O, Corvetta D, Dews M, Caccamo AE, Piotrowska I, Santilli G, Gibson S, Sebire NJ, Himoudi N, Hogarty MD, Anderson J, Bettuzzi S, Thomas-Tikhonenko A, Sala A. Clusterin, a haploinsufficient tumor suppressor gene in neuroblastomas. Journal of the National Cancer Institute 2009;101(9) 663-677.

[28] Reddy MC, Majumdar S, Harris ED. Evidence for a Menkes-like protein with a nuclear targeting sequence. The Biochemical Journal 2000;350 Pt 3 855-863.

[29] Swart M. Localisation of the COMMD1 and COMMD3 proteins in the kidney and mammalian cells. M.S. thesis. University of Otago, Dunedin, New Zealand; 2010.

[30] van de Sluis B, Mao X, Zhai Y, Groot AJ, Vermeulen JF, van der Wall E, van Diest PJ, Hofker MH, Wijmenga C, Klomp LW, Cho KR, Fearon ER, Vooijs M, Burstein E. COMMD1 disrupts HIF-1alpha/beta dimerization and inhibits human tumor cell invasion. The Journal of Clinical Investigation 2010;120(6) 2119-2130.

[31] Vonk WI, Wijmenga C, Berger R, van de Sluis B, Klomp LW. Cu,Zn superoxide dismutase maturation and activity are regulated by COMMD1. The Journal of Biological Chemistry 2010;285(37) 28991-29000.

[32] Materia S, Cater MA, Klomp LW, Mercer JF, La Fontaine S. Clusterin and COMMD1 independently regulate degradation of the mammalian copper ATPases ATP7A and ATP7B. The Journal of Biological Chemistry 2012;287(4) 2485-2499.

[33] Deveraux QL, Takahashi R, Salvesen GS, Reed JC. X-linked IAP is a direct inhibitor of cell-death proteases. Nature 1997;388(6639) 300-304.

[34] Shiozaki EN, Chai J, Rigotti DJ, Riedl SJ, Li P, Srinivasula SM, Alnemri ES, Fairman R, Shi Y. Mechanism of XIAP-mediated inhibition of caspase-9. Molecular Cell 2003;11(2) 519-527.

[35] Hao Z, Mak TW. Type I and type II pathways of Fas-mediated apoptosis are differentially controlled by XIAP. Journal of Molecular Cell Biology 2010;2(2) 63-64.

[36] Burstein E, Ganesh L, Dick RD, van De Sluis B, Wilkinson JC, Klomp LW, Wijmenga C, Brewer GJ, Nabel GJ, Duckett CS. A novel role for XIAP in copper homeostasis through regulation of MURR1. The EMBO Journal 2004;23(1) 244-254.

[37] Eschenburg G, Eggert A, Schramm A, Lode HN, Hundsdoerfer P. Smac mimetic LBW242 sensitizes XIAP-overexpressing neuroblastoma cells for TNF-α-independent apoptosis. Cancer Research 2012;72(10) 2645-2656.

[38] Mufti AR, Burstein E, Csomos RA, Graf PC, Wilkinson JC, Dick RD, Challa M, Son JK, Bratton SB, Su GL, Brewer GJ, Jakob U, Duckett CS. XIAP Is a copper binding protein deregulated in Wilson's disease and other copper toxicosis disorders. Molecular Cell 2006;21(6) 775-785.

[39] Paramasivam A, Sambantham S, Shabnam J, Raghunandhakumar S, Anandan B, Rajiv R, Vijayashree Priyadharsini J, Jayaraman G. Anti-cancer effects of thymoquinone in mouse neuroblastoma (Neuro-2a) cells through caspase-3 activation with downregulation of XIAP. Toxicology Letters 2012;213(2) 151-159.

[40] Kayama T, Yoshimoto T, Fujimoto S, Sakurai Y. Intratumoral oxygen pressure in malignant brain tumor. Journal of Neurosurgery 1991;74(1) 55-59.

[41] Holmquist-Mengelbier L, Fredlund E, Löfstedt T, Noguera R, Navarro S, Nilsson H, Pietras A, Vallon-Christersson J, Borg A, Gradin K, Poellinger L, Påhlman S. Recruitment of HIF-1 alpha and HIF-2 alpha to common target genes is differentially regulated in neuroblastoma: HIF-2 alpha promotes an aggressive phenotype. Cancer Cell 2006;10(5) 413-423.

[42] Warburg O. On respiratory impairment in cancer cells. Science 1956;124(3215) 269-270.

[43] Wang GL, Jiang BH, Rue EA, Semenza GL. Hypoxia-inducible factor 1 is a basic-helix-loop-helix-PAS heterodimer regulated by cellular O2 tension. Proceedings of the National Academy of Sciences of the United States of America 1995;92(12) 5510-5514.

[44] Wiesener MS, Turley H, Allen WE, Willam C, Eckardt KU, Talks KL, Wood SM, Gatter KC, Harris AL, Pugh CW, Ratcliffe PJ, Maxwell PH. Induction of endothelial PAS protein-1 by hypoxia: characterization and comparison with hypoxia-inducible factor-1alpha. Blood 1998;92(7) 2260-2268.

[45] Beasley NJ, Leek R, Alam M, Turley H, Cox GJ, Gatter K, Millard P, Fuggle S, Harris AL. Hypoxia-inducible factors HIF-1alpha and HIF-2alpha in head and neck cancer: relationship to tumor biology and treatment outcome in surgically resected patients. Cancer Research 2002;62(9) 2493-2497.

[46] Qing G, Skuli N, Mayes PA, Pawel B, Martinez D, Maris JM, Simon MC. Combinatorial regulation of neuroblastoma tumor progression by N-Myc and hypoxia inducible factor HIF-1alpha. Cancer Research 2010;70(24):10351-10361.

[47] Martin F, Linden T, Katschinski DM, Oehme F, Flamme I, Mukhopadhyay CK, Eckhardt K, Tröger J, Barth S, Camenisch G, Wenger RH. Copper-dependent activation of hypoxia-inducible factor (HIF)-1: implications for ceruloplasmin regulation. Blood 2005;105(12) 4613-4619.

[48] Mukhopadhyay CK, Mazumder B, Fox PL. Role of hypoxia-inducible factor-1 in transcriptional activation of ceruloplasmin by iron deficiency. The Journal of Biological Chemistry 2000;275(28) 21048-21054.

[49] Tang N, Wang L, Esko J, Giordano FJ, Huang Y, Gerber HP, Ferrara N, Johnson RS. Loss of HIF-1alpha in endothelial cells disrupts a hypoxia-driven VEGF autocrine loop necessary for tumorigenesis. Cancer Cell 2004;6(5) 485-495.

[50] Gerber HP, Condorelli F, Park J, Ferrara N. Differential transcriptional regulation of the two vascular endothelial growth factor receptor genes. Flt-1, but not Flk-1/KDR, is up-regulated by hypoxia. The Journal of Biological Chemistry 1997;272(38) 23659-23667.

[51] White C, Kambe T, Fulcher YG, Sachdev SW, Bush AI, Fritsche K, Lee J, Quinn TP, Petris MJ. Copper transport into the secretory pathway is regulated by oxygen in macrophages. Journal of Cell Science 2009;122(Pt 9) 1315-1321.

[52] Pietras A, Gisselsson D, Ora I, Noguera R, Beckman S, Navarro S, Påhlman S. High levels of HIF-2alpha highlight an immature neural crest-like neuroblastoma cell cohort located in a perivascular niche. The Journal of Pathology 2008;214(4) 482–488.

[53] Xie L, Collins JF. Transcriptional regulation of the Menkes copper ATPase (Atp7a) gene by hypoxia-inducible factor (HIF2{alpha}) in intestinal epithelial cells. American Journal of Physiology. Cell Physiology 2011;300(6) C1298-C1305.

[54] Pourvali K, Matak P, Latunde-Dada GO, Solomou S, Mastrogiannaki M, Peyssonnaux C, Sharp PA. Basal expression of copper transporter 1 in intestinal epithelial cells is regulated by hypoxia-inducible factor 2α. FEBS Letters 2012;586(16) 2423-2427.

[55] Li QQ, Sun YP, Ruan CP, Xu XY, Ge JH, He J, Xu ZD, Wang Q, Gao WC. Cellular prion protein promotes glucose uptake through the Fyn-HIF-2α-Glut1 pathway to support colorectal cancer cell survival. Cancer Science 2011;102(2) 400-406.

[56] McLennan NF, Brennan PM, McNeill A, Davies I, Fotheringham A, Rennison KA, Ritchie D, Brannan F, Head MW, Ironside JW, Williams A, Bell JE. Prion protein accumulation and neuroprotection in hypoxic brain damage. The American Journal of Pathology 2004;165(1) 227-235.

[57] Pan Y, Zhao L, Liang J, Liu J, Shi Y, Liu N, Zhang G, Jin H, Gao J, Xie H, Wang J, Liu Z, Fan D. Cellular prion protein promotes invasion and metastasis of gastric cancer. FASEB Journal 2006;20(11) 1886-1888.

[58] Pauly P, Harris DA. Copper stimulates endocytosis of the prion protein. The Journal of Biological Chemistry 1998 273(50) 33107–33110.

[59] Perera WS, Hooper NM. Ablation of the metal ion-induced endocytosis of the prion protein by disease-associated mutation of the octarepeat region. Current Biology 2001;11(7) 519–523.

[60] Bohlken A, Cheung BB, Bell JL, Koach J, Smith S, Sekyere E, Thomas W, Norris M, Haber M, Lovejoy DB, Richardson DR, Marshall GM. ATP7A is a novel target of retinoic acid receptor beta2 in neuroblastoma cells. British Journal of Cancer 2009;100(1) 96-105.

[61] Vogelstein B, Lane D, Levine AJ. Surfing the p53 network. Nature 2000;408(6810): 307-310.

[62] Carr-Wilkinson J, O'Toole K, Wood KM, Challen CC, Baker AG, Board JR, Evans L, Cole M, Cheung NK, Boos J, Köhler G, Leuschner I, Pearson AD, Lunec J, Tweddle DA. High Frequency of p53/MDM2/p14ARF Pathway Abnormalities in Relapsed Neuroblastoma. Clinical Cancer Research 2010;16(4) 1108-1118.

[63] Keshelava N, Zuo JJ, Waidyaratne NS, Triche TJ, Reynolds CP. p53 mutations and loss of p53 function confer multidrug resistance in neuroblastoma. Medical and Pediatric Oncology 2000;35(6) 563-568.

[64] Moll UM, Ostermeyer AG, Haladay R, Winkfield B, Frazier M, Zambetti G. Cytoplasmic sequestration of wild-type p53 protein impairs the G1 checkpoint after DNA damage. Molecular and Cellular Biology 1996;16(3) 1126-1137.

[65] Moll UM, LaQuaglia M, Bénard J, Riou G. Wild-type p53 protein undergoes cytoplasmic sequestration in undifferentiated neuroblastomas but not in differentiated tumors. Proceedings of the National Academy of Sciences of the United States of America 1995;92(10) 4407-4411.

[66] Matoba S, Kang JG, Patino WD, Wragg A, Boehm M, Gavrilova O, Hurley PJ, Bunz F, Hwang PM. p53 regulates mitochondrial respiration. Science 2006;312(5780) 1650-1653.

[67] Turski ML, Thiele DJ. New roles for copper metabolism in cell proliferation, signaling, and disease. The Journal of Biological Chemistry 2009;284(2) 717-721.

[68] Finkel T, Holbrook NJ. Oxidants, oxidative stress and the biology of ageing. Nature 2000;408(6809) 239–247.

[69] Filomeni G, Aquilano K, Rotilio G, Ciriolo MR. Antiapoptotic response to induced GSH depletion: involvement of heat shock proteins and NF-kappaB activation. Antioxidants & Redox Signaling 2005;7(3-4) 446–455.

[70] Lombardo MF, Ciriolo MR, Rotilio G, Rossi L. Prolonged copper depletion induces expression of antioxidants and triggers apoptosis in SH-SY5Y neuroblastoma cells. Cellular and Molecular Life Sciences 2003;60(8) 1733-1743.

[71] Rossi L, Marchese E, Lombardo MF, Rotilio G, Ciriolo MR. Increased susceptibility of copper-deficient neuroblastoma cells to oxidative stress-mediated apoptosis. Free Radical Biology & Medicine 2001;30(10) 1177-1187.

[72] Arciello M, Capo CR, D'Annibale S, Cozzolino M, Ferri A, Carrì MT, Rossi L. Copper depletion increases the mitochondrial-associated SOD1 in neuronal cells. Biometals 2011;24(2) 269-278.

[73] Rossi L, Ciriolo MR, Marchese E, De Martino A, Giorgi M, Rotilio G. Differential decrease of copper content and copper binding to superoxide dismutase in liver, heart and brain of copper-deficient rats. Biochemical and biophysical research communications 1994;203(2) 1028-1034.

[74] Aquilano K, Vigilanza P, Rotilio G, Ciriolo MR. Mitochondrial damage due to SOD1 deficiency in SH-SY5Y neuroblastoma cells: a rationale for the redundancy of SOD1. FASEB Journal 2006;20(10) 1683-1685.

[75] Vijayvergiya C, Beal MF, Buck J, Manfredi G. Mutant superoxide dismutase 1 forms aggregates in the brain mitochondrial matrix of amyotrophic lateral sclerosis mice. The Journal of Neuroscience 2005;25(10) 2463–2470.

[76] Klamt F, Dal-Pizzol F, Conte da Frota ML, Walz R, Andrades ME, da Silva EG, Brentani RR, Izquierdo I, Fonseca Moreira JC. Imbalance of antioxidant defense in mice lacking cellular prion protein. Free Radical Biology & Medicine 2001;30(10) 1137-1144.

[77] Brown DR, Besinger A. Prion protein expression and superoxide dismutase activity. The Biochemical Journal 1998;334(Pt 2) 423-429.

[78] Brown DR, Schulz-Schaeffer WJ, Schmidt B, Kretzschmar HA. Prion protein-deficient cells show altered response to oxidative stress due to decreased SOD-1 activity. Experimental Neurology 1997;146(1) 104-112.

[79] Salès N, Rodolfo K, Hässig R, Faucheux B, Di Giamberardino L, Moya KL. Cellular prion protein localization in rodent and primate brain. The European Journal of Neuroscience 1998;10(7) 2464-2471.

[80] Brown DR, Besinger A, Herms JW, Kretzschmar HA. Microglial expression of the prion protein. Neuroreport 1998;9(7) 1425-1429.

[81] Jakovljević G, Culić S, Stepan J, Bonevski A, Seiwerth S. Vascular endothelial growth factor in children with neuroblastoma: a retrospective analysis. Journal of Experimental & Clinical Cancer Research 2009;28 143-1-143-11.

[82] Sen CK, Khanna S, Venojarvi M, Trikha P, Ellison EC, Hunt TK, Roy S. Copper-induced vascular endothelial growth factor expression and wound healing. American journal of physiology. Heart and Circulatory Physiology. 2002;282(5) H1821-H1827.

[83] Soncin F, Guitton JD, Cartwright T, Badet J. Interaction of human angiogenin with copper modulates angiogenin binding to endothelial cells. Biochemical and Biophysical Research Communications 1997;236(3) 604-610.

[84] Badet J, Soncin F, Guitton JD, Lamare O, Cartwright T, Barritault D. Specific binding of angiogenin to calf pulmonary artery endothelial cells. Proceedings of the National Academy of Sciences of the United States of America 1989;86(21) 8427-8431.

[85] Landriscina M, Bagalá C, Mandinova A, Soldi R, Micucci I, Bellum S, Prudovsky I, Maciag T. Copper induces the assembly of a multiprotein aggregate implicated in the release of fibroblast growth factor 1 in response to stress. The Journal of Biological Chemistry 2001;276(27) 25549-25557.

[86] Lowndes SA, Harris AL. The role of copper in tumour angiogenesis. Journal of mammary gland biology and neoplasia 2005;10(4) 299-310.

[87] Bar-Or D, Thomas GW, Yukl RL, Rael LT, Shimonkevitz RP, Curtis CG, Winkler JV. Copper stimulates the synthesis and release of interleukin-8 in human endothelial cells: a possible early role in systemic inflammatory responses. Shock 2003;20(2) 154-158.

[88] Finney L, Mandava S, Ursos L, Zhang W, Rodi D, Vogt S, Legnini D, Maser J, Ikpatt F, Olopade OI, Glesne D. X-ray fluorescence microscopy reveals large-scale relocalization and extracellular translocation of cellular copper during angiogenesis. Proceedings of the National Academy of Sciences of the United States of America 2007;104(7) 2247-2252.

[89] Ashino T, Sudhahar V, Urao N, Oshikawa J, Chen GF, Wang H, Huo Y, Finney L, Vogt S, McKinney RD, Maryon EB, Kaplan JH, Ushio-Fukai M, Fukai T. Unexpected role of the copper transporter ATP7A in PDGF-induced vascular smooth muscle cell migration. Circulation Research 2010;107(6) 787-799.

[90] Lemaire-Vieille C, Schulze T, Podevin-Dimster V, Follet J, Bailly Y, Blanquet-Grossard F, Decavel JP, Heinen E, Cesbron JY. Epithelial and endothelial expression of the green fluorescent protein reporter gene under the control of bovine prion protein (PrP) gene regulatory sequences in transgenic mice. Proceedings of the National Academy of Sciences of the United States of America 2000;97(10) 5422-5427.

[91] Sivakumaran M. The expression of prion protein (PrPc) by endothelial cells: an in vitro culture-induced artefactual phenomenon? British journal of haematology 2003;121(4) 673-674.

[92] Krupinski J, Turu MM, Luque A, Badimon L, Slevin M. Increased PrPC expression correlates with endoglin (CD105) positive microvessels in advanced carotid lesions. Acta Neuropathologica 2008;116(5) 537-545.

[93] Weise J, Crome O, Sandau R, Schulz-Schaeffer W, Bähr M, Zerr I. Upregulation of cellular prion protein (PrPc) after focal cerebral ischemia and influence of lesion severity. Neuroscience Letters 2004;372(1-2) 146-150.

[94] Shyu WC, Lin SZ, Chiang MF, Ding DC, Li KW, Chen SF, Yang HI, Li H. Overexpression of PrPC by adenovirus-mediated gene targeting reduces ischemic injury in a stroke rat model. The Journal of Neuroscience 2005;25(39) 8967-8977.

[95] Massimino ML, Griffoni C, Spisni E, Toni M, Tomasi V. Involvement of caveolae and caveolae-like domains in signalling, cell survival and angiogenesis. Cellular Signalling 2002;14(2) 93-98.

[96] Feng Y, Venema VJ, Venema RC, Tsai N, Behzadian MA, Caldwell RB. VEGF-induced permeability increase is mediated by caveolae. Investigative ophthalmology & visual science 1999;40(1) 157-167.

[97] Yoshizawa J, Mizuno R, Yoshida T, Hara A, Ashizuka S, Kanai M, Kuwashima N, Kurobe M, Yamazaki Y. Inhibitory effect of TNP-470 on hepatic metastasis of mouse neuroblastoma. The Journal of Surgical Research 2000;93(1) 82-87.

[98] Nagabuchi E, VanderKolk WE, Une Y, Ziegler MM. TNP-470 antiangiogenic therapy for advanced murine neuroblastoma. Journal of Pediatric Surgery 1997;32(2) 287-293.

[99] Matsuoka S, Uchino J, Une Y, Ishimura H, Tsuchimoto S, Kamiyama T. Effects of tnp-470 (agm-1470) on tumor-growth, angiogenesis and serum copper levels in liver-cancer bearing rats. Oncology Reports 1995;2(4) 583-589.

[100] Ribatti D, Alessandri G, Baronio M, Raffaghello L, Cosimo E, Marimpietri D, Montaldo PG, De Falco G, Caruso A, Vacca A, Ponzoni M. Inhibition of neuroblastoma-induced angiogenesis by fenretinide. International Journal of Cancer 2001;94(3) 314-321.

[101] Dorr RT, Von Hoff DD. Cancer Chemotherapy Handbook. Appleton & Lange: Norwalk; 1994. p286-298.

[102] Qiu YY, Mirkin BL, Dwivedi RS. Inhibition of DNA methyltransferase reverses cisplatin induced drug resistance in murine neuroblastoma cells. Cancer Detection and Prevention 2005;29(5) 456-463.

[103] Tabata K, Sakai H, Nakajima R, Saya-Nishimura R, Motani K, Okano S, Shibata Y, Abiko Y, Suzuki T. Acute application of cisplatin affects methylation status in neuro-blastoma cells. Oncology Reports 2011;25(6) 1655-1660.

[104] Haber M, Bordow SB, Gilbert J, Madafiglio J, Kavallaris M, Marshall GM, Mechetner EB, Fruehauf JP, Tee L, Cohn SL, Salwen H, Schmidt ML, Norris MD. Altered expression of the MYCN oncogene modulates MRP gene expression and response to cyto-toxic drugs in neuroblastoma cells. Oncogene 1999;18(17) 2777-2782.

[105] Liang ZD, Stockton D, Savaraj N, Tien Kuo M. Mechanistic comparison of human high-affinity copper transporter 1-mediated transport between copper ion and cispla-tin. Molecular Pharmacology 2009;76(4) 843-853.

[106] Safaei R, Howell SB. Copper transporters regulate the cellular pharmacology and sensitivity to Pt drugs. Critical Reviews in Oncology/Hematology 2005;53(1) 13-23.

[107] Song IS, Savaraj N, Siddik ZH, Liu P, Wei Y, Wu CJ, Kuo MT. Role of human copper transporter Ctr1 in the transport of platinum-based antitumor agents in cisplatin-sen-sitive and cisplatin-resistant cells. Molecular Cancer Therapeutics 2004;3(12) 1543-1549.

[108] Sinani D, Adle DJ, Kim H, Lee J. Distinct mechanisms for Ctr1-mediated copper and cisplatin transport. The Journal of Biological Chemistry 2007;282(37) 26775-26785.

[109] Guo Y, Smith K, Petris MJ. Cisplatin stabilizes a multimeric complex of the human Ctr1 copper transporter: requirement for the extracellular methionine-rich clusters. The Journal of Biological Chemistry 2004;279(45) 46393-46399.

[110] Kuo MT, Chen HH, Song IS, Savaraj N, Ishikawa T. The roles of copper transporters in cisplatin resistance. Cancer Metastasis Reviews 2007;26(1) 71-83.

[111] Harvey HM, Bray IM, Stallings RL. Functional analysis of miRNA in chemotherapy resistant neuroblastoma. In: Proceedings of the 103rd Annual Meeting of the Ameri-can Association for Cancer Research, AACR, 31 March-4 April 2012, Chicago, Illinois. Philadelphia (PA): AACR; Cancer Res 2012;72(8 Suppl).

[112] Samimi, G, Safaei, R, Katano, K, Holzer, A. K, Rochdi, M, Tomioka, M, Goodman, M, & Howell, S. B. Increased expression of the copper efflux transporter ATP7A medi-ates resistance to cisplatin, carboplatin, and oxaliplatin in ovarian cancer cells. Clini-cal Cancer Research (2004)., 10(14), 4661-4669.

[113] Ishida, S, McCormick, F, Smith-McCune, K, & Hanahan, D. Enhancing tumor-specific uptake of the anticancer drug cisplatin with a copper chelator. Cancer Cell (2010)., 17(6), 574-583.

[114] Yasuno, T, Matsumura, T, Shikata, T, Inazawa, J, Sakabe, T, Tsuchida, S, Takahata, T, Miyairi, S, Naganuma, A, & Sawada, T. Establishment and characterization of a cis-platin-resistant human neuroblastoma cell line. Anticancer Research (1999)., 19(5B), 4049-4057.

[115] Kasahara, K, Fujiwara, Y, Nishio, K, Ohmori, T, Sugimoto, Y, Komiya, K, Matsuda, T, & Saijo, N. Metallothionein content correlates with the sensitivity of human small cell lung cancer cell lines to cisplatin. Cancer Res. (1991)., 51(12), 3237-3242.

[116] Siddik, Z. H. Cisplatin: Mode of cytotoxic action and molecular basis of resistance. Oncogene (2003)., 22(47), 7265-7279.

[117] Zimnicka, A. M, Ivy, K, & Kaplan, J. H. Acquisition of dietary copper: a role for anion transporters in intestinal apical copper uptake. American Journal of Physiology. Cell Physiology (2011)., 300(3), C588-C599.

[118] Petris, M. J. The SLC31 (Ctr) copper transporter family. Pflugers Archiv (2004)., 447(5), 752-755.

[119] van den Berghe, P. V, Folmer, D. E, Malingré, H.E, van Beurden, E, Klomp, A. E, van de Sluis, B, Merkx, M, Berger, R, Klomp, L. W. Human copper transporter 2 is localized in late endosomes and lysosomes and facilitates cellular copper uptake. The Biochemical Journal (2007)., 407(1), 49-59.

[120] Bertinato, J, Iskandar, M, & L'Abbé, M. R. Copper deficiency induces the upregulation of the copper chaperone for Cu/Zn superoxide dismutase in weanling male rats. The Journal of Nutrition (2003)., 133(1), 28-31.

[121] Amaravadi, R, Glerum, D. M, & Tzagoloff, A. Isolation of a cDNA encoding the human homolog of COX17, a yeast gene essential for mitochondrial copper recruitment. Human Genetics (1997)., 99(3), 329-333.

[122] Klomp, L. W, Lin, S. J, Yuan, D. S, Klausner, R. D, Culotta, V. C, & Gitlin, J. D. Identification and functional expression of HAH1, a novel human gene involved in copper homeostasis. The Journal of Biological Chemistry (1997)., 272(14), 9221-9226.

[123] Suzuki, K. T, Imura, N, & Kimura, M. Metallothionein III. Birkhäuser Verlag: Basel; (1993).

Chapter 12

Novel Therapeutic Approaches for Neuroblastoma

Shweta Joshi, Alok R. Singh, Lisa L.R. Hartman,
Muamera Zulcic, Hyunah Ahn and Donald L. Durden

Additional information is available at the end of the chapter

1. Introduction

Neuroblastoma (NB) is the most common pediatric extracranial solid tumor of childhood, and 45% of patients have high-risk tumors, nearly all of which are metastatic (stage 4) when diagnosed [1]. Patients with neuroblastoma are risk stratified based on presenting factors including age, stage and location of disease, and specific biologic molecular markers of the tumor, including NMYC status and ploidy [1-3]. Treatment given is tailored to whether a patient has low, intermediate or high-risk disease. The overall prognosis for those with high risk or relapsed disease remains poor despite the standard therapies of surgery, radiation, and high dose chemotherapy followed by stem cell rescue. Additionally, many patients who survive suffer from complications related to their treatment. In this chapter, we review the literature that provides a rationale for the use of novel targeted agents to improve the treatment and survival while lessening toxicity of patients with neuroblastoma who have failed standard therapies.

In particular, we focus our discussion on a few specific signaling pathways. The central role of the phosphatidylinositol 3-kinase-Akt-phosphatase and tensin homolog (PI3K-Akt-PTEN) axis and RAF-MEK-ERK as potential molecular targets to control downstream effectors of coordinated cell division, tumor growth, angiogenesis, apoptosis, invasion and cellular metabolism in the tumor and surrounding stromal compartments. The PI3K and RAF-MEK-ERK pathways have also been implicated in modulating p53, the hypoxia-inducible factor 1 (HIF1α), mycN and others.

NMYC is known to play a role in the tumorigenesis of certain high-risk neuroblastoma tumors and its control has many implications in targeting therapy. Additional pathways and targets explored in this chapter are the RAS/Raf/MEK/ERK pathway, specific angiogenesis inhibitors including VEGF, ALK 1 mutations and inhibitors, and control of apoptosis through caspase 8.

We also discuss the idea of synthetic lethality and the concepts of sequential versus simulta-neous inhibition. We will discuss the emerging importance of genomic and metabolomic profiling in tumor interrogation with therapeutic considerations.

We will review the literature supporting a role for cancer stem cells (CSCs) in the pathogenesis of neuroblastoma and the signaling pathways that define the CSC phenotype. We discuss the role targeted therapies in CSC related therapeutics and the adaptive responses that such cells have when exposed to targeted therapeutic agents.

Lastly, the emerging role of immunotherapeutics into both standard and targeted therapies for neuroblastoma is explored. This includes areas of T cell and macrophage infiltration of tumors, interleukin and cytokine involvement, and anti-GD2 human and mouse monoclonal antibodies.

2. PTEN and PI-3 kinase and mycN signaling as targets for NB therapeutics — The intercept node hypothesis

The idea that some signaling pathways are more central to tumorigenesis than others was suggested by our laboratory and others [4]. From connectivity map analysis, some signaling proteins appear connected to a large number of upstream and downstream effector pathways. These are considered central "intercept nodes" [4, 5] which provide coordinate control over the output of a large number of cell surface receptor input. The specificity of signaling downstream of such intercept nodes is generally fine tuned by more specialized signaling effector proteins e.g. Rac2, HIF1α, NFκB or mycN which encode more specific signaling content. Two such central pathways, PTEN-PI-3-AKT and Raf-MEK-ERK are critical for NB survival, proliferation, invasion and angiogenesis *in vivo* [6-9]. A large number of small and large pharmaceutical companies have developed small molecule inhibitors which block these two pathways. Considering the importance of mycN amplification in the pathogenesis of NB, and the role of PI-3K and MAP kinase in the GSK3β dependent regulation of mycN a number of investigators have determined the efficacy of PI-3 kinase inhibitors in NB models [9]. Despite evidence of efficacy no PI-3 kinase inhibitors have entered pediatric oncology clinical trials to date. One pan PI-3 kinase inhibitor, SF1126 is slated to enter pediatric oncology Phase I clinical trials in early 2013 [10]. Importantly, the tumor and stromal compartment share many of the same signaling pathways to regulate the process of tumorigenesis *in vivo*.

3. Role of angiogenesis in tumorigenicity of neuroblastoma / PI3 kinase and VEGF inhibitors in treatment of neuroblastoma

Work from a number of laboratories indicates that the angiogenic response is coordinately and highly regulated physiologic response to hypoxia and inflammation. Hence it is not surprising to learn that central node in mammalian cells control output from many cell surface receptors

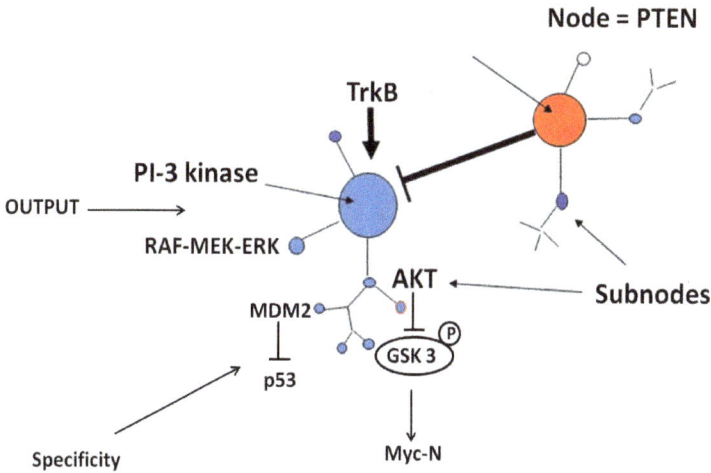

Figure 1. The PI3K–Akt–PTEN intercept node. As shown, a large number of growth factor receptors (GFR) of which TrkB is an oncogene in NB would feed into the central node to activate PI-3 kinase, AKT and/or Raf-MEK-ERK pathways. Downstream subnodes encode specificity e.g. GSK3b, MDM2, mycN, Rac2, etc. Major tumor suppressors like PTEN and p53 control output from these two central nodes. MDM2 regulates p53 in an AKT dependent manner; RAF-MEK-ERK and AKT regulate GSK3b to control mycN stability and transcriptional activity.

to regulate this response [11]. We and others have shown that PTEN a major tumor suppressor protein regulates angiogenesis and loss of PTEN results in deregulation of PTEN and multiple downstream signaling pathways shown in Fig. 1 and 2 which have all been implicated in the literature to exert coordinate control of angiogenesis *in vivo* [4, 5, 12, 13].

In general, angiogenesis plays an important role in the progression and metastasis of malignant tumors [14]. In neuroblastoma, tumor vascularity is correlated with an aggressive phenotype [15, 16]. Pro-angiogenic factors are differentially expressed in high-risk neuroblastoma [17, 18]. Vascular endothelial growth factor (VEGF) is a specific endothelial cell mitogen that stimulates angiogenesis and plays a crucial role in tumor growth [19]. Over expression of VEGF has been demonstrated in neuroblastoma, nephroblastoma, as well as in various other cancers [20-22]. Recent studies have validated inhibition of VEGF as an effective antiangiogenic therapy in some of these cancers [23-25]. Although several preliminary studies have demonstrated that expression of angiogenic growth factors, including VEGF, correlate with a high-risk phenotype in neuroblastoma, clinical data are still insufficient to draw conclusions [17, 21, 26, 27]. Therefore, further clinical studies, are needed to evaluate the possible significance of these factors for use in a routine clinical practice. Preclinical studies also suggest that antiangiogenic strategies may be effective in the treatment of neuroblastoma [28]. In addition, phase I clinical trials (COG study) using the human anti-VEGF antibody, bevacizumab, in pediatric patients with refractory solid tumors reported promising results [29]. Recently, Jakovljevic *et al.* has determined VEGF expression by immunohistochemistry using antiVEGF antibody in paraffin embedded primary tumor tissue from 56 neuroblastoma patients and reported that VEGF expression correlated with disease stage and survival in neuroblastoma patients [30]. Whether inhibition of angiogenesis is a realistic approach for preventing dissemination of neuroblastoma remains to be determined, but we can suggest that inhibitors of VEGF can be used in the treatment of neuroblastoma. Finally, we suggest that the more global inhibition of PI3 kinase or combined PI3K/MEK inhibition would provide a more potent antiangiogenic modality to block tumor induced angiogenesis in this disease.

4. Cancer stem cells in neuroblastoma tumorigenicity

The Cancer Stem Cell Theory postulates that tumors contain a subset of cells that are capable of increased self-renewal and differentiation, can propagate tumor growth and are resistant to apoptosis [31, 32]. These stem-like cancer cells are analogous to normal stem cells [33] but differentiate into diverse cancer cells that form the major portion of the tumor. Recent evidence suggests the presence of stem cells in various cancers including those of the blood [34], breast [35], prostrate [36] and brain [37].

Evidence for the presence of cancer stem cells in brain tumors first came from the observation that human medulloblastoma, astrocytomas, and ependymomas contain cells that express the neural stem cell marker CD133 [38] [39]. Singh et al. [37] have shown that human brain tumors contain CD133+ stem-like cells that are capable of growing tumors in immune-deficient mice. Cournoyer et al.[40] have shown that CD133 high neuroblastoma (NB) cells have high tumor initiating cell properties, and Coulon et al.[41] suggest that CD133, ABC transporter, Wnt and NOTCH genes are sphere markers in NB cells. Overall, 19–29 % of cells in glioblastomas and 6–21 % of cells of medulloblastomas are reported to be CD133+ and tumorigenic [33]. Recently, several groups have suggested that CD15 (stage specific embryonic antigen 1 or SSEA-1), which is expressed on neural progenitor and stem cells, may be a better marker than CD133 of tumor-initiating cells in MB, glioma, and ependymoma [42-44]. Hansford et al has recently identified tumor initiating cells from NB bone marrow metastases that have several properties of cancer stem cells including the expression of stem cell markers, the ability to self renew and the capability to form metastatic NB in immunodeficient animals with as few as 10 cells [45]. Kaplan's laboratory has further defined the NB tumor initiating cell (TIC) with stem cell like properties to express, CD133 and CD44. These cells isolated from NB bone marrow have tumor initiating activity and upon profiling display sensitivity to a number of targeted therapeutic agents.

A key aspect of the tumor stem cell (TSC) niche is the balance of signals received, and over recent years considerable attention has been directed towards understanding the role of signaling pathways, which are critical mediators of normal stem cell biology, in cancers. The embryonic signaling pathways most commonly implicated in tumorigenesis include Hedgehog, Notch, and Wnt pathways. Sonic Hedgehog (SHH) signaling is important in embryonic cell development and proliferation and aberrant pathway activation can lead to tumor formation, tumor cell self-renewal and the development of metastatic disease [48].Similarly,

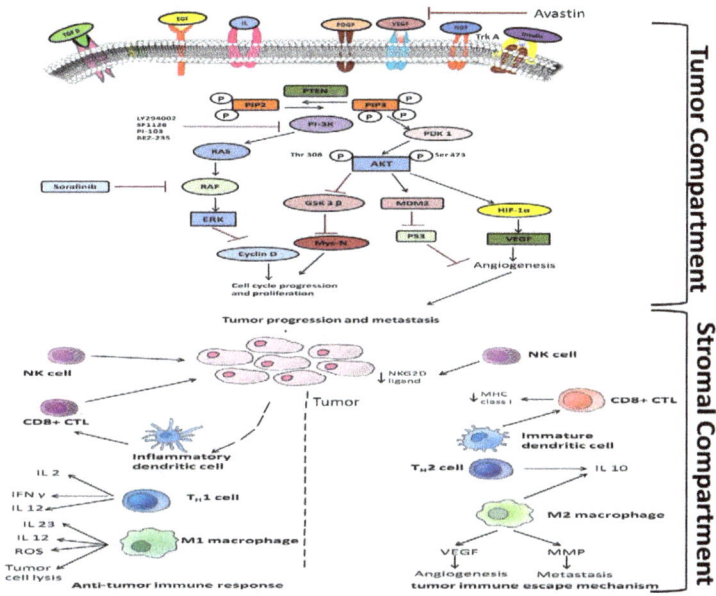

Figure 2. Signaling and cellular pathways controlling tumorigenicity of Neuroblastoma. In tumor compartment PI3K–Akt–PTEN intercept node is a central regulator of survival, proliferation, invasion and angiogenesis in Neuroblastoma. PI3K controls PIP3 levels, thereby regulating lipid-associated second messenger output from upstream effectors. PI3K and Akt can be activated by many cell surface receptors. Akt becomes locked in an active conformation and phosphorylates numerous proteins involved in growth and survival, cellular metabolism, stress response and angiogenesis. Akt modulates phosphorylation of GSK3β and relieves tonic inhibition of c-Myc and cyclin D to promote cell survival [46]. Akt contributes to the Warburg effect by inducing HIF1α transcription and stimulating aerobic glycolysis. Intratumoral hypoxia also drives angiogenesis through transcription of proangiogenic genes including *VEGF* and *PDGF*. Tumor angiogenesis is promoted by Akt-mediated phosphorylation of MDM2. Activated MDM2 translocates from the cytoplasm to the nucleus, where it binds p53, targeting it for ubiquitination and degradation. This process prevents p53 from exerting its antiangiogenic effect. A more effective strategy might be to modulate tumor growth and angiogenesis by targeting major signaling nodes such as the p53–MDM2 or PI3K–Akt–PTEN nodes with agents such as Nutlin 3A or with PI3K inhibitors (e.g. PI-103, BEZ-235 or SF1126), respectively. Abbreviations: GSK3β, glycogen synthase kinase 3 β; HIF1α, hypoxia inducible factor 1α; MDM2, mammalian double minute 2; PDGF, platelet-derived growth factor; PI3K, phosphatidylinositol 3-kinase; In stromal compartment, the major cellular pathways of the immune response which may have anti- or pro-tumor effects are shown. NK cells and CD8+ CTLs may directly target tumor cells for lysis; however this may be countered by decreased tumor expression of NKG2D ligands or MHC class I. Dendritic cells are important for priming an anti-tumor immune response, although immature DCs and IDO-expressing DCs may instead lead to the induction of tolerance. Myeloid-derived suppressor cells and regulatory T cells (Treg) may also suppress the anti-tumor CTL response. TH1 cells and M1 macrophages produce proinflammatory cytokines which help to stimulate the anti-tumor immune response, whilst TH2 cells (and other cell types) produce IL-10 which may have a predominantly inhibitory effect on the anti-tumor response. Tumor-associated M2 macrophages may promote tumor growth and metastases *via* a number of different mechanisms. Figure adopted from Morgenstern et al [47].

Notch plays a crucial role in biological functions of development and cell fate including cell differentiation and proliferation [49]. Constitutive activation of Notch can lead to tumorigenesis and cell survival, and Notch activity is involved in tumor angiogenesis [50]. The Wnt family proteins help direct a wide range of developmental processes including cell fate, proliferation, motility, and polarity [51]. Dysregulation of the Wnt pathways has been implicated in tumor formation, proliferation, and maintenance [52]. All of the current pediatric studies demonstrating that progenitor and stem cells can respond to embryonic signaling have been in MB or primitive neuroectodermal tumors (PNET). Aberrant SHH signaling has been implicated in MB, and recently was used to define one of four distinct molecular variants of MB [53].

In order to identify pathways required for proliferation and cell survival characteristics of TIC in neuroblastoma, Grinshtein et al. has performed drug screen on bone marrow derived tumor initiating cells (TICs) with a unique collection of pharmacological inhibitors. They identified that PI3K (phosphoinositide 3 kinase)/AKT, PKC (protein kinase C), Aurora, ErbB2, Trk and Polo-like kinase 1 (PLK1) are the potential kinase targets for survival of TIC [54]. Their studies demonstrated that PLK1 inhibitors are an attractive candidate therapy for metastatic NB. Another group suggested that both PI-3 kinase as well as Ras-RAF-MEK-Erk signaling pathways promote the tumorigenicity of the glioblastoma cancer stem like cells, and combined treatment with MEK and PI-3 kinase inhibitors can block the differentiation of glioblastoma cancer stem like cell into non tumor initiating status [55].

The therapeutic resistance of cancer stem cell to current treatment modalities such as chemotherapy and radiation make these cells clinically relevant irrespective of their origin. Resistance to chemotherapeutic agents has been demonstrated in neuroblastoma stem cells and sarcoma stem cells including Ewing's sarcoma and osteosarcoma. Recent work by Hambardzumyan suggests that the PI-3 kinase pathway activity promotes post-radiation survival in cancer stem cells in medulloblastoma [67]. Although lots of literatures are available on the cancer stem cell in neuroblastoma but yet the novel signaling pathways controlling the proliferation and survival of cancer stem cell and the mechanism behind resistance developed due to chemotherapy needs to be investigated.

5. Neuroblastoma and cancer metabolism

It has been known from a long time that cancer cells take up and metabolize glucose and glutamine to a degree that far exceeds their needs for these molecules in anabolic macromolecular synthesis [56]. Commonly occurring oncogenic signal transduction pathways initiated by receptor tyrosine kinases or Ras engage PI3K-Akt signaling to directly stimulate glycolytic metabolism under aerobic conditions a condition termed the Warburg and Pasteur effects [56-58]. Myc-activation/amplification is one of the most common oncogenic events observed in cancer and is known to drive the progression of a certain subgroup of neuroblastoma [59]. The activation of mycN could occur through amplification of the mycN gene or through upstream activation of signaling pathways that would stabilize mycN e.g. trkB, IGF-1 or the activation of Raf and/or PI-3K-AKT stimulation. Oncogenic levels of Myc have recently been linked to increased glutaminolysis through a coordinated transcriptional program program [60-62]. Quantitative RTPCR and ChIP experiments support Myc's binding and transcriptional activation of two high affinity glutamine transporters: SLC38A5 (also called SN2) and SLC1A5 (ASCT2), the transporter required for glutamine-dependent mTORC1 activation [60, 63]. In addition to facilitating glutamine uptake, Myc promotes the metabolism of imported gluta-mine into glutamic acid and ultimately into lactic acid [60]. Whether the tendency of Myc to complement Ras and PI3K-Akt [64, 65] is related to the interdependence of glutamine and glucose metabolism in support of cell growth remains an open question. The work of C. Dang and other points to a potential important metabolic requirement for glutamine in c-myc and mycN driven tumors where glutamine can serve a role in promoting tumor growth [58, 66]. This might suggest a role of agents which deplete glutamine (glutaminases) as a therapeutic target for mycN driven malignancies like neuroblastoma and the SHH subtype of medullo-blastoma.

6. Role of tumor infiltrating immune cells in tumorigenicity of neuroblastoma

Solid tumors are composed of tumor stromal cells, blood vessels, infiltrating immune cells and tumor cells themselves. Over the last decade, a growing body of literature has highlighted the importance of the tumor microenvironment for the prognosis of different types of cancer [68]. The tumor microenvironment contains many resident cell types, such as adipocytes and fibroblasts, but it is also populated by migratory hematopoietic cells, including lymphoid cells, granulocytes, mast cells, dendritic cells, natural killer cells, neutrophils and macrophages. These haematopoietic cells have pivotal roles in the progression and metastasis of tumors [69, 70]. The significance of tumor stroma for the overall prognosis may be in part due to the fact that several components of the tumor-microenvironment have been shown to compromise immune effect functions against tumor cells [71]. The concept of tumor-promoting inflamma-tion is a recognized enabling characteristic of cancers [72].

The first evidence suggesting immune responses to neuroblastoma was provided in 1968 when blood leukocytes, which were 50–70% lymphocytes, were reported to inhibit colony formation by neuroblastoma cells [73]. These lymphocytes inhibited colony formation by both autologous and allogeneic neuroblastoma cells but did not affect growth of fibroblasts from the same donors. Plasma from these patients also was reported to inhibit tumor cell colony formation in the presence of complement. In this same time, primary tumors were reported to contain leukocytes [74, 75], and some localized and metastatic neuroblastomas were reported to regress spontaneously [76, 77]. Together, these studies suggest that the immune system could develop an anti-neuroblastoma response. In this section, we will highlight the role of tumor infiltrating immune cells in progression of this disease and how blocking the function of these infiltrating cells may prove beneficial in its treatment of NB.

a. Tumor infiltrating Lymphocytes

Tumor-associated lymphocyte population includes CD8+ cytotoxic T cells, CD4+ T helper cells, regulatory T cells (Tregs), NKT or γδT cells. Tregs are immunosuppressive regulatory T cells. Tregs are able to suppress the activity of CTLs by direct cell-cell contact and also secrete immunoregulatory cytokines such as transforming growth factor β (TGF-β) and interleukin-10 (IL-10). However, the role of Tregs is much less clear and to our knowledge there are no published data on the presence (or otherwise) of Tregs in pediatric tumors.

CD8⁺ cytotoxic T lymphocytes (CTL) are a primary source of anti-tumor activity in the immune system [1, 3]. In many adult cancers the presence of significant numbers of tumor-infiltrating lymphocytes, potentially represents the host immune response against the tumor and is associated with improved prognosis [78-80]. In neuroblastoma, Martin *et al.* [81] suggested a correlation between lymphocyte infiltration and improved survival, although these data are confounded by tumor grade since lymphocytic infiltrates were seen more frequently in low grade, differentiating tumors. In a separate examination of 26 high-risk neuroblastoma tumor samples, there was minimal or undetectable infiltration of CD8+ or CD4+ T cells, CD20+ B cells or CD56+ NK cells within tumor nests [82], although in most patients CD8+ or CD4+ lymphocytes were present within the peritumoral stroma. Interestingly, the majority of patients had evidence of small numbers of circulating cytotoxic T cells against the tumor antigen survivin (expressed by all of the tumors in this study) and these CTLs were highly functional in *in vitro* assays [82]. The experiments conducted by another group in NXS2 murine neuroblastoma model have shown that oral vaccination with a survivin DNA minigene was associated with increased target cell lysis, increased presence of CD8(+) T-cells at the primary tumor site, and enhanced production of pro-inflammatory cytokines [83]. Another pre-clinical study have demonstrated that tyrosine hydroxylase and MYCN proteins, which are relatively specific for neuroblastoma cells compared to normal cells, include peptides that can be targets for CTL. Vaccination of mice with tyrosine hydroxylase DNA minigenes can induce CTLs, eradicate established primary NXS2 neuroblastoma tumors, and inhibit spontaneous metastases without induction of autoimmunity [84, 85].

However, despite these cellular responses to NB, the presence of tumor-infiltrating CTL is rare, suggesting a block in T cell trafficking that may protect the tumor from CTL-mediated cytotoxicity. Therefore, strategies aiming to generate CTLs must take into account mechanisms by which neuroblastoma cells may avoid immune elimination. These include decreased expression of peptide presenting HLA class I molecules by tumor cells, which can impair target peptide recognition by CTLs [82, 86, 87]. Also, neuroblastoma cells express low levels of antigen processing genes, including LMP-2, LMP-7, and TAP-1, which are necessary for preparation of peptides from proteins for presentation by HLA class I molecules to CTLs [88, 89]. Neuroblastoma cells also induce monocytes to release HLA-G, which suppresses both CTL and NK mediated cytotoxicity by interacting with inhibitory receptors or inducing apoptosis via CD8 ligation or the Fas-FasL pathway [90]. Thus, effective CTL anti-tumor responses require that these escape mechanisms be evaluated and, if present, be overcome.

b.   Natural Killer Cells

Natural Killer (NK) cells represent a particular subset of T lymphocytes, which express both T cell markers, such as the αβ T-cell receptor (TCR) and associated CD3 complex, and NK cell markers, such as NK1.1[91]. These cells recognize glycolipids presented by the MHC class I-like molecule CD1d and are believed to play an important role at the interface between the innate and adaptive immune responses to infection and malignancy [92]. Two main subtypes of NKT cell are recognised, with Type I NKT cells expressing an invariant α-TCR chain and being implicated in antitumor immunity, whilst Type II NKT cells express a variety of TCR molecules (in addition to CD1d) and appear to have a more immune inhibitory role [91]. The presence of these immune effector cells within tumors has been examined in a number of different malignancies, including, neuroblastoma. Type I NKT cells were found in 53% of 98 untreated primary stage 4 neuroblastoma samples [93] and their infiltration correlated with favorable outcome, with expression of the chemokine CCL2 and with absence of MYCN amplification (indicating less aggressive disease). Subsequent investigations have confirmed that expression of CCL2 is repressed in MYCN amplified tumors, leading to a failure of NKT cell infiltration and potentially contributing to tumor immune escape [94].

Recent studies have suggested anti-tumor role of NK cells in high risk neuroblastoma NK cells are activated to be cytotoxic and secrete IFNγ by IL-2. IL-2 alone has been tested in phase I and II trials for patients with neuroblastoma, and, although immune effects were documented, no objective tumor responses were observed [95, 96]. Lenalidomide is an immune modulating drug that activates T cells to secrete IL-2, which in turn activates NK cell cytotoxicity and ADCC [97, 98]. Clinical trials in children and adults demonstrated increased numbers of NK cells and cytotoxicity, decreased T regulatory cells, and increased secretion of IL-2, IL-15, and GM-CSF after 21 days of lenalidomide treatment [99, 100]. Thus, lenalidomide may be useful for activating NK cells to enhance mAb immunotherapy of neuroblastoma.

c.   Role of tumor associated macrophages

Macrophages represent a further important cellular component of the tumor stroma. Far from being mere bystanders to tumor development, there is increasing evidence that tumor-associated macrophages (TAMs) promote and facilitate tumor growth [101, 102]. Of key importance is the concept of distinct macrophage phenotypes, mirroring the dichotomy between T_H1 and T_H2 T helper cells and type I and type II immune responses. Alternatively activated M2-macrophages are involved in polarized Th2 inflammatory reactions and characterized by expression of arginase-1 and mannose and scavenger receptors [103, 104]. On the other extreme, classically activated M1 macrophages are IL-12 high, IL-23 high, IL-10 low; produce high levels of inducible nitric oxide synthetase (iNOS); secrete inflammatory cytokines such as IL-1β, IL-6, and TNF; and are inducer and effector cells in Th1 type inflammatory responses [105]. It has been suggested that tumor-associated macrophages (TAMs) display an M2-like phenotype [106].

TAMs are recruited to tumors when stimulated by growth factors and chemokines, produced by the tumor cells [107, 108]. The conventional wisdom about TAM function is that they are recruited to reject the tumor, which has been recognized as foreign because tumors express unique antigens. However, there is a growing body of evidence that the tumor microenvironment is immunosuppressive [109], perhaps as a result of selection for such an environment a process recently termed 'immunoediting. Recent data indicate that TGF-β1 has an important role in suppressing these local responses and that inhibiting this molecule can result in tumor rejection [110, 111]. It is noteworthy that TAMs can both produce TGF-β1 and process latent

TGF-βs to produce their active forms[111]. In addition, the local cytokine milieu in the tumor tends to block the immunological functions of these newly recruited mononuclear phagocytes such as antigen presentation and cytotoxicity towards tumors, and diverts them towards specialized TAMs that are immunosuppressed and trophic [112]. A principal component of this cytokine mixture is CSF-1, which locally blocks the maturation of dendritic cells so that they are unable to present antigens and promotes the development of immunosuppressed trophic TAMs. TAMs promote tumor growth by affecting angiogenesis, immune suppression, invasion and metastasis [101, 102]. Existing literature suggests that tumor associated macrophages secrete several genes including matrix metalloproteinases-9 (MMP-9) [113], urokinase-type plasminogen activator (uPA) [114], vascular endothelial growth factor (VEGF) [115], and cyclooxygenase-2 (Cox-2) [116] which promotes tumor growth by breaking down extracellular matrix. The role of TAMs in tumor growth and progression is highlighted in Figure 3.

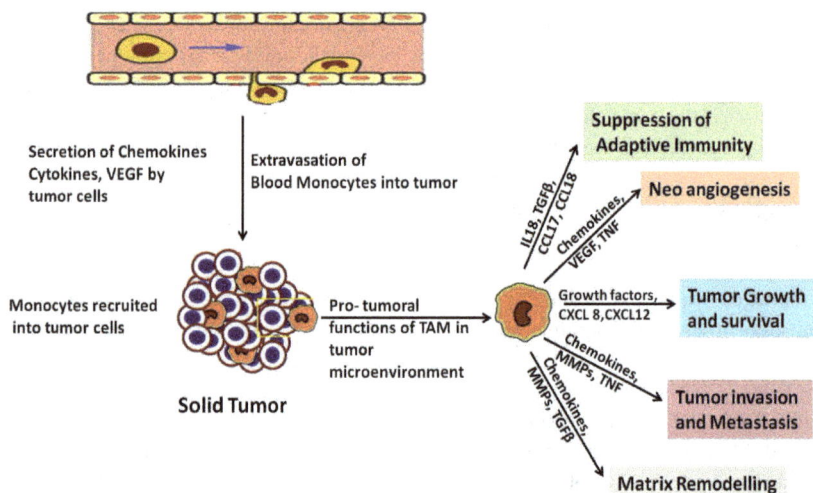

Figure 3. The role of TAMs in tumor growth, invasion and metastasis: Tumor-derived chemokines, cytokines and vascular endothelial growth factor (VEGF), actively recruit circulating blood monocytes at the tumor site In the tumor micro-environment monocytes differentiate into tumor-associated macrophages (TAM), where they promote tumor growth and metastasis and establish a symbiotic relationship with tumor cells. The above tumor-derived factors positively modulate TAM survival. TAMs also secrete growth factors, which promote tumor cell proliferation and survival, regulate matrix deposition and remodeling and activate neo-angiogenesis. Figure modified and adapted from Sica et al. [106]

Clinical studies have, on balance, shown a correlation between an abundance of TAMs and poor prognosis [108]. These data are particularly strong for breast, prostate, pancreatic, ovarian and cervical cancers; the data for stomach and lung cancers are contradictory [108, 117, 118], and in a small study in colorectal cancer, their presence was associated with good prognosis [119]. However, taking all reports into account regardless of method and sample number more than 80% show a significant correlation between TAM density and poor prognosis, whereas less than 10% associate TAM density with a good prognosis [108]. So, increased TAM density is usually associated with advanced tumor progression and metastasis in most of the cancers. However the prognostic significance of tumor associated inflammatory cells in metastatic disease and in childhood cancers is mostly unknown.

Recent reports suggest that interaction between tumor and inflammatory cells contribute to the clinical metastatic neuroblastoma phenotype [120]. It has been reported that metastatic neuro-blastomas had higher infiltration of TAMs than loco regional tumors, and metastatic tumors diagnosed in patients at age ≥ 18 months had higher expression of inflammation related genes than those in patients diagnosed at age < 18 months. They identified 14 genes, out of which nine were tumor cell related and five were inflammation related that comprises a prognostic signature for neuroblastoma. Expression of inflammation related genes representing TAMs (*CD33/CD16/IL6R/IL10/FCGR3*) contributed to 25% of the accuracy of a novel 14-gene tumor classification score [120]. Another study by Song et al., demonstrated that CD1d+ TAMs promote neuroblasto-ma growth via IL-6 production and that expression of monocyte/macrophage markers, CD14/CD16, and IL-6 or IL-6R inversely correlates with long-term disease-free survival in patients with stage 4 *MYCN*–non-amplified neuroblastoma [121]. They suggested that cotransfer of human monocytes and NKTs to tumor-bearing NOD/SCID mice decreased monocyte number at the tumor site and suppressed tumor growth compared with mice transferred with monocytes alone. Thus killing of TAMs can be suggested as a novel mechanism of NKT antitumor activity that relates to the disease outcome. Although less is known about the role of stromal compartment in tumorigenecity in neuroblastoma and other childhood tumors but recent reports suggesting infiltration of macrophages in metastatic neuroblastoma opened new opportunities to target tumor associated immune system cells in childhood cancer. It is unclear whether these TAMs represent M2 macrophages and the mechanisms that control macrophage differentiation along the M1 vs the M2 lineage in tumor biology.

7. Multiple 'Omics' analysis an emerging concept in treatment of neuroblastoma

The "Omics" is a neologism widely adopted by scientists to refer to large scale analysis of genes (genomic), proteins (proteomics) and lately small metabolites (metabolomics). Modern molecu-lar achievements over the last decade have seen the increase and implementation of multiple 'omics technologies in oncology that promises to provide for a deeper comprehension of complex tumor pathways. It is believed that an integration of multiple "omics" technologies is likely to provide even further insight into the holistic view of the biology networks [122]. The studies of global expression profiles of both mRNA and protein are necessary to reveal the important pathways for an enigmatic disease such as neuroblastoma. During the past several years many studies utilized microarray-based high throughput technologies to investigate gene expres-sion profiles and DNA copy number alterations in neuroblastoma [123, 124]. Guo *et al.* has performed exon array profiling to investigate global alternative splicing pattern of 47 neuroblas-toma samples in stage 1 and stage 4 with normal or amplified MYCN copy number (stage 1-, 4-and 4+) Their results demonstrated a significant role of alternative splicing in high stage neuroblastoma and suggested a MYCN-associated splicing regulation pathway in stage 4+

tumors [125]. Studies from other group has measured copy number alterations in a representative set of 82 diagnostic tumors on a customized high-resolution BAC array based CGH platform supplemented with additional clones across 1p36, 2p24, 3p21-22, 11q14-24, and 16p12-13, and integrated these data with RNA expression data[126]. They used an unbiased statistical method to define a set of minimal common regions (MCRs) of aberration and on the basis of unsupervised hierarchal clustering they identified four distinct genomic subclasses. These genomic subsets were highly correlated with patient outcome, and individual MCRs remained prognostic in a multivariable model. These studies mentioned above identified prognostic markers and genomic alterations specific to high-risk neuroblastoma, and showed the capability of identifying signatures which predict patient outcome. Since mRNA expression is not always indicative of corresponding protein expression because the abundance of specific proteins can be controlled by post-transcriptional translation and post-translational modifications, therefore the use of proteomics will help in detecting directly the actual biological effector molecules and should provide more accurate functional information about biological systems. With this idea, Chen *et al.* has performed parallel global protein and mRNA expression profiling on NB tumors of stage4 *MYCN*-amplified (4+) and stage1 *MYCN*-not-amplified (1-) using isotope-coded affinity tags (ICAT) and Affymetrix U133plus2 microarray respectively [127]. Pathway analysis of the differentially expressed proteins conducted by this group showed the enrichment of glycolysis, DNA replication and cell cycle processes in the upregulated proteins and cell adhesion, nervous system development and cell differentiation processes in the down-regulated proteins in 4+ tumors; suggesting a less mature neural and a more invasive phenotype of 4+ tumor.

Metabolomics falls behind its predecessor genomics and proteomics, but represent a burgeoning field with potential to fill up the gap between genotype and phenotype [128] The high throughput nature of metabolomics makes it an attractive tool for scientists involved in the process of drug development. The reason for that lies in the principle that a patients response to drugs and toxicities do not depend only on a person genetic make-up, but it is rather a factorial outcome of interactions between intrinsic factors and environment [128]. Therefore, metabolomics technology is a powerful tool that can accurately measure the entire spectrum of biochemical changes and mapping these changes to metabolic pathways [128, 129]. In 1995, Florian et al. [130] determined the metabolic characteristics of three types of human brain and nervous system tumors by high-resolution in vitro MRS and chromatographic analysis. Signals from leucine, isoleucine, glycine, valine, threonine, lactate, acetate, glutamate, and choline-containing compounds were similarly detected in meningiomas, glioblastomas, and NB. In 2007, Peet et al. [131] reported the results of in vitro 1H high-resolution magic angle spinning NMR spectroscopy (HRMAS) investigations performed on cell suspension of 13 lines of NB possessing multiple genetic alterations. In their study, a specific metabolite profile associated with *MYCN*-amplified and non-amplified tumor subtypes was described. Phosphocholine and taurine concentration ratios relative to total choline were found to be significantly more elevated in the *MYCN*-amplified as compared to the *MYCN*-non-amplified cell lines, and suggested that choline and taurine molecular pathways could be potential therapeutic targets in NB[131]. Recently, Imperiale *et al.* has characterized the metabolic content of intact biopsy samples obtained from 12 patients suffering from neuroblastoma by using (HRMAS) [132].

Their studies suggested that NB patients younger than 12 months contained a higher level of acetate and lysine. Conversely, higher amounts of glutathione, glutamate, myoinositol glycine, serine and ascorbic acid were detected in NB samples belonging to younger children.

Overall, the emerging concept of analyzing NB-specific 'omics profiles to better understand and define the behavior of advanced-stage tumors along with providing direct and targeted therapy may ultimately translate into improved outcomes for high-risk NB.

8. Antibody dependent cellular toxicity (ADCC) / Role of ITAM and ITIM signaling in neuroblastoma

The Fcγ receptors (FcγRs) expressed on hematopoietic cells play a key role in immune defenses by linking humoral and cellular immunity [133]. FcγRs display coordinate and opposing roles in immune responses depending on their cytoplasmic region and/or their associated chains. Indeed, the activating receptors contain an immunoreceptor tyrosine-based activation motif (ITAM) and initiate inflammatory, cytolytic, and phagocytic activities of immune effector cells. In contrast, the inhibitory receptors that downmodulate the immune responses contain an immunoreceptor tyrosine-based inhibitory motif (ITIM) [134, 135]. There are numerous Fc receptors for IgG (FcγR) that are widely expressed on immune cells. The FcγR family consists of four classes of receptors, FcγRI, FcγRII, FcγRIII, and FcγRIV, that have been identified in both mice and humans. There are significant similarities in the functions of the FcγR receptors between mice and humans, but there is limited homology in receptors themselves [136]. To date, only one inhibitory FcγR, FcγRIIb, has been identified and is the only receptor to have complete homology between mice and humans [136]. FcγRs can be found on virtually all hematopoietic cells except T cells; in most cases, cells coexpress activating and inhibitory FcγR, allowing for the balance between activating and inhibitory receptors to dictate their response [136]. NK cells are an exception to this rule and express only the activating FcγRIIIa. NK cells do not express the inhibitory FcγRIIb.

Antibodies directed against neoplastic cells provide new therapeutic approaches against various malignancies, including lymphoma, leukemia, melanoma, and breast and colorectal carcinoma [137, 138] There is increasing evidence that the Fc portion of the anti-tumor IgG is a major component of their therapeutic activity, along with other mechanisms such as activation of apoptosis, blockade of signaling pathways, or masking of tumor antigens. Thus, by binding to activating FcγRs expressed by immune effector cells, such as macrophages, monocytes, neutrophils, or NK cells, tumor-specific antibodies trigger the destruction of malignant cells via antibody-dependent cellular cytotoxicity (ADCC) or phagocytosis [139, 140].

Because of their rapid and unopposed responses to mAb, NK cells play a major role in the anti-tumor response elicited by tumor-specific mAbs. Multiple clinically successful mAbs utilize NK-mediated ADCC as a mechanism of action. Rituximab (anti-CD20), Herceptin (anti-Her-2/ neu), Cetuximab (anti-EGFR), and the anti-GD2-mAbs 3F8 and ch14.18 are examples of tumor-specific mAbs whose clinical activity can be attributed, at least in part, to NK cells. Natural killer (NK) cells are powerful effector cells that can be directed to eliminate tumor cells through tumor-targeted monoclonal antibodies (mAbs). Some tumor-targeted mAbs have been successfully applied in the clinic and are included in the standard of care for certain malignancies. Strategies to augment the antitumor response by NK cells have led to an increased understanding of how to improve their effector responses. Next-generation reagents, such as molecularly modified mAbs and mAb-cytokine fusion proteins (immunocytokines, ICs) designed to augment NK-mediated killing, are showing promise in preclinical and some clinical settings. Continued research into the antitumor effects induced by NK cells and tumor-targeted mAbs suggests that additional intrinsic and extrinsic factors may influence the antitumor response. Therefore more research is needed that focuses on evaluating which NK cell and tumor criteria are best predictive of a clinical response and which combination immunotherapy regimens to pursue for distinct clinical settings.

9. Tumor associated gangliosides / GD2 monoclonal antibodies

Gangliosides (GD) are membrane-associated glycosphingolipids which have important regulatory roles during embryogenesis and have also been implicated in tumor development. Particular gangliosides, which show restricted patterns of expression in normal tissue, may be expressed at high levels by tumor cells (e.g. GD3 by melanoma) and are implicated both in tumorigenesis and as mediators of metastatic spread [141]. There is also evidence that gangliosides secreted by tumor cells can modulate the immune response and, in particular, act to inhibit dendritic cell differentiation and function. Neuroblastoma (and other neuroendocrine) tumor cells ubiquitously express the ganglioside GD2, whilst expression in normal tissues is restricted to neurons. Thus, GD2 is an attractive antigen for neuroblastoma immunotherapy strategies [142] including humanized anti-GD2 monoclonal antibodies such as ch14.18 [143], or GD2-directed cytotoxic lymphocytes. A chimeric human–murine anti-GD2 monoclonal antibody [144] called ch14.18 has shown activity against neuroblastoma in preclinical studies [145] and early-phase clinicaltrials[146, 147], this activity could be enhanced when ch14.18 is used in combination with granulocyte–macrophage colony-stimulating factor (GM-CSF) [148] or interleukin-2 [149, 150] to augment antibody-dependent cell-mediated cytotoxicity. The feasibility of administering ch14.18 in combination with GM-CSF, interleukin-2, and isotretinoin during the early post-transplantation period has been shown in two sequential pilot phase 1 studies [143, 151]. This progression of clinical trials culminated in the recently completed phase III randomized study of isotretinoin together with ch14.18, IL-2, and GMCSF vs. isotretinoin only for children with high-risk neuroblastoma who had a clinical response to induction therapy and myeloablative consolidation therapy/AHSCT. Immunotherapy after consolidation significantly improve event free survival (EFS) (66 ±5% vs. 46 ±5% at 2 years, P = 0.01) and overall survival (86 ± 4% vs. 75 ± 5% at 2 years, P = 0.02). This was the first demonstration that antibody based therapy improves EFS and overall survival. Although EFS was improved by adding immunotherapy to isotretinoin, approximately 40% of patients still relapsed during or after this therapy [152]. Additionally, the combination of ch14.18 with IL-2 and GM-CSF has significant toxicities, including neuropathic pain, fever without neutropenia, infection, hypokalemia, hypotension, and capillary leak syndrome. Thus, a search for new agents to combine with ch14.18 to improve efficacy and decrease toxicity is justified.

Immunocytokines commonly known as antibody-cytokine fusion proteins combine the targeting ability of antibodies with the functional activity of cytokines, and are known to improve antibody-based therapy by delivering cytokines to the microenvironment to both activate effector cells and modulate the microenvironment. To date, immunocytokine research has focused on ADCC mediated by NK cells and on induction of CTL. An anti-GD2/IL-2 immunocytokine eradicated hepatic metastases of neuroblastomas in SCID mice that had been reconstituted with human lymphokine (IL-2) activated killer cells [153, 154]. In contrast, the combination of monoclonal anti-GD2 antibody and IL-2 at doses equivalent to the immuno-cytokine only reduced tumor load. In a syngeneic murine model of GD2 expressing melanoma, targeting with an anti-GD2 antibody/IL-2 immunocytokine resulted in generation of CD8+ T lymphocytes that could eradicate tumor as well as prevent tumor growth [154]. Based upon these data, phase I and II studies have tested a humanized anti-GD2/IL-2 immunocytokine (hu14.18/IL-2) in patients with refractory or relapsed neuroblastoma. In the phase I study of 27 patients, treatment with hu14.18/IL2 caused elevated serum levels of soluble IL-2 receptor alpha (sIL2R_) and lymphocytosis. There were no measurable complete or partial responses to hu14.18/IL2; however, three patients showed evidence of antitumor activity [155]. In the phase II study, 39 patients with recurrent or refractory neuroblastoma were enrolled (36 evaluable). No responses were seen for patients with disease measurable by standard radio-graphic criteria (stratum 1) (n = 13). Of 23 patients with disease evaluable only by 123I-metaiodobenzylguanidine (MIBG) scintigraphy and/or bone marrow histology (stratum 2), five patients (21.7%) responded; all had a complete response of 9, 13, 20, 30, and 35+ months duration. Grade 3 and 4 non-hematologic toxicities included capillary leak, hypoxia, pain, rash, allergic reaction, elevated transaminases, and hyperbilirubinemia, which were reversible within a few days of completing a treatment course. These results support further testing of hu14.18/IL2 in children with non-bulky high-risk neuroblastoma [156].

10. Summary

Herein, we have reviewed a number of important areas of basic and translational research related to emerging novel therapies for the pediatric solid tumor, neuroblastoma. These include: 1) Signaling pathways within the tumor cell itself e.g. oncogenes and tumor suppres-sor proteins 2) Signaling pathways that regulate the tumor stromal compartment to control angiogenesis and the immune system and 3) Elements of cancer metabolism related to the oncogene addiction hypothesis.

Future studies will tap into these areas of basic science investigation to illuminate new avenues for therapeutics. We hereby advocate the need to genotype and perform molecular profiling by multi "omic" analysis on the tumor and stromal cells within the tumor and metastatic sites. Moreover, we suggest that we should examine the adaptive responses to targeted therapeutic agents in mouse models and patients treated with these agents in search of most potent combinations and mechanisms for resistance. This will be required to affect a cure of this difficult to treat disease.

Author details

Shweta Joshi[1], Alok R. Singh[1], Lisa L.R. Hartman[1,2], Muamera Zulcic[1], Hyunah Ahn[2] and Donald L. Durden[1]

*Address all correspondence to: ddurden@ucsd.edu

1 Department of Pediatrics, Moores Cancer Center, University of California San Diego, La Jolla, CA, USA

2 Department of Pediatrics, Rady Children's Hospital-San Diego/UCSD, MC San Diego CA, USA

References

[1] Shimada H, Stram DO, Chatten J, Joshi VV, Hachitanda Y, Brodeur GM, et al. Identi‐ fication of subsets of neuroblastomas by combined histopathologic and N-myc analy‐ sis. J Natl Cancer Inst. 1995 Oct 4;87(19):1470-6.

[2] Seeger RC, Brodeur GM, Sather H, Dalton A, Siegel SE, Wong KY, et al. Association of multiple copies of the N-myc oncogene with rapid progression of neuroblastomas. N Engl J Med. 1985 Oct 31;313(18):1111-6.

[3] Schmidt ML, Lal A, Seeger RC, Maris JM, Shimada H, O'Leary M, et al. Favorable prognosis for patients 12 to 18 months of age with stage 4 nonamplified MYCN neu‐ roblastoma: a Children's Cancer Group Study. J Clin Oncol. 2005 Sep 20;23(27): 6474-80.

[4] Castellino RC, Durden DL. Mechanisms of disease: the PI3K-Akt-PTEN signaling node--an intercept point for the control of angiogenesis in brain tumors. Nat Clin Pract Neurol. 2007 Dec;3(12):682-93.

[5] Castellino RC, Muh CR, Durden DL. PI-3 kinase-PTEN signaling node: an intercept point for the control of angiogenesis. Curr Pharm Des. 2009;15(4):380-8.

[6] Chesler L, Schlieve C, Goldenberg DD, Kenney A, Kim G, McMillan A, et al. Inhibi‐ tion of phosphatidylinositol 3-kinase destabilizes Mycn protein and blocks malignant progression in neuroblastoma. Cancer Res. 2006 Aug 15;66(16):8139-46.

[7] Kang J, Rychahou PG, Ishola TA, Mourot JM, Evers BM, Chung DH. N-myc is a novel regulator of PI3K-mediated VEGF expression in neuroblastoma. Oncogene. 2008 Jun 26;27(28):3999-4007.

[8] Chanthery YH, Gustafson WC, Itsara M, Persson A, Hackett CS, Grimmer M, et al. Paracrine signaling through MYCN enhances tumor-vascular interactions in neuroblastoma. Sci Transl Med. 2012 Jan 4;4(115):115ra3.

[9] Peirce SK, Findley HW, Prince C, Dasgupta A, Cooper T, Durden DL. The PI-3 kinase-Akt-MDM2-survivin signaling axis in high-risk neuroblastoma: a target for PI-3 kinase inhibitor intervention. Cancer Chemother Pharmacol. 2011 Aug;68(2):325-35.

[10] Garlich JR, De P, Dey N, Su JD, Peng X, Miller A, et al. A vascular targeted pan phosphoinositide 3-kinase inhibitor prodrug, SF1126, with antitumor and antiangiogenic activity. Cancer Res. 2008 Jan 1;68(1):206-15.

[11] Wen S, Stolarov J, Myers MP, Su JD, Wigler MH, Tonks NK, et al. PTEN controls tumor-induced angiogenesis. Proc Natl Acad Sci U S A. 2001 Apr 10;98(8):4622-7.

[12] Fang J, Ding M, Yang L, Liu LZ, Jiang BH. PI3K/PTEN/AKT signaling regulates prostate tumor angiogenesis. Cell Signal. 2007 Dec;19(12):2487-97.

[13] Tian T, Nan KJ, Wang SH, Liang X, Lu CX, Guo H, et al. PTEN regulates angiogenesis and VEGF expression through phosphatase-dependent and -independent mechanisms in HepG2 cells. Carcinogenesis. 2010 Jul;31(7):1211-9.

[14] Hanahan D, Folkman J. Patterns and emerging mechanisms of the angiogenic switch during tumorigenesis. Cell. 1996 Aug 9;86(3):353-64.

[15] Meitar D, Crawford SE, Rademaker AW, Cohn SL. Tumor angiogenesis correlates with metastatic disease, N-myc amplification, and poor outcome in human neuroblastoma. J Clin Oncol. 1996 Feb;14(2):405-14.

[16] Ribatti D, Vacca A, Nico B, De Falco G, Giuseppe Montaldo P, Ponzoni M. Angiogenesis and anti-angiogenesis in neuroblastoma. Eur J Cancer. 2002 Apr;38(6):750-7.

[17] Eggert A, Ikegaki N, Kwiatkowski J, Zhao H, Brodeur GM, Himelstein BP. High-level expression of angiogenic factors is associated with advanced tumor stage in human neuroblastomas. Clin Cancer Res. 2000 May;6(5):1900-8.

[18] Chlenski A, Liu S, Crawford SE, Volpert OV, DeVries GH, Evangelista A, et al. SPARC is a key Schwannian-derived inhibitor controlling neuroblastoma tumor angiogenesis. Cancer Res. 2002 Dec 15;62(24):7357-63.

[19] Goldberg MA, Schneider TJ. Similarities between the oxygen-sensing mechanisms regulating the expression of vascular endothelial growth factor and erythropoietin. J Biol Chem. 1994 Feb 11;269(6):4355-9.

[20] Rossler J, Taylor M, Geoerger B, Farace F, Lagodny J, Peschka-Suss R, et al. Angiogenesis as a target in neuroblastoma. Eur J Cancer. 2008 Aug;44(12):1645-56.

[21] Drozynska E, Izycka-Swieszewska E, Balcerska A, Bodalski J, Bohosiewicz J, Brozyna A, et al. [Analysis of microvascular density and the expression of vascular-endothelial growth factor (VEGF) and its membrane receptor Flk-1 in neuroblastoma]. Med Wieku Rozwoj. 2006 Jul-Sep;10(3 Pt 1):745-55.

[22] Ghanem MA, van Steenbrugge GJ, Sudaryo MK, Mathoera RB, Nijman JM, van der Kwast TH. Expression and prognostic relevance of vascular endothelial growth factor (VEGF) and its receptor (FLT-1) in nephroblastoma. J Clin Pathol. 2003 Feb;56(2): 107-13.

[23] Yang JC, Haworth L, Sherry RM, Hwu P, Schwartzentruber DJ, Topalian SL, et al. A randomized trial of bevacizumab, an anti-vascular endothelial growth factor antibody, for metastatic renal cancer. N Engl J Med. 2003 Jul 31;349(5):427-34.

[24] Hurwitz H, Fehrenbacher L, Novotny W, Cartwright T, Hainsworth J, Heim W, et al. Bevacizumab plus irinotecan, fluorouracil, and leucovorin for metastatic colorectal cancer. N Engl J Med. 2004 Jun 3;350(23):2335-42.

[25] Herbst RS, Johnson DH, Mininberg E, Carbone DP, Henderson T, Kim ES, et al. Phase I/II trial evaluating the anti-vascular endothelial growth factor monoclonal antibody bevacizumab in combination with the HER-1/epidermal growth factor receptor tyrosine kinase inhibitor erlotinib for patients with recurrent non-small-cell lung cancer. J Clin Oncol. 2005 Apr 10;23(11):2544-55.

[26] Fukuzawa M, Sugiura H, Koshinaga T, Ikeda T, Hagiwara N, Sawada T. Expression of vascular endothelial growth factor and its receptor Flk-1 in human neuroblastoma using in situ hybridization. J Pediatr Surg. 2002 Dec;37(12):1747-50.

[27] Rossler J, Breit S, Havers W, Schweigerer L. Vascular endothelial growth factor expression in human neuroblastoma: up-regulation by hypoxia. Int J Cancer. 1999 Mar 31;81(1):113-7.

[28] Shusterman S, Maris JM. Prospects for therapeutic inhibition of neuroblastoma angiogenesis. Cancer Lett. 2005 Oct 18;228(1-2):171-9.

[29] Glade Bender JL, Adamson PC, Reid JM, Xu L, Baruchel S, Shaked Y, et al. Phase I trial and pharmacokinetic study of bevacizumab in pediatric patients with refractory solid tumors: a Children's Oncology Group Study. J Clin Oncol. 2008 Jan 20;26(3): 399-405.

[30] Jakovljevic G, Culic S, Stepan J, Bonevski A, Seiwerth S. Vascular endothelial growth factor in children with neuroblastoma: a retrospective analysis. J Exp Clin Cancer Res. 2009;28:143.

[31] Huntly BJ, Gilliland DG. Cancer biology: summing up cancer stem cells. Nature. 2005 Jun 30;435(7046):1169-70.

[32] Reya T, Morrison SJ, Clarke MF, Weissman IL. Stem cells, cancer, and cancer stem cells. Nature. 2001 Nov 1;414(6859):105-11.

[33] Cho RW, Clarke MF. Recent advances in cancer stem cells. Curr Opin Genet Dev. 2008 Feb;18(1):48-53.

[34] Bonnet D, Dick JE. Human acute myeloid leukemia is organized as a hierarchy that originates from a primitive hematopoietic cell. Nat Med. 1997 Jul;3(7):730-7.

[35] Al-Hajj M, Wicha MS, Benito-Hernandez A, Morrison SJ, Clarke MF. Prospective identification of tumorigenic breast cancer cells. Proc Natl Acad Sci U S A. 2003 Apr 1;100(7):3983-8.

[36] O'Brien CA, Pollett A, Gallinger S, Dick JE. A human colon cancer cell capable of initiating tumour growth in immunodeficient mice. Nature. 2007 Jan 4;445(7123):106-10.

[37] Singh SK, Hawkins C, Clarke ID, Squire JA, Bayani J, Hide T, et al. Identification of human brain tumour initiating cells. Nature. 2004 Nov 18;432(7015):396-401.

[38] Hemmati HD, Nakano I, Lazareff JA, Masterman-Smith M, Geschwind DH, Bronner-Fraser M, et al. Cancerous stem cells can arise from pediatric brain tumors. Proc Natl Acad Sci U S A. 2003 Dec 9;100(25):15178-83.

[39] Singh SK, Clarke ID, Terasaki M, Bonn VE, Hawkins C, Squire J, et al. Identification of a cancer stem cell in human brain tumors. Cancer Res. 2003 Sep 15;63(18):5821-8.

[40] Cournoyer S, Nyalendo C, Addioui A, Belounis A, Beaunoyer M, Aumont A, et al. Genotype analysis of tumor-initiating cells expressing CD133 in neuroblastoma. Genes Chromosomes Cancer. 2012 Aug;51(8):792-804.

[41] Coulon A, Flahaut M, Muhlethaler-Mottet A, Meier R, Liberman J, Balmas-Bourloud K, et al. Functional sphere profiling reveals the complexity of neuroblastoma tumor-initiating cell model. Neoplasia. 2011 Oct;13(10):991-1004.

[42] Mao XG, Zhang X, Xue XY, Guo G, Wang P, Zhang W, et al. Brain Tumor Stem-Like Cells Identified by Neural Stem Cell Marker CD15. Transl Oncol. 2009 Dec;2(4): 247-57.

[43] Ward RJ, Lee L, Graham K, Satkunendran T, Yoshikawa K, Ling E, et al. Multipotent CD15+ cancer stem cells in patched-1-deficient mouse medulloblastoma. Cancer Res. 2009 Jun 1;69(11):4682-90.

[44] Read TA, Fogarty MP, Markant SL, McLendon RE, Wei Z, Ellison DW, et al. Identification of CD15 as a marker for tumor-propagating cells in a mouse model of medulloblastoma. Cancer Cell. 2009 Feb 3;15(2):135-47.

[45] Hansford LM, McKee AE, Zhang L, George RE, Gerstle JT, Thorner PS, et al. Neuroblastoma cells isolated from bone marrow metastases contain a naturally enriched tumor-initiating cell. Cancer Res. 2007 Dec 1;67(23):11234-43.

[46] Cantley LC. The phosphoinositide 3-kinase pathway. Science. 2002 May 31;296(5573): 1655-7.

[47] Anderson DAMaJ. The Immune Response in Paediatric Cancer. The Open Pathology Journal. 2010;4:45-59.

[48] Dahmane N, Sanchez P, Gitton Y, Palma V, Sun T, Beyna M, et al. The Sonic Hedgehog-Gli pathway regulates dorsal brain growth and tumorigenesis. Development. 2001 Dec;128(24):5201-12.

[49] Artavanis-Tsakonas S, Matsuno K, Fortini ME. Notch signaling. Science. 1995 Apr 14;268(5208):225-32.

[50] Rehman AO, Wang CY. Notch signaling in the regulation of tumor angiogenesis. Trends Cell Biol. 2006 Jun;16(6):293-300.

[51] van Amerongen R, Nusse R. Towards an integrated view of Wnt signaling in development. Development. 2009 Oct;136(19):3205-14.

[52] Reya T, Clevers H. Wnt signalling in stem cells and cancer. Nature. 2005 Apr 14;434(7035):843-50.

[53] Northcott PA, Korshunov A, Witt H, Hielscher T, Eberhart CG, Mack S, et al. Medulloblastoma comprises four distinct molecular variants. J Clin Oncol. 2011 Apr 10;29(11):1408-14.

[54] Grinshtein N, Datti A, Fujitani M, Uehling D, Prakesch M, Isaac M, et al. Small molecule kinase inhibitor screen identifies polo-like kinase 1 as a target for neuroblastoma tumor-initiating cells. Cancer Res. 2011 Feb 15;71(4):1385-95.

[55] Sunayama J, Sato A, Matsuda K, Tachibana K, Suzuki K, Narita Y, et al. Dual blocking of mTor and PI3K elicits a prodifferentiation effect on glioblastoma stem-like cells. Neuro Oncol. 2010 Dec;12(12):1205-19.

[56] Kroemer G, Pouyssegur J. Tumor cell metabolism: cancer's Achilles' heel. Cancer Cell. 2008 Jun;13(6):472-82.

[57] Vander Heiden MG, Cantley LC, Thompson CB. Understanding the Warburg effect: the metabolic requirements of cell proliferation. Science. 2009 May 22;324(5930):1029-33.

[58] Dang CV. Links between metabolism and cancer. Genes Dev. 2012 May 1;26(9):877-90.

[59] Schwab M, Alitalo K, Klempnauer KH, Varmus HE, Bishop JM, Gilbert F, et al. Amplified DNA with limited homology to myc cellular oncogene is shared by human neuroblastoma cell lines and a neuroblastoma tumour. Nature. 1983 Sep 15-21;305(5931):245-8.

[60] Wise DR, DeBerardinis RJ, Mancuso A, Sayed N, Zhang XY, Pfeiffer HK, et al. Myc regulates a transcriptional program that stimulates mitochondrial glutaminolysis and leads to glutamine addiction. Proc Natl Acad Sci U S A. 2008 Dec 2;105(48):18782-7.

[61] Yuneva M, Zamboni N, Oefner P, Sachidanandam R, Lazebnik Y. Deficiency in glu-tamine but not glucose induces MYC-dependent apoptosis in human cells. J Cell Biol. 2007 Jul 2;178(1):93-105.

[62] Gao P, Tchernyshyov I, Chang TC, Lee YS, Kita K, Ochi T, et al. c-Myc suppression of miR-23a/b enhances mitochondrial glutaminase expression and glutamine metabo-lism. Nature. 2009 Apr 9;458(7239):762-5.

[63] Nicklin P, Bergman P, Zhang B, Triantafellow E, Wang H, Nyfeler B, et al. Bidirec-tional transport of amino acids regulates mTOR and autophagy. Cell. 2009 Feb 6;136(3):521-34.

[64] Land H, Parada LF, Weinberg RA. Tumorigenic conversion of primary embryo fibro-blasts requires at least two cooperating oncogenes. Nature. 1983 Aug 18-24;304(5927): 596-602.

[65] Kauffmann-Zeh A, Rodriguez-Viciana P, Ulrich E, Gilbert C, Coffer P, Downward J, et al. Suppression of c-Myc-induced apoptosis by Ras signalling through PI(3)K and PKB. Nature. 1997 Feb 6;385(6616):544-8.

[66] Dang CV. MYC on the path to cancer. Cell. 2012 Mar 30;149(1):22-35.

[67] Hambardzumyan D, Becher OJ, Rosenblum MK, Pandolfi PP, Manova-Todorova K, Holland EC. PI3K pathway regulates survival of cancer stem cells residing in the per-ivascular niche following radiation in medulloblastoma in vivo. Genes Dev. 2008 Feb 15;22(4):436-48.

[68] Marx J. Cancer biology. All in the stroma: cancer's Cosa Nostra. Science. 2008 Apr 4;320(5872):38-41.

[69] Balkwill F, Mantovani A. Inflammation and cancer: back to Virchow? Lancet. 2001 Feb 17;357(9255):539-45.

[70] Lin EY, Nguyen AV, Russell RG, Pollard JW. Colony-stimulating factor 1 promotes progression of mammary tumors to malignancy. J Exp Med. 2001 Mar 19;193(6): 727-40.

[71] Duluc D, Corvaisier M, Blanchard S, Catala L, Descamps P, Gamelin E, et al. Interfer-on-gamma reverses the immunosuppressive and protumoral properties and prevents the generation of human tumor-associated macrophages. Int J Cancer. 2009 Jul 15;125(2):367-73.

[72] Hanahan D, Weinberg RA. Hallmarks of cancer: the next generation. Cell. 2011 Mar 4;144(5):646-74.

[73] Hellstrom IE, Hellstrom KE, Pierce GE, Bill AH. Demonstration of cell-bound and humoral immunity against neuroblastoma cells. Proc Natl Acad Sci U S A. 1968 Aug; 60(4):1231-8.

[74] Bill AH. The implications of immune reactions to neuroblastoma. Surgery. 1969 Aug; 66(2):415-8.

[75] Bill AH, Morgan A. Evidence for immune reactions to neuroblastoma and future possibilities for investigation. J Pediatr Surg. 1970 Apr;5(2):111-6.

[76] D'Angio GJ, Evans AE, Koop CE. Special pattern of widespread neuroblastoma with a favourable prognosis. Lancet. 1971 May 22;1(7708):1046-9.

[77] Evans AE, Gerson J, Schnaufer L. Spontaneous regression of neuroblastoma. Natl Cancer Inst Monogr. 1976 Nov;44:49-54.

[78] Katz SC, Pillarisetty V, Bamboat ZM, Shia J, Hedvat C, Gonen M, et al. T cell infiltrate predicts long-term survival following resection of colorectal cancer liver metastases. Ann Surg Oncol. 2009 Sep;16(9):2524-30.

[79] Hornychova H, Melichar B, Tomsova M, Mergancova J, Urminska H, Ryska A. Tumor-infiltrating lymphocytes predict response to neoadjuvant chemotherapy in patients with breast carcinoma. Cancer Invest. 2008 Dec;26(10):1024-31.

[80] Zhang L, Conejo-Garcia JR, Katsaros D, Gimotty PA, Massobrio M, Regnani G, et al. Intratumoral T cells, recurrence, and survival in epithelial ovarian cancer. N Engl J Med. 2003 Jan 16;348(3):203-13.

[81] Martin RF, Beckwith JB. Lymphoid infiltrates in neuroblastomas: their occurrence and prognostic significance. J Pediatr Surg. 1968 Feb;3(1):161-4.

[82] Coughlin CM, Fleming MD, Carroll RG, Pawel BR, Hogarty MD, Shan X, et al. Immunosurveillance and survivin-specific T-cell immunity in children with high-risk neuroblastoma. J Clin Oncol. 2006 Dec 20;24(36):5725-34.

[83] Fest S, Huebener N, Bleeke M, Durmus T, Stermann A, Woehler A, et al. Survivin minigene DNA vaccination is effective against neuroblastoma. Int J Cancer. 2009 Jul 1;125(1):104-14.

[84] Huebener N, Fest S, Strandsby A, Michalsky E, Preissner R, Zeng Y, et al. A rationally designed tyrosine hydroxylase DNA vaccine induces specific antineuroblastoma immunity. Mol Cancer Ther. 2008 Jul;7(7):2241-51.

[85] Huebener N, Fest S, Hilt K, Schramm A, Eggert A, Durmus T, et al. Xenogeneic immunization with human tyrosine hydroxylase DNA vaccines suppresses growth of established neuroblastoma. Mol Cancer Ther. 2009 Aug;8(8):2392-401.

[86] Lampson LA, Fisher CA. Weak HLA and beta 2-microglobulin expression of neuronal cell lines can be modulated by interferon. Proc Natl Acad Sci U S A. 1984 Oct; 81(20):6476-80.

[87] Reid GS, Shan X, Coughlin CM, Lassoued W, Pawel BR, Wexler LH, et al. Interferon-gamma-dependent infiltration of human T cells into neuroblastoma tumors in vivo. Clin Cancer Res. 2009 Nov 1;15(21):6602-8.

[88] Raffaghello L, Prigione I, Airoldi I, Camoriano M, Morandi F, Bocca P, et al. Mecha-
      nisms of immune evasion of human neuroblastoma. Cancer Lett. 2005 Oct
      18;228(1-2):155-61.

[89] Raffaghello L, Prigione I, Bocca P, Morandi F, Camoriano M, Gambini C, et al. Multi-
      ple defects of the antigen-processing machinery components in human neuroblasto-
      ma: immunotherapeutic implications. Oncogene. 2005 Jul 7;24(29):4634-44.

[90] Morandi F, Levreri I, Bocca P, Galleni B, Raffaghello L, Ferrone S, et al. Human neu-
      roblastoma cells trigger an immunosuppressive program in monocytes by stimulat-
      ing soluble HLA-G release. Cancer Res. 2007 Jul 1;67(13):6433-41.

[91] Godfrey DI, MacDonald HR, Kronenberg M, Smyth MJ, Van Kaer L. NKT cells:
      what's in a name? Nat Rev Immunol. 2004 Mar;4(3):231-7.

[92] Terabe M, Berzofsky JA. The role of NKT cells in tumor immunity. Adv Cancer Res.
      2008;101:277-348.

[93] Metelitsa LS, Wu HW, Wang H, Yang Y, Warsi Z, Asgharzadeh S, et al. Natural killer
      T cells infiltrate neuroblastomas expressing the chemokine CCL2. J Exp Med. 2004
      May 3;199(9):1213-21.

[94] Song L, Ara T, Wu HW, Woo CW, Reynolds CP, Seeger RC, et al. Oncogene MYCN
      regulates localization of NKT cells to the site of disease in neuroblastoma. J Clin In-
      vest. 2007 Sep;117(9):2702-12.

[95] Truitt RL, Piaskowski V, Kirchner P, McOlash L, Camitta BM, Casper JT. Immuno-
      logical evaluation of pediatric cancer patients receiving recombinant interleukin-2 in
      a phase I trial. J Immunother (1991). 1992 May;11(4):274-85.

[96] Marti F, Pardo N, Peiro M, Bertran E, Amill B, Garcia J, et al. Progression of natural
      immunity during one-year treatment of residual disease in neuroblastoma patients
      with high doses of interleukin-2 after autologous bone marrow transplantation. Exp
      Hematol. 1995 Dec;23(14):1445-52.

[97] Bartlett JB, Dredge K, Dalgleish AG. The evolution of thalidomide and its IMiD de-
      rivatives as anticancer agents. Nat Rev Cancer. 2004 Apr;4(4):314-22.

[98] Hayashi T, Hideshima T, Akiyama M, Podar K, Yasui H, Raje N, et al. Molecular
      mechanisms whereby immunomodulatory drugs activate natural killer cells: clinical
      application. Br J Haematol. 2005 Jan;128(2):192-203.

[99] Berg SL, Cairo MS, Russell H, Ayello J, Ingle AM, Lau H, et al. Safety, pharmacoki-
      netics, and immunomodulatory effects of lenalidomide in children and adolescents
      with relapsed/refractory solid tumors or myelodysplastic syndrome: a Children's
      Oncology Group Phase I Consortium report. J Clin Oncol. 2011 Jan 20;29(3):316-23.

[100] Bartlett JB, Michael A, Clarke IA, Dredge K, Nicholson S, Kristeleit H, et al. Phase I
      study to determine the safety, tolerability and immunostimulatory activity of thali-

domide analogue CC-5013 in patients with metastatic malignant melanoma and other advanced cancers. Br J Cancer. 2004 Mar 8;90(5):955-61.

[101] Pollard JW. Tumour-educated macrophages promote tumour progression and metastasis. Nat Rev Cancer. 2004 Jan;4(1):71-8.

[102] Lin EY, Li JF, Gnatovskiy L, Deng Y, Zhu L, Grzesik DA, et al. Macrophages regulate the angiogenic switch in a mouse model of breast cancer. Cancer Res. 2006 Dec 1;66(23):11238-46.

[103] Gordon S, Taylor PR. Monocyte and macrophage heterogeneity. Nat Rev Immunol. 2005 Dec;5(12):953-64.

[104] Mosser DM. The many faces of macrophage activation. J Leukoc Biol. 2003 Feb;73(2): 209-12.

[105] Mantovani A, Sica A, Locati M. Macrophage polarization comes of age. Immunity. 2005 Oct;23(4):344-6.

[106] Sica A, Schioppa T, Mantovani A, Allavena P. Tumour-associated macrophages are a distinct M2 polarised population promoting tumour progression: potential targets of anti-cancer therapy. Eur J Cancer. 2006 Apr;42(6):717-27.

[107] Leek RD, Harris AL. Tumor-associated macrophages in breast cancer. J Mammary Gland Biol Neoplasia. 2002 Apr;7(2):177-89.

[108] Bingle L, Brown NJ, Lewis CE. The role of tumour-associated macrophages in tumour progression: implications for new anticancer therapies. J Pathol. 2002 Mar; 196(3):254-65.

[109] Elgert KD, Alleva DG, Mullins DW. Tumor-induced immune dysfunction: the macrophage connection. J Leukoc Biol. 1998 Sep;64(3):275-90.

[110] Gorelik L, Flavell RA. Immune-mediated eradication of tumors through the blockade of transforming growth factor-beta signaling in T cells. Nat Med. 2001 Oct;7(10): 1118-22.

[111] Chong H, Vodovotz Y, Cox GW, Barcellos-Hoff MH. Immunocytochemical localization of latent transforming growth factor-beta1 activation by stimulated macrophages. J Cell Physiol. 1999 Mar;178(3):275-83.

[112] Menetrier-Caux C, Montmain G, Dieu MC, Bain C, Favrot MC, Caux C, et al. Inhibition of the differentiation of dendritic cells from CD34(+) progenitors by tumor cells: role of interleukin-6 and macrophage colony-stimulating factor. Blood. 1998 Dec 15;92(12):4778-91.

[113] Giraudo E, Inoue M, Hanahan D. An amino-bisphosphonate targets MMP-9-expressing macrophages and angiogenesis to impair cervical carcinogenesis. J Clin Invest. 2004 Sep;114(5):623-33.

[114] Marconi C, Bianchini F, Mannini A, Mugnai G, Ruggieri S, Calorini L. Tumoral and macrophage uPAR and MMP-9 contribute to the invasiveness of B16 murine melanoma cells. Clin Exp Metastasis. 2008;25(3):225-31.

[115] Schoppmann SF, Fenzl A, Nagy K, Unger S, Bayer G, Geleff S, et al. VEGF-C expressing tumor-associated macrophages in lymph node positive breast cancer: impact on lymphangiogenesis and survival. Surgery. 2006 Jun;139(6):839-46.

[116] Nakao S, Kuwano T, Tsutsumi-Miyahara C, Ueda S, Kimura YN, Hamano S, et al. Infiltration of COX-2-expressing macrophages is a prerequisite for IL-1 beta-induced neovascularization and tumor growth. J Clin Invest. 2005 Nov;115(11):2979-91.

[117] DeNardo DG, Brennan DJ, Rexhepaj E, Ruffell B, Shiao SL, Madden SF, et al. Leukocyte complexity predicts breast cancer survival and functionally regulates response to chemotherapy. Cancer Discov. 2011 Jun;1(1):54-67.

[118] Kurahara H, Shinchi H, Mataki Y, Maemura K, Noma H, Kubo F, et al. Significance of M2-polarized tumor-associated macrophage in pancreatic cancer. J Surg Res. 2011 May 15;167(2):e211-9.

[119] Nakayama Y, Nagashima N, Minagawa N, Inoue Y, Katsuki T, Onitsuka K, et al. Relationships between tumor-associated macrophages and clinicopathological factors in patients with colorectal cancer. Anticancer Res. 2002 Nov-Dec;22(6C):4291-6.

[120] Asgharzadeh S, Salo JA, Ji L, Oberthuer A, Fischer M, Berthold F, et al. Clinical significance of tumor-associated inflammatory cells in metastatic neuroblastoma. J Clin Oncol. 2012 Oct 1;30(28):3525-32.

[121] Song L, Asgharzadeh S, Salo J, Engell K, Wu HW, Sposto R, et al. Valpha24-invariant NKT cells mediate antitumor activity via killing of tumor-associated macrophages. J Clin Invest. 2009 Jun;119(6):1524-36.

[122] Cavill R, Kamburov A, Ellis JK, Athersuch TJ, Blagrove MS, Herwig R, et al. Consensus-phenotype integration of transcriptomic and metabolomic data implies a role for metabolism in the chemosensitivity of tumour cells. PLoS Comput Biol. 2011 Mar; 7(3):e1001113.

[123] Wei JS, Greer BT, Westermann F, Steinberg SM, Son CG, Chen QR, et al. Prediction of clinical outcome using gene expression profiling and artificial neural networks for patients with neuroblastoma. Cancer Res. 2004 Oct 1;64(19):6883-91.

[124] Ohira M, Oba S, Nakamura Y, Isogai E, Kaneko S, Nakagawa A, et al. Expression profiling using a tumor-specific cDNA microarray predicts the prognosis of intermediate risk neuroblastomas. Cancer Cell. 2005 Apr;7(4):337-50.

[125] Guo X, Chen QR, Song YK, Wei JS, Khan J. Exon array analysis reveals neuroblastoma tumors have distinct alternative splicing patterns according to stage and MYCN amplification status. BMC Med Genomics. 2011;4:35.

[126] Mosse YP, Diskin SJ, Wasserman N, Rinaldi K, Attiyeh EF, Cole K, et al. Neuroblastomas have distinct genomic DNA profiles that predict clinical phenotype and regional gene expression. Genes Chromosomes Cancer. 2007 Oct;46(10):936-49.

[127] Chen QR, Song YK, Yu LR, Wei JS, Chung JY, Hewitt SM, et al. Global genomic and proteomic analysis identifies biological pathways related to high-risk neuroblastoma. J Proteome Res. 2010 Jan;9(1):373-82.

[128] Dettmer K, Hammock BD. Metabolomics--a new exciting field within the "omics" sciences. Environ Health Perspect. 2004 May;112(7):A396-7.

[129] Griffin JL, Shockcor JP. Metabolic profiles of cancer cells. Nat Rev Cancer. 2004 Jul; 4(7):551-61.

[130] Florian CL, Preece NE, Bhakoo KK, Williams SR, Noble M. Characteristic metabolic profiles revealed by 1H NMR spectroscopy for three types of human brain and nervous system tumours. NMR Biomed. 1995 Sep;8(6):253-64.

[131] Peet AC, McConville C, Wilson M, Levine BA, Reed M, Dyer SA, et al. 1H MRS identifies specific metabolite profiles associated with MYCN-amplified and non-amplified tumour subtypes of neuroblastoma cell lines. NMR Biomed. 2007 Nov;20(7): 692-700.

[132] Imperiale A, Elbayed K, Moussallieh FM, Neuville A, Piotto M, Bellocq JP, et al. Metabolomic pattern of childhood neuroblastoma obtained by (1)H-high-resolution magic angle spinning (HRMAS) NMR spectroscopy. Pediatr Blood Cancer. 2011 Jan; 56(1):24-34.

[133] Ravetch JV, Bolland S. IgG Fc receptors. Annu Rev Immunol. 2001;19:275-90.

[134] Amigorena S, Bonnerot C, Drake JR, Choquet D, Hunziker W, Guillet JG, et al. Cytoplasmic domain heterogeneity and functions of IgG Fc receptors in B lymphocytes. Science. 1992 Jun 26;256(5065):1808-12.

[135] Van den Herik-Oudijk IE, Capel PJ, van der Bruggen T, Van de Winkel JG. Identification of signaling motifs within human Fc gamma RIIa and Fc gamma RIIb isoforms. Blood. 1995 Apr 15;85(8):2202-11.

[136] Nimmerjahn F, Ravetch JV. Fcgamma receptors as regulators of immune responses. Nat Rev Immunol. 2008 Jan;8(1):34-47.

[137] White CA, Weaver RL, Grillo-Lopez AJ. Antibody-targeted immunotherapy for treatment of malignancy. Annu Rev Med. 2001;52:125-45.

[138] Safa MM, Foon KA. Adjuvant immunotherapy for melanoma and colorectal cancers. Semin Oncol. 2001 Feb;28(1):68-92.

[139] Clynes R, Takechi Y, Moroi Y, Houghton A, Ravetch JV. Fc receptors are required in passive and active immunity to melanoma. Proc Natl Acad Sci U S A. 1998 Jan 20;95(2):652-6.

[140] van de Winkel JG, Bast B, de Gast GC. Immunotherapeutic potential of bispecific antibodies. Immunol Today. 1997 Dec;18(12):562-4.

[141] Birkle S, Zeng G, Gao L, Yu RK, Aubry J. Role of tumor-associated gangliosides in cancer progression. Biochimie. 2003 Mar-Apr;85(3-4):455-63.

[142] Modak S, Cheung NK. Disialoganglioside directed immunotherapy of neuroblastoma. Cancer Invest. 2007 Feb;25(1):67-77.

[143] Gilman AL, Ozkaynak MF, Matthay KK, Krailo M, Yu AL, Gan J, et al. Phase I study of ch14.18 with granulocyte-macrophage colony-stimulating factor and interleukin-2 in children with neuroblastoma after autologous bone marrow transplantation or stem-cell rescue: a report from the Children's Oncology Group. J Clin Oncol. 2009 Jan 1;27(1):85-91.

[144] Gillies SD, Lo KM, Wesolowski J. High-level expression of chimeric antibodies using adapted cDNA variable region cassettes. J Immunol Methods. 1989 Dec 20;125(1-2): 191-202.

[145] Mueller BM, Romerdahl CA, Gillies SD, Reisfeld RA. Enhancement of antibody-dependent cytotoxicity with a chimeric anti-GD2 antibody. J Immunol. 1990 Feb 15;144(4):1382-6.

[146] Yu AL, Uttenreuther-Fischer MM, Huang CS, Tsui CC, Gillies SD, Reisfeld RA, et al. Phase I trial of a human-mouse chimeric anti-disialoganglioside monoclonal antibody ch14.18 in patients with refractory neuroblastoma and osteosarcoma. J Clin Oncol. 1998 Jun;16(6):2169-80.

[147] Handgretinger R, Anderson K, Lang P, Dopfer R, Klingebiel T, Schrappe M, et al. A phase I study of human/mouse chimeric antiganglioside GD2 antibody ch14.18 in patients with neuroblastoma. Eur J Cancer. 1995;31A(2):261-7.

[148] Barker E, Mueller BM, Handgretinger R, Herter M, Yu AL, Reisfeld RA. Effect of a chimeric anti-ganglioside GD2 antibody on cell-mediated lysis of human neuroblastoma cells. Cancer Res. 1991 Jan 1;51(1):144-9.

[149] Albertini MR, Hank JA, Schiller JH, Khorsand M, Borchert AA, Gan J, et al. Phase IB trial of chimeric antidisialoganglioside antibody plus interleukin 2 for melanoma patients. Clin Cancer Res. 1997 Aug;3(8):1277-88.

[150] Kendra K, Malkovska V, Allen M, Guzman J, Albertini M. In vivo binding and antitumor activity of Ch14.18. J Immunother. 1999 Sep;22(5):423-30.

[151] Ozkaynak MF, Sondel PM, Krailo MD, Gan J, Javorsky B, Reisfeld RA, et al. Phase I study of chimeric human/murine anti-ganglioside G(D2) monoclonal antibody (ch14.18) with granulocyte-macrophage colony-stimulating factor in children with neuroblastoma immediately after hematopoietic stem-cell transplantation: a Children's Cancer Group Study. J Clin Oncol. 2000 Dec 15;18(24):4077-85.

[152] Yu AL, Gilman AL, Ozkaynak MF, London WB, Kreissman SG, Chen HX, et al. Anti-GD2 antibody with GM-CSF, interleukin-2, and isotretinoin for neuroblastoma. N Engl J Med. 2010 Sep 30;363(14):1324-34.

[153] Sabzevari H, Gillies SD, Mueller BM, Pancook JD, Reisfeld RA. A recombinant antibody-interleukin 2 fusion protein suppresses growth of hepatic human neuroblastoma metastases in severe combined immunodeficiency mice. Proc Natl Acad Sci U S A. 1994 Sep 27;91(20):9626-30.

[154] Becker JC, Varki N, Gillies SD, Furukawa K, Reisfeld RA. Long-lived and transferable tumor immunity in mice after targeted interleukin-2 therapy. J Clin Invest. 1996 Dec 15;98(12):2801-4.

[155] Osenga KL, Hank JA, Albertini MR, Gan J, Sternberg AG, Eickhoff J, et al. A phase I clinical trial of the hu14.18-IL2 (EMD 273063) as a treatment for children with refractory or recurrent neuroblastoma and melanoma: a study of the Children's Oncology Group. Clin Cancer Res. 2006 Mar 15;12(6):1750-9.

[156] Shusterman S, London WB, Gillies SD, Hank JA, Voss SD, Seeger RC, et al. Antitumor activity of hu14.18-IL2 in patients with relapsed/refractory neuroblastoma: a Children's Oncology Group (COG) phase II study. J Clin Oncol. 2010 Nov 20;28(33): 4969-75.

miRNAs as Essential Mediators of the Actions of Retinoic Acid in Neuroblastoma Cells

Salvador Meseguer, Juan-Manuel Escamilla and
Domingo Barettino

Additional information is available at the end of the chapter

1. Introduction

The discovery of microRNAs (miRNAs, miRs) led to a profound change on our vision about the regulation of gene expression in eukaryotes. MicroRNAs are an emerging class of small non-coding endogenous RNAs that participate on the fine tuning of gene expression at the post-transcriptional level. First discovered at the early 90s in the nematode *C. elegans* [1], microRNAs have been involved in multiple important biological processes both in animal as in plant cells. These regulatory RNAs are transcribed as primary longer transcripts, which are then processed into 19-23-nt mature miRNAs. One strand of the mature miRNA is then incorporated into the RNA-induced silencing complex (RISC) to regulate gene expression by targeting the 3′-untranslated region (3′UTR) of mRNAs with consequent translational repression and/or target mRNA degradation. This mode of action demonstrates the great regulatory potential of miRNAs, since a unique mRNA can be targeted by diverse miRNAs and conversely each miRNA may have hundreds of different target mRNAs. In recent years miRNAs have been established as important regulators of tumor development, progression and metastasis, and have demonstrated to be useful for tumor diagnosis and classification. Moreover, miRNA regulation might represent a new avenue for cancer treatment in a near future.

Neuroblastoma is the most common extracranial solid tumor in childhood and the most common tumor in infants, which originates from aberrant development of primordial neural crest cells. Several lines of evidence support the idea that microRNA deregulation could contribute to neuroblastoma pathogenesis and progression [2, 3], and the usefulness of miRNA profiles for neuroblastoma diagnostics, classification and prognosis has been recently reported [4]. Neuroblastoma cell lines can be induced to differentiate *in vitro* by several agents, including Retinoic Acid (RA) [5, 6], the biologically active form of vitamin A. RA treatments lead to proliferative arrest and neuronal differentiation [5, 7] and to a reduction of the biological aggressiveness of neuroblastoma cells, by reducing their migratory and invasive abilities [8-10]. As a consequence of this, RA and its derivatives have been introduced into therapeutic protocols for neuroblastoma patients [11-13].

In this article we want to review the evidences supporting the contribution of miRNA regulation to RA-induced differentiation of neuroblastoma cells. We will show that miRNA contribute to the gene-expression changes associated with neuroblastoma cell differentiation and that specific RA-induced miRNAs target the expression of relevant genes in the context of neural differentiation. In addition RA-regulated miRNAs contribute to the reduction in the biological aggressiveness elicited by RA *in vitro*. We put forward the idea that miRNA regulation is part of the RA signaling pathway, and that miRNAs are essential mediators of the actions of RA in neuroblastoma cells.

2. The molecular bases of miRNA action

2.1. Biogenesis of miRNAs

miRNAs use complementary base pairing and the RNA induced silencing complex (RISC) to bind and either block translation and/or promote degradation of their target mRNAs. miRNAs are 19-22 nt-long RNA molecules transcribed mainly from non-coding regions of the genome, although some are embedded within genes, primarily as part of intronic sequences [14]. In addition, clusters of miRNAs were also found in the genome [15]. miRNAs are transcribed as large hairpin-containing molecules, called pri-miRNA, that are cleaved in the nucleus by the microprocessor complex, involving Drosha and Pasha/DGCR8 proteins [16, 17]. The result of this cleavage is a shorter precursor hairpin (approx. 70 nt), called pre-miRNA. Pre-miRNAs are exported through RAN GTPase and exportin-5 to the cytoplasm [18] where undergo further cleavage by Dicer to yield a transient intermediate imperfect duplex of approx 19-22 bp miRNA [19]. Subsequently, the duplex unwinds and miRNA strand is loaded into RISC complex together with proteins of the Argonaute (Ago) family [20]. The miRNA strand in RISC acts as a guide strand to find the complementary site in mRNA, and thereby suppressing the translational activity of the target mRNA. The complementary strand (known as miRNA* or as passenger strand) is degraded when the duplex is unwound, although recent evidences show that in some cases miRNA* accumulated at physiological levels and support the idea of a role for miRNA* on gene regulation [21]. (see Figure 1)

2.2. miRNA target binding

miRNAs interact primarily with the 3'-untranslated (3'UTR) region of their target mRNAs, although recent evidences show that miRNAs can also associate with sites located within the coding region of target genes [22]. In fact, complex arrays of multiple binding sites for either the same or different miRNAs located both in the 3'UTR as well as in the coding region of the target genes have been reported [23]. The base pairing of miRNA and mRNA in vertebrates requires only partial homology, with a preference for contiguous pairing occurring only at the *seed* region, located at nucleotides 2-7 of the guide strand. The lack of stringency results in a many-to-many relationship between miRNAs and mRNA targets, with the consequence that a high percentage of the genome may be regulated post-transcriptionally by a comparatively small set of miRNAs. A consequence of that is also that bioinformatic prediction of miRNA target mRNAs becomes relatively inaccurate. The guide strand binds to its complementary region in the 3'UTR of its target mRNA through Watson–Crick base pairing of the seed residues. Several alternative seed binding arrangements have been observed that involved different number of residues and therefore could have different binding affinity [24].

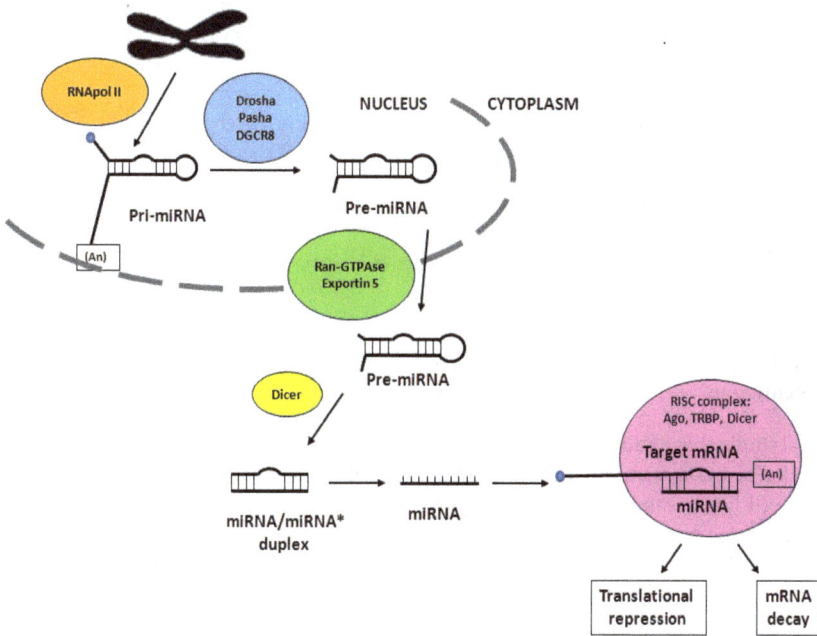

Figure 1. miRNA Biogenesis. The scheme depicts the different steps in the biogenesis of miRNAs, the enzymes involved and the intermediate miRNA forms.

2.3. Suppression of mRNA translation and/or mRNA degradation mediated by miRNAs

The binding of miRNA-RISC complex to its cognate mRNA target leads to mRNA silencing through suppression of mRNA translation and/or mRNA decay. [25, for review] Several mechanisms involving different protein complexes have been proposed. mRNA translation could be blocked at initiation step as well as post-initiation stages. The miRNA-RISC complex inhibits translation initiation by interfering with eIF4F-cap recognition and 40S small ribosomal subunit recruitment or by antagonizing 60S subunit joining and preventing 80S ribosomal complex formation. The interaction of the GW182 protein with the poly(A)-binding protein (PABP) might interfere with the closed-loop formation mediated by the eIF4G-PABP interaction and thus contribute to the repression of translation initiation. The miRNA-RISC might inhibit also translation at post-initiation steps by inhibiting ribosome elongation, inducing ribosome drop-off, or promoting proteolysis of nascent polypeptides. To promote mRNA degradation, the miRNA-RISC complex interacts with the CCR4-NOT1 deadenylase complex to facilitate deadenylation of the mRNA poly(A) tail. Deadenylation requires the direct interaction of the GW182 protein with PABP. Following deadenylation, the 5'-terminal cap (m^{7}G) is removed by the DCP1-DCP2 decapping complex. Although miRNA-mediated deadenylation followed by mRNA degradation appear to be widespread events, not all miRNA-targeted mRNAs are destabilized. miRNA-targeted translationally repressed mRNAs can accumulate in discrete cytoplasmic foci, such as P or GW bodies, or stress granules. A fraction of GW bodies co-localizes with multivesicular bodies (MVBs), membrane structures that play a role in miRNA-mediated repression. Compelling evidences support a role for miRNAs at the nucleus, acting on transcriptional regulation via chromatin remodeling and epigenetic mechanisms [26].

3. Profiling miRNA expression during retinoic-acid-induced neuroblastoma cell differentiation

3.1. Profiling miRNA expression during retinoic-acid induced neuroblastoma cell differentiation

Several studies have addressed the changes in the expression of miRNAs upon RA-dependent induction of differentiation of neuroblastoma cells, with somewhat different results depending on the cell line, treatment duration, analysis platform used, etc. [2, 27-30]. To analyze the contribution of microRNA regulation to RA-induced differentiation of neuroblastoma cells, we have studied the changes in the pattern of expression of 667 different human miRNAs upon RA treatment of SH-SY5Y neuroblastoma cells. We used miRNA profiling with TaqMan RT-PCR Low Density Arrays, and we found that 452 miRNAs were expressed above detection level. From them, 42 specific miRNAs change significatively their expression levels (26 upregulated and 16 downregulated) during RA-induced differentiation (Figure 2). This suggests miRNAs as an additional post-transcriptional regulatory layer under RA control [30].

3.2. A role for miRNAs-10a and -10b in RA-dependent regulation of neuroblastoma differentiation

We have focused our study on the closely related miR-10a and -10b, that showed the most prominent expression changes in SH-SY5Y cell line. Similar results have been reported for other neuroblastoma cell lines, like LA-N-1, LAN5 and SK-N-BE [29, 30].

Loss of function experiments with anti-sense anti-miRs antagonists could show that miR-10a and -10b contribute to the regulation of RA-induced differentiation. RA-induced neurite outgrowth was impaired in cells with experimentally reduced levels of miR-10a or -10b, and

the expression of several neural differentiation markers like Tyrosine Kinase receptors *NTRK2*

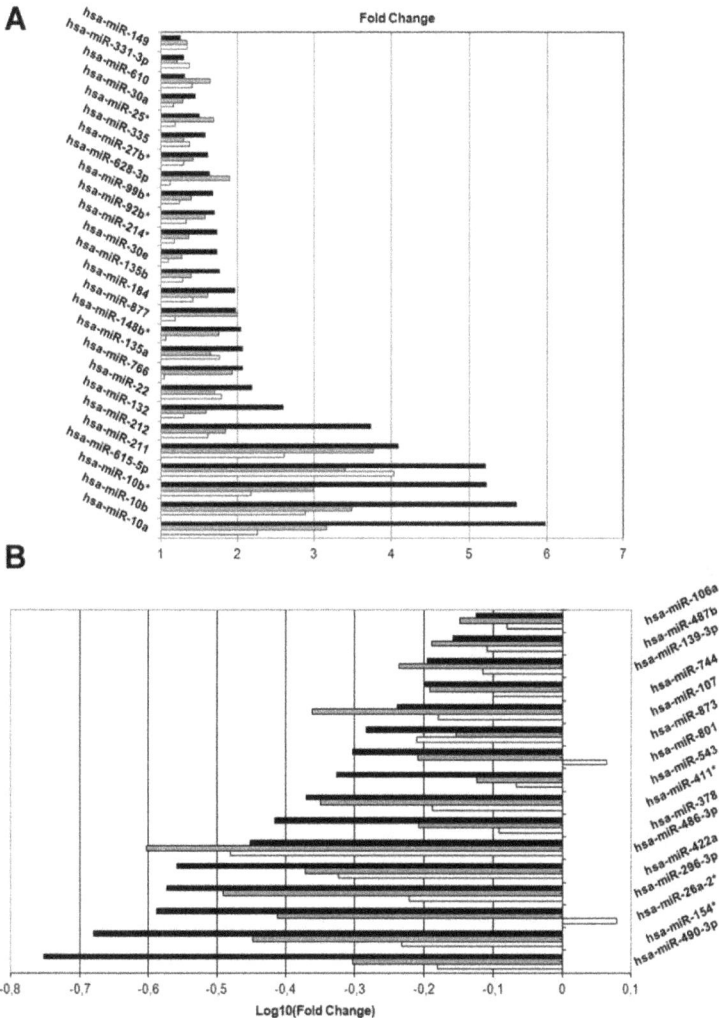

Figure 2. miRNA expression profiling in differentiating SH-SY5Y cells. Relative expression values detected in Taq-Man microRNA Low Density Arrays for microRNAs with FDR<0.05 at least in two of the three treated versus non-treated comparisons, for upregulated **(A)** and downregulated miRNAs **(B)**. The values for 24 (empty bars), 48 (grey bars) and 96 (black bars) h of RA treatment are represented.

(*trkB*) and *RET, GAP43,* Neuron-specific Enolase (*ENO2*), medium-size neurofilament protein NEFM and the enzyme Tyrosine Hydroxylase (TH) was abrogated or severely impaired after suppression of miR-10a or -10b (Figure 3).

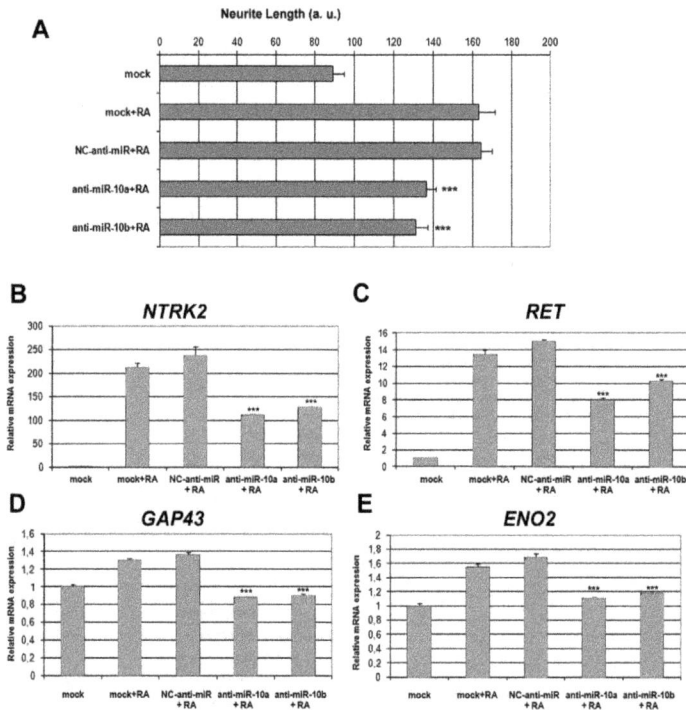

Figure 3. Knock-down of miR-10a and -10b impaired RA-induced differentiation. Blocking the action of miR-10a and -10b by transfection of their cognate anti-miRs diminished neurite outgrowth (A) and reduced the expression of neuronal differentiation markers *NTRK2* (B), *RET* (C), *GAP43* (D) and *ENO2* (E), as shown by quantitative RT-PCR. (Statistical signification in the Figures: *: $p<0.05$; **: $p<0.01$; ***: $p<0,001$; ns: non significative)

Conversely, the downregulation of the members of the ID gene family, *ID1, ID2* and *ID3* was abolished in RA-treated cells transfected with anti-miR-10a and anti-miR-10b. However, miR-10a and -10b did not appear to play a relevant role in RA-induced proliferation arrest, because the strong reduction of the incorporation of ^{3}H-Thymidine (to approximately 30% of the control values) and the decrease in the percentage of cells in S- phase (to 50% of the control) induced by RA treatment, was equivalent in neuroblastoma cells transfected with anti-miR-10a and anti-miR-10b [30]. However, a reduction in the cell growth in SK-N-BE neuroblastoma cells when transfected with pre-miR-10a and -10b has been reported [29]. Overexpression of miR-10 and -10b by transfecting synthetic precursor pre-miRs could not trigger full differentiation itself and although the mRNA levels of *RET, NTRK2, GAP43* and *ENO2* or the protein levels of NEFM and TH were slightly enhanced by transfection of pre-miR-10a and -10b, the attained expression levels for all the markers analyzed were far below those obtained by RA treatment. Similarly, ectopic expression of miR-10a and -10b led to certain increase in neurite outgrowth, but lower to that obtained for RA treatment [30]. Therefore, miR-10a and-10b appeared to be necessary but not sufficient for full neural differentiation, and consequently additional actions of RA must contribute to differentiation.

3.3. miRNAs-10a and -10b contribute to the reduction on the biological aggressiveness of neuroblastoma cells induced by RA

It has been reported that RA treatment of neuroblastoma cells results in a reduction in their biological aggressiveness, by decreasing their migratory and invasive abilities [8-10]. We wanted to analyze whether RA-induced expression of miR-10a and -10b could be related to the reduction in migratory and invasive potential of neuroblastoma cells. To test the migratory potential of SH-SY-5Y cells we used a modified, light-opaque Boyden chamber assay (Falcon HTS FluoroBlok, 8 μm pore size). Cells were transfected with anti-miR-10a or -10b or the corresponding Negative Control anti-miR, treated with 1 μM RA or vehicle in culture medium during 96 h, and labeled in the plate with Calcein AM. Labeled cells were counted and added to the upper chamber of the Boyden chamber, and allow to migrate towards de lower chamber, filled with medium containing 10% FBS as chemoattractant. The results show that indeed RA-treatment reduced the migration of neuroblastoma cells. However suppressing miR-10a or -10b expression not only abolished that reduction but increased migration over basal levels, supporting a contribution of RA-induced miR-10a and 10b to the reduction of migratory activity produced by RA [30]. (Figure 4A)

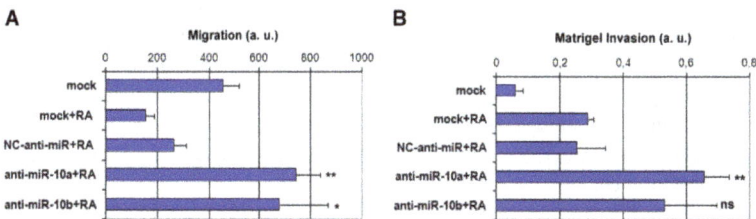

Figure 4. Involvement of miR-10a and -10b on the effects of RA in migratory and invasive potential of neuro-blastoma cells. Mock-transfected cells and cells transfected with Negative Control (NC) anti-miR, anti-miR-10a or anti-miR-10b were treated with 1 μM RA or vehicle for 96 h and used in migration **(A)** or matrigel invasion **(B)** transwell assays. The graph shows a representative experiment performed in triplicate (mean ± SD). Statistical significance was analyzed by comparing samples transfected with anti-miR-10a and -10b with those transfected with NC-anti-miR.

For invasion assays we used a similar assay, with the difference that the porous membrane separating the upper and lower chambers of the Boyden chamber was covered with BD *Matrigel* matrix (5 μg/cm^2 in serum-free medium). The lower chamber contained 10% FBS as chemoattractant to promote cell invasion. In this case RA treatment results in increased invasive potential, whereas in cells transfected with anti-miR-10a or 10b the same treatment the increase in invasion induced by RA treatment is even larger, supporting the idea that the expression of miR-10a and -10b contributes to a reduction in the invasive potential [30]. (Figure 4B)

To analyze the effects of RA treatment on the metastatic potential of neuroblastoma cells we used the chicken embryo chorioallantoic membrane assays (also known as CAM assay; [31]). This assay is useful to study intravasation and metastasis *in vivo*, since it recapitulates all the steps of the metastatic process. In the CAM assay the cells to be tested are inoculated on the chorioallantoic membrane of 10-day-old chicken embryos. After a week, the egg is opened, the embryo is obtained and secondary organs like the lungs were dissected. The presence of human cells in the chicken organ is evaluated and quantified after obtaining their genomic DNA, by detecting the presence of human-specific *Alu*-sequences by Real-Time PCR (Figure 3). As this is a complex technique that requires a higher number of replicate experiments we have simplified the study to analyze only the effects of miR-10a suppression. Neuroblastoma cells could be detected in the chicken lungs after 7 days incubation. Suppression of miR-10a expression with its cognate anti-miR resulted in an increase of the metastatic cells. As expected, RA treatment led to a reduction of the number of neuroblastoma cells reaching the lungs. However this inhibitory effect of RA was abolished in cells having a reduced amount of miR-10a by transfecting the corresponding anti-miR-10a [30].

In good agreement with our results, it has been reported that miR-10a and -10b reduces the ability of neuroblastoma cells to form colonies in soft agar [29], a phenotype that is characteristic of malignant cells. All these results support the idea that miR-10a and -10b expression contribute to reduction of migratory, invasive and metastatic activities induced by RA. In a recent report it has been shown that a protein involved in cell migration, Tiam1, is targeted by miR-10b in mammary tumor cells. Overexpression of miR-10b suppresses the ability of breast carcinoma cells to migrate and invade [32]. Consistent to that, it has been reported an association between lower miR-10a expression and lower overall survival for a subclass of neuroblastoma tumors (11q- tumor cohort) [29]. However other reports seem to involve the members of the miR-10 family as promoters of migration and metastasis in different tumors [33-40]. This apparent controversy may suggest that the role of the microRNAs from the miR-10 family in tumorigenesis and metastasis would depend on their molecular targets and therefore would depend on the cellular context.

4. Molecular targets of miR-10a and -10b in the differentiation of neuroblastoma cells

4.1. The search for the molecular targets for miRNAs

The identification of molecular targets for miRNAs is a crucial step towards the understanding of miRNA function. Because an ever growing number of experimentally validated targets for miRNAs are being reported, a simple way to identify miRNA targets is to search for validated targets in the literature or in databases as TarBase [41]. A validated target for miR-10b in breast cancer cells is the homeobox gene *HOXD10* [34, 42]. However, we could not find regulation of *HOXD10* in SH-SY5Y neuroblastoma cells, when treated with RA or when the levels of miR-10a and -10b were experimentally altered [30].

A lot of effort has been made to generate computational miRNA target prediction tools [reviewed in 43], mainly based on the search for complementary sequences in the genome.

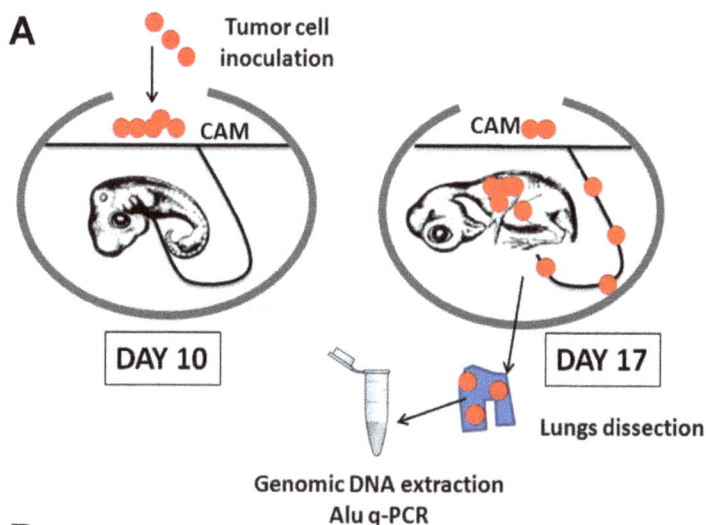

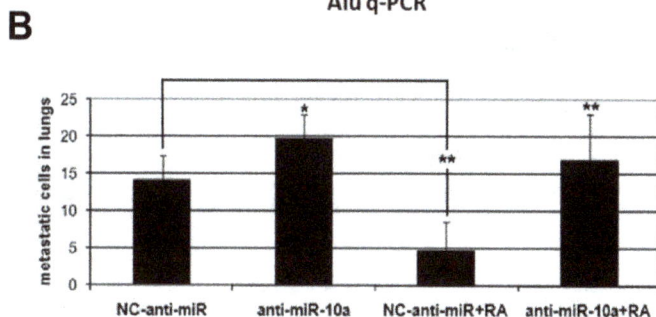

Figure 5. Chorioallantoic Membrane Metastasis Assay. (A) Schematic representation of the experiment. Cells from the different treatment groups were transferred to the upper chorioallantoic membrane of 10-day-old chicken embryos and the number of metastatized cells into the lungs evaluated 7 days later. (B) Cells transfected with Negative Control (NC) anti-miR or anti-miR-10a were treated with 1 µM RA or vehicle for 96 h as indicated in the figure. The graph represents the values obtained from six parallel assays (mean ± SD). Statistical significance was analyzed by comparing samples transfected with anti-miR-10a with those transfected with NC-anti-miR. In addition samples transfected with NC-anti-miR treated with vehicle were compared to those treated with RA.

However, that is not an easy task, because short sequences are problematic for the algorithms usually developed for complementarity analysis. As indicated in 2.2, the base pairing of miRNA and mRNA in vertebrates requires only partial homology, with a preference for contiguous pairing occurring only at the "seed" region, located at nucleotides 2-7 of the guide strand, and this makes even more difficult to find the right target sequence in the genome. Several authors have approached this problem from different startpoints, using mainly complementarity analysis of the complete miRNA sequence, complementarity analysis of the seed sequence, or adding thermodynamic stability analysis of duplex sequences or 3'UTR sequence conservation to the complementarity analysis. Nowadays a set of miRNA target prediction resources are available, mainly as web-based tools. However it becomes striking to the new users of these tools how different results can be obtained when using the same sequence with different prediction tools. In addition, prediction tools generate lists of hundreds of genes for each of the miRNAs, and the fact of having sequence diversity at the 3'UTR by alternative polyadenylation sites could also complicate the analysis [for discussion, see 44].

To find relevant targets for miR-10a and-10b in neuroblastoma cells we choose to combine bioinformatic prediction tools together with experimental analysis. We created a list of potential miR-10a and -10b targets by including the common predicted genes using three different prediction resources: miRbase targets [45], TargetScan [46] and PicTar [47]. Only mRNAs that contained evolutionarily conserved miRNA binding sequences on their 3'UTR were considered. This list was crossed with the dataset of an Affymetrix microarray experiment containing the genes downregulated after 48 h RA treatment. In the resulting list, two members of the Arginine/serine-rich splicing factors, *SFRS1* (SF2/ASF) and *SFRS10* (TRA2B), as well as the nuclear receptor co-repressor *NCOR2* (SMRT) were on top [30].

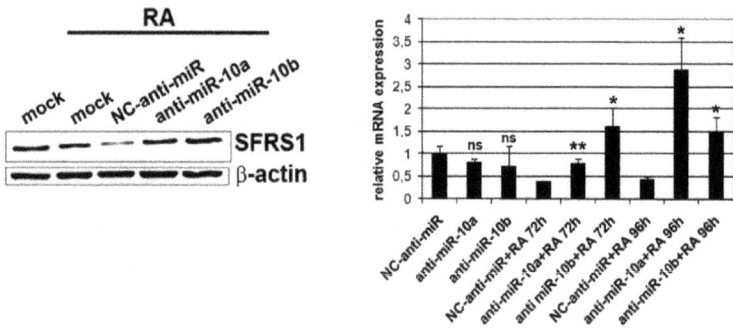

Figure 6. miR-10a/-10b knockdown leads to increased SFRS1 protein and mRNA levels in SH-SY5Y cells. (Left panel) Western blot of SFRS1 protein expression after anti-miR-10a, -10b and negative control NC-anti-miR transfection of SH-SY5Y cells followed by 1μM RA treatment. The blot was reprobed with actin beta antibodies as loading control. (Right panel). RT-qPCR analysis of SFRS1 mRNA levels in same conditions. The graph shows expression levels relative to that of RA untreated, NC-anti-miR transfected cells (mean ± SD of a triplicate experiment). Statistical analysis for right panel was made by comparing the values from cells transfected with anti-miR-10a or -10b to those from cells transfected with NC-anti-miR; ns= non significative.

4.2. Regulation of *SFRS1* (SF2/ASF) by miR-10a and -10b

The regulation of *SFRS1* (SF2/ASF) by miR-10a and-10b was experimentally validated at mRNA and protein levels in HeLa and SH-SY5Y cells (Figure 6). In addition regulation by miR-10a and -10b was shown in transfection experiments with reporter plasmids containing *SFRS1* 3'UTR sequences linked to the Luciferase gene. miR-10a and -10b are new players in the complex regulation of *SFRS1* protein through a mechanism involving enhanced mRNA cleavage. In addition, we showed how changes in miR-10a and -10b expression levels may influence some molecular activities in which the product of *SFRS1* is involved, such as translation enhancement of certain mRNAs and alternative splicing, that could have importance in the neural differentiation process [30] (Figure 7). We have reported that the activation of signaling pathways by RA treatment results in rapid changes in the phosphorylation pattern of SR proteins, including SFRS1 and subsequently, changes in alternative splicing selection and an increase of the translation of mRNAs containing SFRS1 binding sites take place [48]. In this context, the reduction in *SFRS1* levels through miR-10a and -10b regulation could be interpreted as the closing of the feedback regulatory loop of RA on the activities of *SFRS1*.

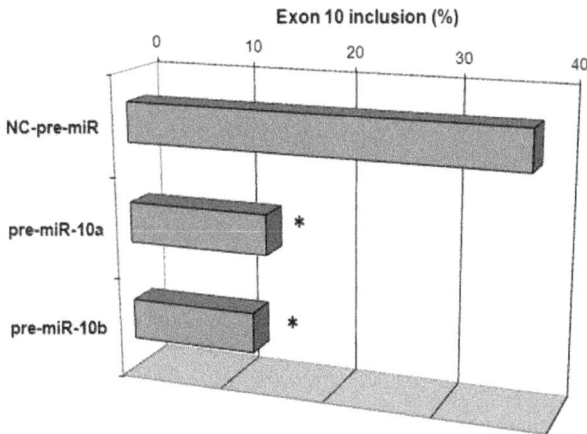

Figure 7. Experimental alteration of miR-10a and -10b levels resulted in an impairment of SFRS1 functions in the regulation of alternative splicing. Alternative splicing of *tau* protein exon 10 is altered by transfection of anti-miR-10a and -10b. RT-PCR was performed on RNA extracted from anti-miR-10a, -10b or negative control (NC) anti-miR transfected SH-SY5Y cells. *tau* Exon 10 flanking primers were used in RT-PCR reaction according to [49]. Quantification of the percentage of exon 10 inclusion. The graph shows the average from 3 independent experiments. Statistical analysis was made by comparing the values from cells transfected with pre-miR-10a or -10b to those from cells transfected with NC-pre-miR.

4.3. Regulation of *NCOR2* (SMRT) by miR-10a and -10b

The regulation of *NCOR2* by miR-10a and-10b was experimentally validated at mRNA and protein levels in SK-N-BE neuroblastoma cells. Moreover, a luciferase reporter construct containing the *NCOR2* 3'UTR showed a significant decrease in luciferase activity when co-transfected with mature miR-10a, -10b or 10a/10b mimics in SK-N-BE cells. This decrease in luciferase activity was completely abolished when the putative miR-10a and -10b target site was mutated in its seed sequence. Knock-down of *NCOR2* expression through transfection of siRNAs to SK-N-BE cells recapitulates most of the changes induced by RA, like neurite outgrowth, proliferative arrest, expression of neural markers, downregulation of *MYCN* and expression of miR-10a [29]. *NCOR2* acts as co-repressor in the regulation of many genes, especially as co-regulator of nuclear receptor-regulated genes. Bound to the unliganded receptor, *NCOR2* maintains the promoters of nuclear receptor-regulated genes in a repressed state, and its release from the complex with the receptor upon ligand binding allows tran-scriptional activation [50]. It has been reported that *NCOR2* represses expression of the jumonji-domain containing gene *JMJD3*, a direct retinoic-acid-receptor target that functions as a histone H3 trimethyl K27 demethylase and which is capable of activating specific compo-nents of the neurogenic program [51]. Therefore, downregulation of *NCOR2* by miR-10a and -10b would potentiate the actions of RA through RARs and RXRs and could contribute to some of the changes in gene expression associated with neural differentiation.

5. Conclusion

MicroRNAs are essential players in the process on neural differentiation of neuroblastoma cells, and contribute to the transduction of Retinoic Acid signaling. In addition, miRNAs have been reported to participate in the pathogenesis and progression of human neuroblastoma tumors [2, 3], and miRNA profiles have been recently proven to be useful for classification and prognosis [4]. Finally miRNAs open new avenues for the treatment of neuroblastoma cells, and proof of concept experiments showing a therapeutic action of miRNA-based treatments in animal models of neuroblastoma [52-54] and other tumors [33] have been reported. Therefore, we have to expect in the next years an increased interest in the study of microRNAs among the neuroblastoma researchers community.

Acknowledgements

The research work described in this article was financed through grants of the Spanish National Plan for Research, Development and Innovation (SAF2007-60780, SAF2010-15032 and SAF2011-23869), Generalitat Valenciana (ACOMP 09/212) and Genoma España to D. Barettino. S. Meseguer was the recipient of an EACR training and travel fellowship award and a CSIC I3P predoctoral fellowship/contract.

Author details

Salvador Meseguer, Juan-Manuel Escamilla and Domingo Barettino

Instituto de Biomedicina de Valencia, Consejo Superior de Investigaciones Científicas, Valencia, Spain

References

[1] Lee, R.C., Feinbaum, R.L.,Ambros, V. The C. elegans heterochronic gene lin-4 enco- des small RNAs with antisense complementarity to lin-14. Cell 1993; 75(5): 843-54.

[2] Chen, Y.,Stallings, R.L. Differential patterns of microRNA expression in neuroblasto- ma are correlated with prognosis, differentiation, and apoptosis. Cancer Res 2007; 67(3): 976-83.

[3] Welch, C., Chen, Y.,Stallings, R.L. MicroRNA-34a functions as a potential tumor sup- pressor by inducing apoptosis in neuroblastoma cells. Oncogene 2007; 26(34): 5017-22.

[4] De Preter, K., Mestdagh, P., Vermeulen, J., Zeka, F., Naranjo, A., Bray, I., Castel, V., Chen, C., Drozynska, E., Eggert, A., Hogarty, M.D., Izycka-Swieszewska, E., London, W.B., Noguera, R., Piqueras, M., Bryan, K., Schowe, B., van Sluis, P., Molenaar, J.J., Schramm, A., Schulte, J.H., Stallings, R.L., Versteeg, R., Laureys, G., Van Roy, N., Speleman, F.,Vandesompele, J. miRNA expression profiling enables risk stratification in archived and fresh neuroblastoma tumor samples. Clin Cancer Res 2011; 17(24): 7684-92.

[5] Sidell, N. Retinoic acid-induced growth inhibition and morphologic differentiation of human neuroblastoma cells in vitro. J Natl Cancer Inst 1982; 68(4): 589-596.

[6] Pahlman, S., Ruusala, A.I., Abrahamsson, L., Mattsson, M.E.,Esscher, T. Retinoic acid-induced differentiation of cultured human neuroblastoma cells: a comparison with phorbolester-induced differentiation. Cell Differ 1984; 14(2): 135-144.

[7] Thiele, C.J., Reynolds, C.P.,Israel, M.A. Decreased expression of N-myc precedes reti- noic acid-induced morphological differentiation of human neuroblastoma. Nature 1985; 313(6001): 404-406.

[8] Voigt, A.,Zintl, F. Effects of retinoic acid on proliferation, apoptosis, cytotoxicity, mi- gration, and invasion of neuroblastoma cells. Med Pediatr Oncol 2003; 40(4): 205-13.

[9] Joshi, S., Guleria, R., Pan, J., DiPette, D.,Singh, U.S. Retinoic acid receptors and tissue- transglutaminase mediate short-term effect of retinoic acid on migration and inva- sion of neuroblastoma SH-SY5Y cells. Oncogene 2006; 25(2): 240-7.

[10] Escamilla, J.M., Bäuerl, C., López, C.M.R., Pekkala, S.P., Navarro, S.,Barettino, D., Retinoic-Acid-Induced Downregulation of the 67 KDa Laminin Receptor Correlates with Reduced Biological Aggressiveness of Human Neuroblastoma Cells, in Neuroblastoma-Present and Future, H. Shimada, Editor. 2012, InTech: Rijeka. p. 217-232.

[11] Matthay, K.,Reynolds, C. Is there a role for retinoids to treat minimal residual disease in neuroblastoma? Br J Cancer 2000; 83(9): 1121-1123.

[12] Matthay, K.K., Reynolds, C.P., Seeger, R.C., Shimada, H., Adkins, E.S., Haas-Kogan, D., Gerbing, R.B., London, W.B.,Villablanca, J.G. Long-term results for children with high-risk neuroblastoma treated on a randomized trial of myeloablative therapy followed by 13-cis-retinoic acid: a children's oncology group study. J Clin Oncol 2009; 27(7): 1007-13.

[13] Matthay, K.K., Villablanca, J.G., Seeger, R.C., Stram, D.O., Harris, R.E., Ramsay, N.K., Swift, P., Shimada, H., Black, C.T., Brodeur, G.M., Gerbing, R.B.,Reynolds, C.P. Treatment of high-risk neuroblastoma with intensive chemotherapy, radiotherapy, autologous bone marrow transplantation, and 13-cis- retinoic acid. Children's Cancer Group. N Engl J Med 1999; 341(16): 1165-1173.

[14] Zhu, Y., Kalbfleisch, T., Brennan, M.D.,Li, Y. A MicroRNA gene is hosted in an intron of a schizophrenia-susceptibility gene. Schizophr Res 2009; 109(1-3): 86-9.

[15] Rodriguez, A., Griffiths-Jones, S., Ashurst, J.L.,Bradley, A. Identification of mammalian microRNA host genes and transcription units. Genome Res 2004; 14(10A): 1902-10.

[16] Lee, Y., Jeon, K., Lee, J.T., Kim, S.,Kim, V.N. MicroRNA maturation: stepwise processing and subcellular localization. Embo J 2002; 21(17): 4663-70.

[17] Lee, Y., Ahn, C., Han, J., Choi, H., Kim, J., Yim, J., Lee, J., Provost, P., Radmark, O., Kim, S.,Kim, V.N. The nuclear RNase III Drosha initiates microRNA processing. Nature 2003; 425(6956): 415-9.

[18] Yi, R., Qin, Y., Macara, I.G.,Cullen, B.R. Exportin-5 mediates the nuclear export of pre-microRNAs and short hairpin RNAs. Genes Dev 2003; 17(24): 3011-6.

[19] Hutvagner, G., McLachlan, J., Pasquinelli, A.E., Balint, E., Tuschl, T.,Zamore, P.D. A cellular function for the RNA-interference enzyme Dicer in the maturation of the let-7 small temporal RNA. Science 2001; 293(5531): 834-8.

[20] Meister, G., Landthaler, M., Patkaniowska, A., Dorsett, Y., Teng, G.,Tuschl, T. Human Argonaute2 mediates RNA cleavage targeted by miRNAs and siRNAs. Mol Cell 2004; 15(2): 185-97.

[21] Mah, S.M., Buske, C., Humphries, R.K.,Kuchenbauer, F. miRNA*: a passenger stranded in RNA-induced silencing complex? Crit Rev Eukaryot Gene Expr 2010; 20(2): 141-8.

[22] Forman, J.J.,Coller, H.A. The code within the code: microRNAs target coding regions. Cell Cycle 2010; 9(8): 1533-41.

[23] Annibali, D., Gioia, U., Savino, M., Laneve, P., Caffarelli, E.,Nasi, S. A new module in neural differentiation control: two microRNAs upregulated by retinoic acid, miR-9 and -103, target the differentiation inhibitor ID2. PLoS One 2012; 7(7): e40269.

[24] Bartel, D.P. MicroRNAs: target recognition and regulatory functions. Cell 2009; 136(2): 215-33.

[25] Fabian, M.R., Sonenberg, N.,Filipowicz, W. Regulation of mRNA translation and sta-bility by microRNAs. Annu Rev Biochem 2010; 79: 351-79.

[26] Huang, V.,Li, L.C. miRNA goes nuclear. RNA Biol 2012; 9(3): 269-73.

[27] Beveridge, N.J., Tooney, P.A., Carroll, A.P., Tran, N.,Cairns, M.J. Down-regulation of miR-17 family expression in response to retinoic acid induced neuronal differentia-tion. Cell Signal 2009; 21(12): 1837-45.

[28] Chen, H., Shalom-Feuerstein, R., Riley, J., Zhang, S.D., Tucci, P., Agostini, M., Aber-dam, D., Knight, R.A., Genchi, G., Nicotera, P., Melino, G.,Vasa-Nicotera, M. miR-7 and miR-214 are specifically expressed during neuroblastoma differentiation, cortical development and embryonic stem cells differentiation, and control neurite out-growth in vitro. Biochem Biophys Res Commun 2010; 394(4): 921-7.

[29] Foley, N.H., Bray, I., Watters, K.M., Das, S., Bryan, K., Bernas, T., Prehn, J.H.,Stal-lings, R.L. MicroRNAs 10a and 10b are potent inducers of neuroblastoma cell differ-entiation through targeting of nuclear receptor corepressor 2. Cell Death Differ 2011; 18(7): 1089-98.

[30] Meseguer, S., Mudduluru, G., Escamilla, J.M., Allgayer, H.,Barettino, D. Micro-RNAs-10a and -10b Contribute to Retinoic Acid-induced Differentiation of Neuro-blastoma Cells and Target the Alternative Splicing Regulatory Factor SFRS1 (SF2/ASF). J Biol Chem 2011; 286(6): 4150-64.

[31] Zijlstra, A., Mellor, R., Panzarella, G., Aimes, R.T., Hooper, J.D., Marchenko, N.D.,Quigley, J.P. A quantitative analysis of rate-limiting steps in the metastatic cas-cade using human-specific real-time polymerase chain reaction. Cancer Res 2002; 62(23): 7083-92.

[32] Moriarty, C.H., Pursell, B.,Mercurio, A.M. miR-10b targets Tiam1: implications for Rac activation and carcinoma migration. J Biol Chem 2010; 285(27): 20541-6.

[33] Ma, L., Reinhardt, F., Pan, E., Soutschek, J., Bhat, B., Marcusson, E.G., Teruya-Feld-stein, J., Bell, G.W.,Weinberg, R.A. Therapeutic silencing of miR-10b inhibits metasta-sis in a mouse mammary tumor model. Nat Biotechnol 2010; 28(4): 341-7.

[34] Ma, L., Teruya-Feldstein, J.,Weinberg, R.A. Tumour invasion and metastasis initiated by microRNA-10b in breast cancer. Nature 2007; 449(7163): 682-8.

[35] Veerla, S., Lindgren, D., Kvist, A., Frigyesi, A., Staaf, J., Persson, H., Liedberg, F., Chebil, G., Gudjonsson, S., Borg, A., Mansson, W., Rovira, C.,Hoglund, M. MiRNA expression in urothelial carcinomas: important roles of miR-10a, miR-222, miR-125b, miR-7 and miR-452 for tumor stage and metastasis, and frequent homozygous losses of miR-31. Int J Cancer 2009; 124(9): 2236-42.

[36] Weiss, F.U., Marques, I.J., Woltering, J.M., Vlecken, D.H., Aghdassi, A., Partecke, L.I., Heidecke, C.D., Lerch, M.M.,Bagowski, C.P. Retinoic acid receptor antagonists inhibit miR-10a expression and block metastatic behavior of pancreatic cancer. Gastroenterology 2009; 137(6): 2136-45 e1-7.

[37] Sasayama, T., Nishihara, M., Kondoh, T., Hosoda, K.,Kohmura, E. MicroRNA-10b is overexpressed in malignant glioma and associated with tumor invasive factors, uP-AR and RhoC. Int J Cancer 2009; 125(6): 1407-13.

[38] Nakata, K., Ohuchida, K., Mizumoto, K., Kayashima, T., Ikenaga, N., Sakai, H., Lin, C., Fujita, H., Otsuka, T., Aishima, S., Nagai, E., Oda, Y.,Tanaka, M. MicroRNA-10b is overexpressed in pancreatic cancer, promotes its invasiveness, and correlates with a poor prognosis. Surgery 2011; 150(5): 916-22.

[39] Lu, Y.C., Chen, Y.J., Wang, H.M., Tsai, C.Y., Chen, W.H., Huang, Y.C., Fan, K.H., Tsai, C.N., Huang, S.F., Kang, C.J., Chang, J.T.,Cheng, A.J. Oncogenic function and early detection potential of miRNA-10b in oral cancer as identified by microRNA profiling. Cancer Prev Res (Phila) 2012; 5(4): 665-74.

[40] Liu, Z., Zhu, J., Cao, H., Ren, H.,Fang, X. miR-10b promotes cell invasion through RhoC-AKT signaling pathway by targeting HOXD10 in gastric cancer. Int J Oncol 2012; 40(5): 1553-60.

[41] Vergoulis, T., Vlachos, I.S., Alexiou, P., Georgakilas, G., Maragkakis, M., Reczko, M., Gerangelos, S., Koziris, N., Dalamagas, T.,Hatzigeorgiou, A.G. TarBase 6.0: capturing the exponential growth of miRNA targets with experimental support. Nucleic Acids Res 2012; 40(Database issue): D222-9.

[42] Ma, L.,Weinberg, R.A. Micromanagers of malignancy: role of microRNAs in regulating metastasis. Trends Genet 2008; 24(9): 448-56.

[43] Maziere, P.,Enright, A.J. Prediction of microRNA targets. Drug Discov Today 2007; 12(11-12): 452-8.

[44] Clancy, J.L., Wei, G.H., Echner, N., Humphreys, D.T., Beilharz, T.H.,Preiss, T. mRNA isoform diversity can obscure detection of miRNA-mediated control of translation. Rna 2011; 17(6): 1025-31.

[45] John, B., Enright, A.J., Aravin, A., Tuschl, T., Sander, C.,Marks, D.S. Human MicroRNA targets. PLoS Biol 2004; 2(11): e363.

[46] Lewis, B.P., Shih, I.H., Jones-Rhoades, M.W., Bartel, D.P.,Burge, C.B. Prediction of mammalian microRNA targets. Cell 2003; 115(7): 787-98.

[47] Krek, A., Grun, D., Poy, M.N., Wolf, R., Rosenberg, L., Epstein, E.J., MacMenamin, P., da Piedade, I., Gunsalus, K.C., Stoffel, M.,Rajewsky, N. Combinatorial microRNA target predictions. Nat Genet 2005; 37(5): 495-500.

[48] Laserna, E.J., Valero, M.L., Sanz, L., Sánchez del Pino, M.M., Calvete, J.J.,Barettino, D. Proteomic analysis of phosphorylated nuclear proteins underscores novel roles for rapid actions of retinoic acid in the regulation of mRNA splicing and translation. Mol Endocrinol 2009; 23(11): 1799-814.

[49] Kondo, S., Yamamoto, N., Murakami, T., Okumura, M., Mayeda, A.,Imaizumi, K. Tra2 beta, SF2/ASF and SRp30c modulate the function of an exonic splicing enhancer in exon 10 of tau pre-mRNA. Genes Cells 2004; 9(2): 121-30.

[50] Xu, L., Glass, C.K.,Rosenfeld, M.G. Coactivator and corepressor complexes in nuclear receptor function. Curr Opin Genet Dev 1999; 9(2): 140-7.

[51] Jepsen, K., Solum, D., Zhou, T., McEvilly, R.J., Kim, H.J., Glass, C.K., Hermanson, O.,Rosenfeld, M.G. SMRT-mediated repression of an H3K27 demethylase in progression from neural stem cell to neuron. Nature 2007; 450(7168): 415-9.

[52] Tivnan, A., Foley, N.H., Tracey, L., Davidoff, A.M.,Stallings, R.L. MicroRNA-184-mediated inhibition of tumour growth in an orthotopic murine model of neuroblastoma. Anticancer Res 2010; 30(11): 4391-5.

[53] Tivnan, A., Tracey, L., Buckley, P.G., Alcock, L.C., Davidoff, A.M.,Stallings, R.L. MicroRNA-34a is a potent tumor suppressor molecule in vivo in neuroblastoma. BMC Cancer 2011; 11: 33.

[54] Tivnan, A., Orr, W.S., Gubala, V., Nooney, R., Williams, D.E., McDonagh, C., Prenter, S., Harvey, H., Domingo-Fernandez, R., Bray, I.M., Piskareva, O., Ng, C.Y., Lode, H.N., Davidoff, A.M.,Stallings, R.L. Inhibition of neuroblastoma tumor growth by targeted delivery of microRNA-34a using anti-disialoganglioside GD2 coated nanoparticles. PLoS One 2012; 7(5): e38129.

Permissions

The contributors of this book come from diverse backgrounds, making this book a truly international effort. This book will bring forth new frontiers with its revolutionizing research information and detailed analysis of the nascent developments around the world.

We would like to thank Hiroyuki Shimada, MD, PhD, for lending his expertise to make the book truly unique. He has played a crucial role in the development of this book. Without his invaluable contribution this book wouldn't have been possible. He has made vital efforts to compile up to date information on the varied aspects of this subject to make this book a valuable addition to the collection of many professionals and students.

This book was conceptualized with the vision of imparting up-to-date information and advanced data in this field. To ensure the same, a matchless editorial board was set up. Every individual on the board went through rigorous rounds of assessment to prove their worth. After which they invested a large part of their time researching and compiling the most relevant data for our readers. Conferences and sessions were held from time to time between the editorial board and the contributing authors to present the data in the most comprehensible form. The editorial team has worked tirelessly to provide valuable and valid information to help people across the globe.

Every chapter published in this book has been scrutinized by our experts. Their significance has been extensively debated. The topics covered herein carry significant findings which will fuel the growth of the discipline. They may even be implemented as practical applications or may be referred to as a beginning point for another development. Chapters in this book were first published by InTech; hereby published with permission under the Creative Commons Attribution License or equivalent.

The editorial board has been involved in producing this book since its inception. They have spent rigorous hours researching and exploring the diverse topics which have resulted in the successful publishing of this book. They have passed on their knowledge of decades through this book. To expedite this challenging task, the publisher supported the team at every step. A small team of assistant editors was also appointed to further simplify the editing procedure and attain best results for the readers.

Our editorial team has been hand-picked from every corner of the world. Their multi-ethnicity adds dynamic inputs to the discussions which result in innovative outcomes. These outcomes are then further discussed with the researchers and contributors who give their valuable feedback and opinion regarding the same. The feedback is then collaborated with the researches and they are edited in a comprehensive manner to aid the understanding of the subject.

Apart from the editorial board, the designing team has also invested a significant amount of their time in understanding the subject and creating the most relevant covers. They scrutinized every image to scout for the most suitable representation of the subject and create an appropriate cover for the book.

The publishing team has been involved in this book since its early stages. They were actively engaged in every process, be it collecting the data, connecting with the contributors or procuring relevant information. The team has been an ardent support to the editorial, designing and production team. Their endless efforts to recruit the best for this project, has resulted in the accomplishment of this book. They are a veteran in the field of academics and their pool of knowledge is as vast as their experience in printing. Their expertise and guidance has proved useful at every step. Their uncompromising quality standards have made this book an exceptional effort. Their encouragement from time to time has been an inspiration for everyone.

The publisher and the editorial board hope that this book will prove to be a valuable piece of knowledge for researchers, students, practitioners and scholars across the globe.

List of Contributors

Josef Malis
Dept. of Pediatric Oncology, University Hospital Motol and Charles University, Prague, Czech Republic

Shigeki Yagyu, Tomoko Iehara and Hajime Hosoi
Department of Pediatrics, Graduate School of Medical Science, Kyoto Prefectural University of Medicine, Kyoto, Japan

Pierdomenico Ruggeri, Antonietta R. Farina, Lucia Cappabianca, Natalia Di Ianni, Marzia Ragone, Stefania Merolle, and Andrew R. Mackay
Department of Applied Clinical and Biotechnological Science, University of L'Aquila, Coppito II, L'Aquila, Italy

Alberto Gulino
Department of Molecular Medicine, University of Rome "La Sapienza", Rome, Italy
Neuromed Institute, Pozzilli, Italy

Fergal C. Kelleher
Peter MacCallum Cancer Centre, Melbourne, Victoria, Australia

Mandeep Sidhu and Daniel J. Belliveau
Department of Anatomy and Cell Biology, Schulich of Medicine & Dentistry and School of Health Studies, Faculty of Health Sciences, Western University, London, Ontario, Canada

Fieke Lamers
Department of Oncogenomics, Academic Medical Center, University of Amsterdam, AZ Amsterdam, The Netherlands

Aru Narendran
Laboratory for Preclinical and Drug Discovery Studies, Pediatric Oncology Experimental Therapeutics Investigators' Consortium (POETIC), Division of Pediatric Oncology, Alberta Children's Hospital, University of Calgary, Calgary, Alberta, Canada

Enrique Hernández-Lemus
Computational Genomics Department, National Institute of Genomic Medicine, México, D.F, México
Center for Complexity Sciences, National Autonomous University of México, México, D.F, México

Anllely Grizett Gutiérrez, Adriana Vázquez-Aguirre and Carmen Mejía
Genomic Medicine and Environmental Toxicology Department, Institute of Biomedical Research, National Autonomous University of México, México, D.F, México

M. Lourdes Palma-Tirado
Microscopy Unit, Neurobiology Institute, Campus Juriquilla, National Autonomous University of México, Querétaro, México

Lena Ruiz-Azuara
Inorganic and Nuclear Chemistry Department, School of Chemistry, National Autonomous University of México, México, D.F, México

Shanique A. Young, Ryon Graf and Dwayne G. Stupack
Reproductive Medicine Department, UCSD Moores Cancer Center, La Jolla, California, USA

Fabio Morandi, Barbara Carlini and Maria Valeria Corrias
Laboratory of Oncology, IRCCS Giannina Gaslini Institute, Genoa, Italy

Paola Scaruffi and Sara Stigliani
Center of Physiopathology of Human Reproduction, Obstetrics and Gynecology Unit, IRCCS San Martino Hospital-National Cancer Research Institute, Genoa, Italy

Xao X. Tang
Department of Anatomy and Cell Biology, College of Medicine, University of Illinois at Chicago, Chicago, Illinois, USA

Hiroyuki Shimada
Department of Pathology & Laboratory Medicine, Children's Hospital Los Angeles and University of Southern California Keck School of Medicine, Los Angeles, California, USA

Emanuela Urso and Michele Maffia
Department of Biological and Environmental Sciences and Technology, University of Salento, Lecce, Italy

Shweta Joshi, Alok R. Singh, Muamera Zulcic and Donald L. Durden
Department of Pediatrics, Moores Cancer Center, University of California San Diego, La Jolla, CA, USA

Hyunah Ahn
Department of Pediatrics, Rady Children's Hospital-San Diego/UCSD, MC San Diego CA, USA

Lisa L.R. Hartman
Department of Pediatrics, Moores Cancer Center, University of California San Diego, La Jolla, CA, USA
Department of Pediatrics, Rady Children's Hospital-San Diego/UCSD, MC San Diego CA, USA

Salvador Meseguer, Juan-Manuel Escamilla and Domingo Barettino
Instituto de Biomedicina de Valencia, Consejo Superior de Investigaciones Científicas, Valencia, Spain

www.ingramcontent.com/pod-product-compliance
Lightning Source LLC
Chambersburg PA
CBHW070736190326
41458CB00004B/1188